DISORDERS
OF THE FOOT

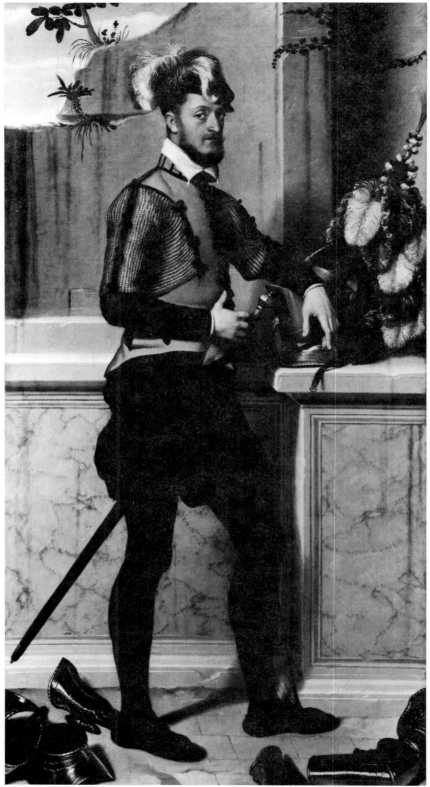

Portrait of a Gentleman by Moroni. The metal brace he is using to overcome his left foot drop is hardly visible. (Courtesy of the National Gallery, London)

DISORDERS OF THE FOOT

ARTHUR J. HELFET

B.Sc. (Cape Town), M.D., M.Ch.Orth. (Liverpool),
F.R.C.S. (England), F.A.C.S.

*Clinical Professor, late Chairman, Department of Orthopaedic Surgery,
Albert Einstein College of Medicine, New York; formerly Consulting
Orthopaedic Surgeon, Hospital for Joint Diseases, New York; formerly
Senior Visiting Orthopaedic Surgeon and Lecturer in Orthopaedic Surgery,
University of Cape Town and Groote Schuur Hospital, Cape Town, R.S.A.;
Hunterian Professor, Royal College of Surgeons*

DAVID M. GRUEBEL LEE

M.B.B.Ch. (Witwatersrand), F.R.C.S. (England),
F.R.C.S. (Edinburgh)

*Senior Consultant Orthopaedic Surgeon, West Surrey/N.E. Hampshire
Health District; Consultant Orthopaedic Surgeon, Rowley Bristow Orthopaedic Centre, Pyrford Hospital, Byfleet, Surrey, England*

With 11 Guest Authors

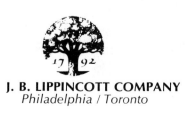

J. B. LIPPINCOTT COMPANY
Philadelphia / Toronto

Copyright © 1980 by J. B. Lippincott Company

This book is fully protected by copyright, and with the exception
of brief extracts for review, no part of it may be reproduced in any
form, by print, photoprint, microfilm, or any other means, without
the written permission of the publishers.

ISBN 0-397-50430-6

Library of Congress Catalog Card Number 79-22830
Printed in the United States of America

5   4   3   2   1

Library of Congress Cataloging in Publication Data

Main entry under title:
Disorders of the foot.

Includes index.
1. Foot—Abnormalities.   2. Foot—Diseases.
I. Helfet, Arthur J.   II. Gruebel Lee, David M.
RD781.D57   617'.585   79-22830
ISBN 0-397-50430-6

Guest Authors

Ralph Ger, M.D., F.R.C.S., F.A.C.S.
Director of Surgery, Professor of Surgery and Anatomy, Albert Einstein College of Medicine, a Division of Montefiore Hospital and Medical Center, New York

J. E. Handelsman, M.D., M.Ch.Orth., F.R.C.S.
Professor of Orthopedic Surgery and Director of Pediatric Orthopedics, Department of Orthopedic Surgery, State University of New York at Stony Brook, Health Sciences Center, Stony Brook, New York

David W. Holmes
Fellow of the British Institute of Surgical Technicians

W. P. U. Jackson, M.A., M.D., F.R.C.P. (London), D.C.H., F.R.S. (South Africa)
Professor, Department of Medicine, University of Cape Town; Chief Physician, Groote Schuur Hospital, Observatory, Cape Town, R.S.A.; Head, Diabetes and Endocrine Service; Director, Endocrine Research Unit (Medical Research Council/UCT)

Lipmann Kessel, M.B.E., M.C., F.R.C.S.
Professor of Orthopaedics, Institute of Orthopaedics, University of London; Director of Clinical Studies, Royal National Orthopaedic Hospital, London

Daniel N. Kuland, M.D.
Assistant Professor of Orthopedic Surgery and Rehabilitation, and Chief of the Foot Clinic, University of Virginia Medical Center; Adjunct Assistant Professor of Physical Education, University of Virginia, Charlottesville, Virginia; Member, American College of Sports Medicine

J. H. Louw, Ch.M., F.R.C.S.
Departments of Medicine and Surgery, University of Cape Town and Groote Schuur Hospital, Observatory, Cape Town, R.S.A.

Michael T. Manley, Ph.D.
Department of Biomedical Engineering, University of Cape Town and Groote Schuur Hospital, Observatory, Cape Town, R.S.A.

H. S. Myers, M.B., Ch.B., M.Med. (Rad. D.)
Departments of Medicine and Radiology, University of Cape Town and Groote Schuur Hospital, Observatory, Cape Town, R.S.A.

Glenn S. Quittell, D.P.M.
Clinical Instructor in Medicine, California College of Podiatric Medicine; Clinical Assistant Professor, Ohio College of Podiatric Medicine; Adjunct Clinical Faculty, Pennsylvania College of Podiatric Medicine; Clinical Instructor, New York College of Podiatric Medicine; Member of the Staff, New Rochelle Hospital Medical Center

Geoffrey Walker, M.B., F.R.C.S.
Consultant Orthopaedic Surgeon, Queen Mary's Hospital for Children, Carshalton, Surrey, England

Foreword

Who wants a book on foot disorders? The simple answer is: nearly everyone. Certainly pediatricians, podiatrists, general practitioners, orthopaedic surgeons, rheumatologists, and shoe designers; though even this list is far from complete. And who better to write it than two such experienced collaborators as Helfet and Gruebel Lee? They showed in their book on back disorders how well they worked together and how they illuminated the dark corners of a difficult subject.

Compared with the hand, the foot has been grossly neglected—by artists, by sculptors, and by poets, as well as by medical authors. This may be the result of a mistaken impression that the foot is much simpler than the hand. In fact it is much more specialized. If you doubt this, think of those unfortunate people without hands; they may become foot and mouth artists. But have you ever heard of anyone who, without feet, learned to walk on his hands?

Anyone with painful feet will tell you the seriousness of the problem. My own approach, as a teacher of orthopaedics, is perhaps somewhat naive. In discussing the subject I first ask the question (in a Socratic sense), "Why do we have feet?" Clearly we need them to stand on, since we have nothing else; and we need

them to walk with, since we can't go everywhere in an automobile; and we have to wear shoes on them, or we get broken glass in our feet. For standing, the ideal is a very broad platform; for walking, we need supple joints and strong muscles; and in order to be able to wear shoes we need feet that are sufficiently standard in shape to be fitted in a shop (we don't break in a new suit; why should we break in a new pair of shoes?).

Broad platforms, supple joints, standard-shape feet—this combination is all we need. But if any single aspect is lacking, we grumble. And how we grumble! Examples of narrow platforms are conditions such as varus feet and pes cavus, on both of which the area bearing the body weight is too small and painful callosities result. Joints that are insufficiently supple occur in hallux rigidus and in arthritis, to say nothing of rarities such as congenital or spasmodic flatfoot; all may lead to painful stiffness. Shoes cannot fit feet with large bunions, with hammer toes, or with heel knobs, so painful pressure areas result. These are, very generally speaking, the main groups of painful feet.

It may be objected that I have omitted Kohler's disease, Freiberg's disease, plantar fasciitis, Severs' disease, Morton's metatarsalgia, stress fracture, gout, diabetic ulcers, and a host of other conditions. But these rarely cause painful feet—they cause a painful foot, which is quite different; and they nearly always display their presence by local tenderness. Nor, for the same reason, have I mentioned my hobby horse, the medial sesamoid of the hallux, that small bone of almost supernatural significance; that treasure-house of pathology readily revealed by careful clinical examination and eminently curable by simple operation.

But I must resist the temptation to write a book instead of a foreword. Helfet and Gruebel Lee have already produced a splendid one, dealing first, as they should, with anatomy, terminology, clinical aspects, and biomechanics, before proceeding to discuss painful conditions of the feet, flatfoot, the foot in athletes (happily not referred to as "athlete's foot") the paralyzed foot, the rheumatoid foot, and a host of other conditions. Indeed they consider virtually every aspect of foot disorders; to achieve such wide coverage they have enlisted the cooperation of a number of eminent authors; moreover, I feel sure I can detect the fine poetic hand of Lydia Gruebel Lee in the more mellifluous passages. The sum total is an enjoyable and a masterly account of a difficult and important subject. I can think of no one in the list of potential readers at the head of this foreword who will not learn a great deal from this book.

A. Graham Apley, M.B., F.R.C.S.

Preface

Feet may not remain supple and comfortable for a lifetime. They tire and ache and swell and stiffen. They may be cold feet or hot feet; may lose sensation or gain unpleasant sensitivity; be white or blue or purple; or be deformed in arch, heel, or toes. They may move with the plod of the plowman or the beauty of a ballet dancer. Symptoms originate locally or may signal disease elsewhere.

We are wont to view the foot as a poor relation of the hand: more realistically, it is, as Wood Jones has written, "the most distinctly human part of the whole anatomical make up, the hallmark which distinguishes him from all other members of the animal kingdom."

The foot should not be considered a lever. It is a torsion spring which, as it winds and unwinds, unleashes power and agility. Its movements, in sinuous synchrony with those of the ankle, knee, and hip, are an essential contribution to the strength and mechanical excellence of the leg.

Due regard to the precepts of the anatomy, physiology, and biomechanics of the foot leads to a clinical view and understanding of the functions and dysfunctions and of ways of healing, *not only by physicians and surgeons, but by all practitioners concerned in the management of patients suffering discomfort, disability, and deformity of the feet.*

In this book, a variety of conditions is examined: to our considerable advantage we have, in addition, a series of contributions by distinguished guest authors:

Ralph Ger presents the anatomy of the foot in the manner in which it may be applied to function, including his original operation to transpose the muscles with their vascular supply intact, to close defects, following injury or infection, of the malleolar region, heel, and dorsum of the foot.

Michael Manley adds the precise language of his laboratory to the clinical interpretation of the biomechanics of the foot, which stresses the crucial role of the torsion spring action of the foot in human locomotion.

Jack Handelsman reports on his researches into the etiology of clubfoot. While the authors feel that the questions are not yet resolved, the finding of histological abnormalities in the muscles of children suffering from the condition must stimulate further studies.

Lipmann Kessel describes the place of arthroplasty of the forefoot in rheumatoid arthritis; a subject on which he first reported as long ago as 1957.

One of man's oldest pursuits, that of running, in danger of obsolescence in the motorized world, has become the pastime of joggers, a discipline for athletes striving for excellence, and an addiction of the elite marathon runner. Dan Kuland relates the interesting problems of the new specialty of sports medicine. Track surfaces should be tuned to the mechanics of running. A compliant surface acts like a spring. "Runners on this track have had fewer injuries and better times, compared to their performance on other tracks."

The changes that may limit the foot of a diabetic, or the person with thyroid or pituitary gland malfunction, and eventually disturb the circulation of the limb, are the subject of a survey by W. P. U. Jackson and J. H. Louw, while H. S. Myers describes comprehensively the radiographic appearances in acromegaly.

The number of children referred with foot problems whose condition is a simple variant of the normal is of concern to Geoffrey Walker. He discusses the features of normality before distinguishing "neurologic" feet in otherwise apparently normal children from those with known neurologic problems.

Glenn Quitell gives us a podiatrist's view of his specialty; a discipline that plays an increasing part in the management of disorders of the feet.

When man walked barefoot, the skin of the sole was thick and tough and could withstand the rough of rocks and jungle. Footwear added protection and warmth. Indifferent footwear exacts a human price. While we approve the old proverb, "Better cut the shoe than pinch the foot," David Holmes discusses the preferred prescription for shoes that fit and devices that bring comfort and support.

We are deeply indebted to our guest authors for splendid contributions; to Stuart Freeman and Suzanne Boyd who, in the Lippincott tradition, eased progress and production; and to our wives, Natalie (H.) and Lydia (G.L.). We should like to thank Mr. David Seaton for his drawings and Mr. Ken Sensom for his photographs.

A.J.H.
D.G.L.

Contents

DISORDERS OF THE FOOT

1 Terminology

Much of the confusion surrounding the diagnosis and treatment of disorders of the feet arises from imprecise use of the terms used to describe them. Many words, used for centuries, have their roots in Latin. Most terms are logical; a few, hallowed by tradition, are obscure. Some words have changed their meaning over the years: for example, in the eighteenth century, *valgus* and *varus* meant the opposite of what they mean now.

In an attempt to clarify, we shall define the terms used in this book—both those used to describe the movements of the foot and ankle, and those defining the shape, normal and abnormal, of the foot.

MOVEMENTS

While each joint has its characteristic range of movements, it is more practical to describe the movements of the foot and ankle as a whole in a clinical context, provided it is borne in mind that these are complex and may be combined at several joints.

Plantar flexion is the movement of the foot and ankle downward; that is, toward the sole of the foot (Fig. 1-1A). It consists, for the most part, of flexion at the ankle joint, but includes some movement of all the joints of the foot.

Dorsiflexion is the opposite movement (Fig. 1-1B). The front of the foot is brought upward, mainly by extension at the ankle joint, accom-

panied by some outward rotation of the foot itself.

Inversion is the movement of the whole foot, inward, until the sole is pointing medially (Fig. 1-2A). It is a complex, rotational movement, in which all the joints of the hindfoot are involved, including the subtalar and midtarsal. During the movement, the sole of the foot is not only rotated medially, but tends to face upward: in other words, there is some degree of supination of the sole.

Eversion is the opposite movement of the whole foot, outward, into a flat-foot or pronated position (Fig. 1-2B). Like inversion, it is a complex, rotational movement, involving all the joints of the hindfoot.

Abduction is a movement away from the midline (Fig. 1-3A,B). The word can also be used to describe a shape: thus it is possible to speak of an *abduction deformity. Abduction* is

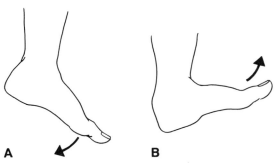

Fig. 1-1. (*A*) Plantarflexion. (*B*) Dorsiflexion.

1

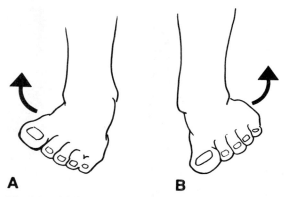

Fig. 1-2. (*A*) Inversion. (*B*) Eversion.

not synonymous with *valgus,* when used to describe a shape, although both terms are used to describe a deformity in the same plane. The difference can be defined precisely: *valgus* (see below) describes a movement of the limb away from the *midline of the body,* whereas *abduction* describes a movement of a distal part of the body away from the *midline axis of the main trunk.*

A consideration of the definition will show the difference. In knock-knee deformity, for example, the foot moves away from the midline of the body. It may be described as *genu valgum* (Latin for a valgus knee) or as *abduction deformity.* In the case of the big toe (*hallux,* in Latin) if it were displaced away from the midline of the body, it would be described as *hallux valgus*: but it is *not* an

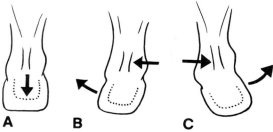

A   B   C

Fig. 1-3. Diagram representing abduction- and adduction deformities of the heel. (*A*) A vertical left heel, viewed from behind. It can be seen (*arrow*) that the heel is in the line of axis of the limb. (*B*) Posterior view of a left heel with an abduction deformity. The heel has tilted away from the axis of the limb to the lateral side, and in so doing, bowstrings the Achilles tendon laterally. (*C*) In a similar way, adduction deformity bowstrings the Achilles tendon medial to the axis of the limb.

abduction deformity, since the toe is displaced toward the axis of the foot, running through the second toe. It is correctly described as an adduction deformity.

Adduction is the opposite movement or displacement to abduction; that is, it is a movement *toward* the central axis of the part of the body proximal to the limb or digit (Fig. 1-3C).

ABNORMALITIES IN THE SHAPE OF THE FOOT

Talipes is a traditional word, of Latin derivation, used to describe a fixed deformity of the whole foot that is present at birth. It remains a useful term, implying, as it does, a true deformity of a child's foot, rather than just a variation in shape. The word is not used to describe deformities with a known etiology; for example, a known disease of the nervous system.

Equinus, the horse-foot deformity, is a condition in which the foot is fixed in plantar flexion, so that the heel cannot be brought to the ground and the patient has to walk on the metatarsal heads (Fig. 1-4A).

Calcaneus is the term used to describe a fixed, dorsiflexed deformity of the foot, in which the heel is said to be presenting for weight bearing (Fig. 1-4B).

Pes planus is Latin for flat foot.

Pes cavus means a foot with a fixed, high arch (Fig. 1-5).

Valgus and Varus. Of all the words used to describe shape of the limbs, *valgus* and *varus* cause the most difficulty. The origin of the

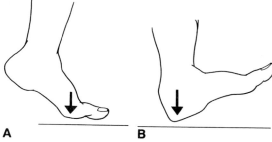

A   B

Fig. 1-4. (*A*) Equinus deformity in which the weight is borne on the front of the foot. (*B*) Calcaneus deformity, where the weight is borne on the presenting heel.

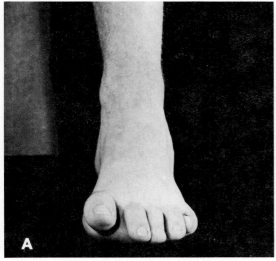

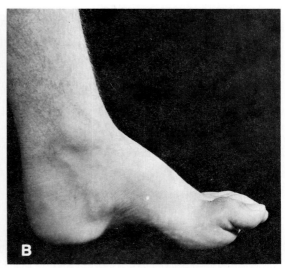

Fig. 1-5. Anterior (*A*) and lateral (*B*) views of a foot with pes cavus, showing a typical fixed high arch and clawing of the toes.

terms is obscure, and if they did not exist, it would not be wise to invent them; but they are used so universally that they cannot be discarded. Provided they are clearly defined, they are useful.

Valgus and *varus* describe angular deformities of the limbs when the patient is viewed from the front; that is, they refer to angulation in the transverse plane of the body. By convention, the position of parts of the body is described with the subject standing with feet together and arms by the sides, palms facing forward (Fig. 1-6). This is known as the anatomical position.

It should be imagined that, with the body in the anatomical position, a vertical line extends

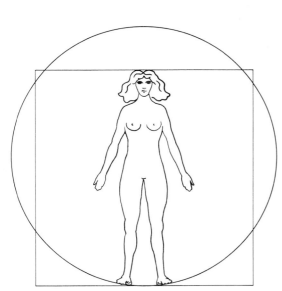

Fig. 1-6. A diagram showing the anatomical position as defined by convention.

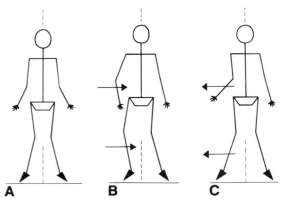

Fig. 1-7. (*A*) "Matchstick" drawing of the anatomical position. (*B*) On the right side of the body, deformities of the right elbow and knee are shown. Arrows indicate that the distal part of the limb is moved toward the midline in each case; that is, there is a varus deformity of the right elbow (cubitus varus) and right knee (genu varum). (*C*) In this diagram, valgus deformities of the right elbow and right knee are shown. It can be seen that the limb distal to the joint is moved away from the midline axis of the body; that is, cubitus valgus and genu valgum.

from the tip of the chin to the ground (Fig. 1-7A). Any deformity of the limb, whether arm or leg, in which the distal extremity is moved nearer the midline of the body, is described as *varus* (Fig. 1-7B). *Valgus* describes a deformity in which the limb distal to the deformity is angulated away from the midline (Fig. 1-7C).

Most valgus or varus deformities occur at the joints, but they may be present in the shaft of a bone, due to breaking or bending. Figure 1-7B represents varus injuries of the right elbow and knee, while Figure 1-7C shows valgus deformities of the elbow and knee on the right side.

2 A Clinical View of the Function of the Foot

When one is standing, the weight is borne principally on the heel and the ball of the foot; in the latter, especially by the heads of the first, fourth, and fifth metatarsals. This essentially three-point, weight-bearing mechanism is converted into a stable tripod by the longitudinal and transverse arches, which add resilience and a springy quality to the foot because of their ligamentous elasticity.

In walking, the weight is borne alternately on this tripod and on a platform composed of the heads of the metatarsals and the extended five toes. In this position, the anterior arch of the foot is flattened. The heads of all the metatarsals, being depressed, share the load evenly. The toes are straightened and the weight distributed on a broad surface.

In the evolution of the foot from a part that was capable of specialized prehension to one that serves the relatively simple functions of locomotion and support, the action of the anterior half of the foot has "fallen into a state of dereliction . . . and relative weakness,"[1] especially when we consider the correlated development of the heel as the new weight-bearing part.

THE CONCEPT OF THE TORSION SPRING

The hand is used to touch, to test, to grasp; the foot is a support, a balance in any posture of the body. It is also a flexible lever, used to promote propulsive action; but this definition is incomplete. Closer examination reveals that the foot behaves like a torsion spring, which propels the body forward actively during walking. The torque is similar in character to that of the other joints of the lower limb and is in sinuous adaptation with them. The helical nature[2] of such joints provides significant advantages over simple hinge joints in the maintenance of posture, in lifting, and in propulsion.

To initiate movement of the body from the standing position, weight is shifted by bringing one foot forward. The foot is raised as it advances, and at this moment the whole weight is shifted to the supporting foot, which remains in contact with the ground. To continue this forward movement of the raised foot, the supporting foot changes its function, first from passive to active support, and then to propulsion. The change is effected by a smooth and orderly translation of the weight-bearing surface. From the stable support of the calcaneus and outer border of the sole, the weight-bearing area moves forward in a single, rolling action, from the heel, through the outer margin, to the stabilized fore-part of the ball of the foot. Finally, the weight is borne on the platform composed of the straightened toes, extended at the metatarsophalangeal joints. To reach this position, the load is transferred across the ball of the foot to the head of the first metatarsal. This platform requires active muscle contraction to stabilize it against the force of gravity by obtaining a grip on the ground. During the act of gripping with the toes, all the digital flexors contract. The interossei are essential to this process. These short muscles straighten the toes while fixing the metatarsophalangeal joints. To this grip is added the pull of the gastrocnemius and soleus muscles, which fixes the raised heel.

The short flexors of the foot, associated with the plantar aponeurosis and the tibialis posterior, brace the longitudinal bony arch, while allowing elasticity in the tread. Wood Jones, with whose writings the above description of the action of the muscles is in agreement, went on to say that obtaining a grip, "was one of the actions to correct walking that is hampered by the wearing of hard-soled footwear, for the toes, which should grip the ground while the foot rises from it, are unable to perform this function properly."[3]

REFERENCES

1. Lake, N. C.: The Foot. London, Bailliere, Tindall & Cox, 1945.
2. Helfet, A. J.: Disorders of the Knee. Philadelphia, J. B. Lippincott, 1974, p. 18.
3. Wood Jones, J.: Structure and Function as Seen in the Foot. London, Bailliere, Tindall & Cox, 1949.

3 The Clinical Anatomy of the Foot

RALPH GER

If the foot lacks the beautiful precision of the hand, the latter has evolved only because man was able to support himself on his feet and so free the upper limbs to carry out his various tasks. The foot, however, should not be thought of merely as a stable base supporting the weight of the body above it. Were this so, walking—not to mention running and jumping—would be awkward and difficult. An understanding of the function of this versatile appendage is well worthwhile, for the benefits of civilization are turning the foot into a semirigid organ with common deformities. It is doubtful whether we shall ever revert to the unshod foot and attempt to compete with the prehensile feet of our nearest rivals, the great apes. The picture, however, of the unfortunate who has lost the use of his upper limbs but yet is able to write and paint with his feet should remind us of their potential and help to dismiss the concept of the foot as merely a sophisticated platform.

THE BONES

The Tibia and Fibula

The lower end of the tibia (Fig. 3-1) is expanded into a large, weight-bearing area, and from its medial aspect a considerable bony process projects downward: the medial malleolus. The lateral aspect of the distal extremity of the tibia has a narrow facet for the fibula, above which is a rough area for a large, interosseous ligament.

The lower end of the fibula, likewise, has an expanded end, the lateral malleolus, which is situated at a level lower than, and posterior to, the medial malleolus. Any disturbance of this relationship of the two malleoli means that displacement has occurred. The medial aspect of the fibula also has a small strip for the tibia, above which is a rough area for the interosseous membrane. Below this strip is a triangular facet which articulates with the talus.

When these two bones are placed together, it will be seen that they form a mortise into which fits the talus.

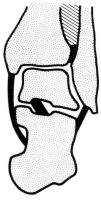

Fig. 3-1. The lower ends of tibia and fibula with their malleoli grasp the talus. The collateral ligaments, interosseus ligament, and membrane are seen.

7

The Talus

The talus, the superiorly placed bone of the tarsus, has a convex upper articular surface continuous with a larger lateral surface and a smaller surface on its medial aspect (Fig. 3-2). The smooth area articulates with the mortise, and the medial and lateral facets are firmly grasped by the respective malleoli. Note that the surface of the talus is broader in front than behind; a point of considerable importance. The talus then narrows anteriorly into a neck, in front of which is the head, which has a large facet to articulate with the succeeding bone of the tarsus (Fig. 3-3). Posteriorly, a tendon occupies a groove which separates the posterior and medial tubercles. The under-surface of the talus articulates with the bone lying inferior to it, the calcaneus, by three facets, the posterior being separated from the two anterior by a deep groove, occupied by a very powerful interosseous ligament joining the two bones. The talus has another facet on its anteromedial aspect, which articulates with the spring ligament.

The Calcaneus

The calcaneus is the largest and the most posteriorly situated bone of the tarsus. The

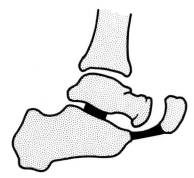

Fig. 3-3. The talus articulates with tibia above, the calcaneus below, and the navicular anteriorly. The interosseous and spring ligaments are outlined.

backward-projecting part of the calcaneus, peculiar to man, is for the insertion of the tendo calcaneus, while inferiorly it bears two large tuberosities to carry the whole weight of the body. Anteriorly, on its upper surface, is an area which articulates superiorly with the talus by three facets. Projecting medially from the middle facet is a shelf of bone called the sustentaculum tali. Beneath this shelf run some of the tendons passing from leg to foot. Anteriorly, the bone ends in an articular facet for the following bone of the foot, the cuboid. Its lateral aspect has two small bosses for ligamentous attachments.

The Cuboid

The cuboid bone articulates behind with the calcaneus and in front with the fourth and fifth metatarsals. The most noteworthy feature is a large groove on its under-surface, which accommodates a tendon.

The Navicular

The anterior aspect of the talus articulates with the navicular, a boat-shaped bone also called the tarsal scaphoid, which ends in a large knob palpable on the medial side of the foot, the tuberosity of the navicular.

The Cuneiforms

The navicular articulates anteriorly with three small bones, the wedge-shaped medial, intermediate and lateral cuneiforms. The latter articulates with the cuboid on its lateral side.

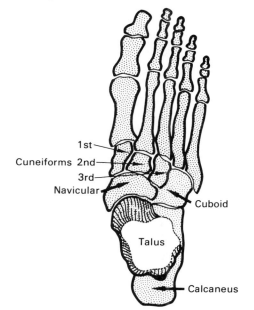

1st
Cuneiforms 2nd
3rd
Navicular
Cuboid
Talus
Calcaneus

Fig. 3-2. The bones of the foot, related to the talus.

The Metatarsals

Anterior to the cuboid and three cuneiforms, which form an irregular horizontal line, are the five metatarsal bones. The first is short and very stout, as it carries a lot of weight, and the remaining four metatarsals are slender, with their heads distal and their bases proximal. The base of the second metatarsal is wedged between the medial and lateral cuneiforms, because the smaller intermediate bone does not project as far distally. The fifth metatarsal is noteworthy in that it has an easily palpable tuberosity at its base.

The Phalanges

Each toe has three phalanges; proximal, middle and distal, except for the big toe, which has only two, each of which is very much stouter than those in the other toes.

THE JOINTS

The Ankle

The bones comprising this mortise joint are the lower ends of the tibia and fibula and the upper surface and sides of the body of the talus. The projecting malleoli of the tibia and fibula grip the talus very firmly. The curved articular surface of the talus is broader in front than behind.

The capsule of the joint is attached to the bones just beyond the articular surfaces. A strong ligament on either side protects the joint, while the ligaments in front and behind are understandably weak, because the joint moves only in these directions.

The medial or deltoid ligament (Fig. 3-4) is a stout, fan-shaped ligament running from the lower border and tip of the medial malleolus in a triangular fashion from front to back to the tuberosity of the navicular and sustentaculum tali. It includes the spring ligament, which joins these two bony points to the medial tubercle and neck of the talus. Compared to the lateral ligament, the medial, being thick and strong, is not often injured.

The lateral ligament (Fig. 3-5) has three separate bands that all run from the fibular

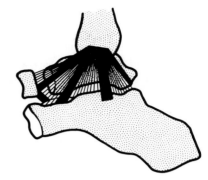

Fig. 3-4. The medial ligament at the ankle joint (deltoid ligament) is seen attached to the malleolus, above, and, inferiorly, to the navicular, spring ligament, sustentaculum tali, and talus from before backward.

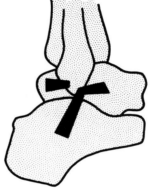

Fig. 3-5. The three bands of the lateral ligament.

malleolus: the anterior talofibular, forward to the neck of the talus; the posterior, backward from the small dimple on the medial aspect of this malleolus to the talus; and the middle band, downward to a small protuberance on the lateral aspect of the calcaneus. Strains of this ligament are common, and it is usually quite simple to diagnose which band has been stretched or ruptured by locating the point of tenderness.

Movements. For practical purposes, the ankle is a simple, hinged joint. In dorsiflexion the toes are raised toward the leg, and in plantar flexion the toes point down, away from the leg. The tight grip of the two malleoli on the talus becomes somewhat looser in extreme plantar flexion, for example in standing on tiptoe, when the narrow part of the talus articulates with the bones. In this position it is possible to rotate the talus slightly and therefore produce abduction, adduction, inversion, and eversion. This means that tiptoe is a rather unstable position, whereas dorsiflexion, where the broad anterior part of the talus is engaged, is a much more solid position.

The Talocalcaneonavicular Joint

This is a separate joint, with its own capsule and synovial membrane, between the head of the talus, fitting into the cup-shaped navicular bone anteriorly, and inferiorly onto the two anteriorly placed calcaneal articular surfaces, one lying on the sustentaculum tali and the other slightly in front of it. Between the sustentaculum tali and the navicular tuberosity is a smooth, polished portion of the talus, which is not engaged by any bony articular surface but by an extremely powerful ligament between these two bony points: the spring or plantar calcaneonavicular ligament. This ligament is extremely thick and actually becomes cartilaginous in part. It is a major support for the talus, and stretching of the ligament, which occurs in advanced flatfoot, allows the head of the talus to drop and project inferiorly.

The Talocalcaneal Joint

It is a simple joint between the posterior facet of the talus and the posterior facet on the upper surface of the calcaneus. Between this joint and the talocalcaneonavicular is a tunnel, narrow medially and widening laterally. This is the sinus tarsi, which has a large interosseous ligament joining the bones. Considerable force is necessary to rupture the ligament and dislocate the talus.

The Calcaneocuboid Joint

This is a simple joint with little movement between the calcaneus and the cuboid.

The Cuneonavicular Joints

In front of the navicular lie the three cuneiform bones, so-called because of their wedged shape: the medial, with wedge in an upward direction, and the two smaller cuneiforms wedged downward. The larger size of the

medial and lateral cuneiforms leaves a small, intermediate one, so that the distal articular surfaces of the three medial metatarsals, which articulate one with each bone, are at different levels, while the base of the second metatarsal is wedged between and articulates to some degree with the medial and lateral cuneiforms. This is of importance during any amputation involving the whole of the second metatarsal bone.

The Tarsometatarsal and Metatarsophalangeal Joints

The first three metatarsal bases articulate with each cuneiform, and the fourth and fifth with the cuboid. The heads of the five metatarsals articulate with the proximal phalanges and have ligaments similar to those in the hand, including the large, volar fibrocartilaginous pads. The first metatarsal is noteworthy in that it is short and stout and also has, on its inferior surface, two articular facets for the two sesamoid bones. These bones act as roller bearings and are normally subdivided into several small parts due to aberrant ossification. As in the fingers, the metatarsophalangeal joints are condyloid in shape and able to flex, extend, abduct, and adduct.

The Interphalangeal Joints

These more distal joints are hinges, flexing and extending only. They are constructed on the same principles as those of the fingers, but are obviously much less important, as they do not perform the same intricate work. They are, however, important in walking.

THE ARCHES

The imprint left by a wet foot shows that the foot touches the ground at the heel and at the fifth and first metatarsals, forming a sort of tripod, with the foot arched between these points, both longitudinally and horizontally.

Bones of the Arches

The medial longitudinal arch (Fig. 3-6) is much higher than the lateral. Posteriorly it consists of the calcaneus and body of the talus and, anteriorly, the navicular, cuneiforms and their attached metatarsals. The head of the talus is the keystone between the posterior and anterior parts of the arch.

The Lateral Longitudinal Arch (Fig. 3-7). The calcaneus lies posteriorly, with the cuboid and its two metatarsals anteriorly. These bones constitute a much lower arch, which almost touches the ground.

The Horizontal Arches. Each arch, when aligned to the opposite foot, forms a complete arch, but in each foot, separately, they are half arches. There are two transverse arches; one formed by the cuneiforms and cuboid (that is, the tarsal bones) and an arch farther forward formed by the five metatarsal bones strung together by ligaments (Figs. 3-8 and 3-9).

Ligaments of the Arches

The ligaments play a substantial part in holding the bones together (Fig. 3-10). If persistently stressed, however, they become stretched and painful. Muscle is much better fitted to take strain, and the contraction of voluntary muscle is unsurpassed in resisting distraction. The following ligaments are important.

The spring ligament (plantarcalcaneo navicular ligament) is a fibrocartilaginous band which joins the navicular and sustentaculum tali; which supports the head of the talus and has itself support from the long tendons running from the leg to the foot beneath it.

The Two Plantar Ligaments. The long plantar ligament is a substantial structure running from the plantar surface of the calcaneus across the ridge of the cuboid, to which it gains attachment, so forming a tunnel for a tendon and continuing as far as the middle three metatarsals. It is an important tie-beam for the longitudinal arch. The short plantar ligament is merely the calcaneocuboid ligament lying deep to the long ligament.

Plantar Aponeurosis. Not a true ligament, this important subcutaneous fibrous tissue structure acts as a strong tie, stretching from the calcaneus to the phalanges.

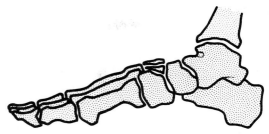

Fig. 3-6. The medial longitudinal arch.

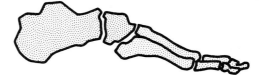

Fig. 3-7. The lateral longitudinal arch.

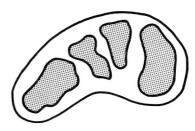

Fig. 3-8. The transverse arch formed by the cuneiforms and the cuboid.

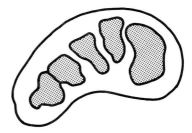

Fig. 3-9. The transverse arch formed by five metatarsals.

Muscles of the Arches

There are two groups of muscles: the extrinsic, which arise in the calf and run to the foot, and the intrinsic, which arise and insert in the sole of the foot. They will be detailed later, and are probably the most important structures in maintaining both the longitudinal and transverse arches.

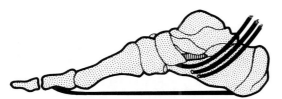

Fig. 3-10. The tendons and ligaments supporting the arch. The plantar fascia is the inferior tie, while, above, the spring ligament is supported by the tibialis posterior and flexor digitorum longus and -hallucis longus from above downward.

MUSCLES ACTING AT THE ANKLE AND FOOT JOINTS

The Anterolateral Group of Muscles

This group of muscles is firmly embraced by the tibia and fibula on each side, the interosseous membrane deeply, and a very strong fascia superficially. These rigid structures prevent appreciable swelling of the muscles, a phenomenon which leads to the anterior compartment syndrome (see p. 68).

The actions and positions of the muscles and tendons passing the ankle joint are simple to determine if it is remembered that those which act on the tarsus are situated peripherally and end in the tarsus, whereas those destined for the digits lie more centrally (that is, the evertors and invertors flank the digitorum muscles; Fig. 3-11). The tibialis anterior arises from the tibia and has a large tendon which passes downward, obliterating the sharp anterior border of the tibia in its lowest part, to cross the bone and insert into the medial side of the medial cuneiform bone and the base of the first metatarsal. (Another muscle, the peroneus longus, inserts into these same two bones but arrives by another route.) The peroneus tertius arises from the fibula and inserts into the fifth metatarsal bone. These two muscles are the invertors and evertors, respectively. Between them lie the muscles to the big toe, the extensor hallucis longus, and to the other four toes, the extensor digitorum longus. These two muscles and the peroneus tertius arise from a narrow area on the fibula between the interosseous and anterior borders. The long extensors are joined by the tendons of the extensor digitorum brevis, which arises

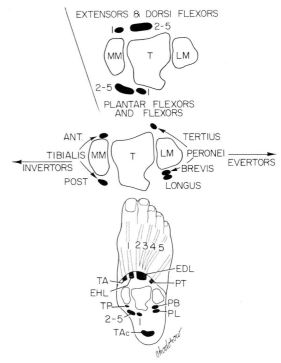

Fig. 3-11. (*Top*) The diagram shows the extensors anteriorly and the flexors posteriorly. (*Middle*) This diagram indicates the invertors medially and the evertors laterally, before and behind the respective malleoli. MM, medial malleolus; LM, lateral malleolus; T, talus. (*Bottom*) This diagram illustrates the invertors and evertors flanking the tendons for the digits.

from the upper surface of the distal part of the calcaneus.

The Peroneal Muscles

The peroneal muscles take origin from the lateral surface of the fibula; the longus, from above and behind the brevis. The two tendons pass behind the fibular malleolus, the brevis going to the fifth metatarsal and the longus running inferiorly to reach the cuboid, where it develops a sesamoid bone that plays on the surface of the cuboid (Fig. 3-12). The tendon enters a deep ridge on the plantar surface of this bone; runs medially across the sole of the foot and inserts into the same bones as the tibialis anterior (Fig. 3-13). The bony ridge is converted into a tunnel for this tendon by the long plantar ligament (Fig. 3-14). The two tendons, which have well-formed synovial

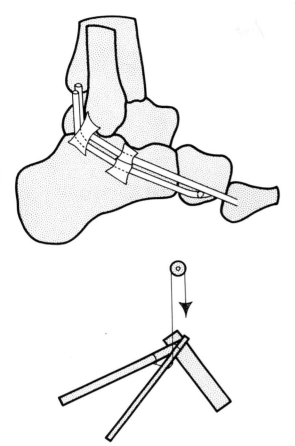

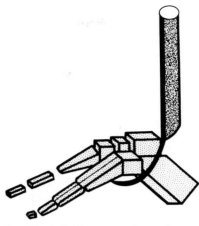

Fig. 3-12. (*Top left*) The peroneal muscles are secured by the two retinacula; the brevis is inserting into the fifth metatarsal tuberosity and the longus is entering the groove on the under-surface of the cuboid, at which point its sesamoid bone is outlined.

Fig. 3-13. (*Top right*) The peroneus longus muscle gives rise to its tendon, which runs across the sole of the foot to its medial side, supporting the longitudinal arch as it does so. (Redrawn from Lee Mc Gregor, A. L.: A Synopsis of Surgical Anatomy. ed. 9. Bristol, John Wright, 1963)

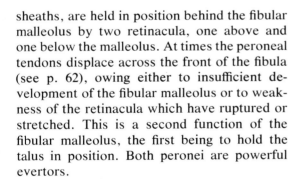

Fig. 3-14. (*Left*) The peroneus longus tendon acts as a pulley for the longitudinal arch. (Redrawn from Lee Mc Gregor, A. L.: A Synopsis of Surgical Anatomy. ed. 9. Bristol, John Wright, 1963)

sheaths, are held in position behind the fibular malleolus by two retinacula, one above and one below the malleolus. At times the peroneal tendons displace across the front of the fibula (see p. 62), owing either to insufficient development of the fibular malleolus or to weakness of the retinacula which have ruptured or stretched. This is a second function of the fibular malleolus, the first being to hold the talus in position. Both peronei are powerful evertors.

The Posterior Muscles of the Calf

The muscles are arranged in a superficial group, the gastrocnemius, soleus, and plantaris, which are separated by a thick sheet of fascia from a deep group, the long flexors of the toes, hallucis and digitorum, and the muscle that is to go to the tarsus, the tibialis posterior.

Gastrocnemius. The two bellies of this muscle arises from the popliteal surface of the femur and join at mid-calf, to be inserted into the tendo calcaneus. This is the largest tendon in the body and is inserted into the posterior surface of the tuberosity of the calcaneus.

The soleus muscle arises from both bones; from the oblique line on the posterior surface of the upper and middle thirds of the medial surface of the tibia, and the upper third of the posterior surface of the fibula. These bellies join together, rather like the flexor digitorum superficialis of the forearm, and insert into the anterior surface of the tendo calcaneus, reaching down almost to the insertion of the latter. The muscle is responsible for more of the bulk of the calf than the gastrocnemius. Running lateromedially between the gastrocnemius and soleus is the plantaris tendon, which eventually appears on the medial side of the tendo calcaneus, to run with it and insert separately into the calcaneus. The tendo calcaneus is surrounded by a loose sheath, often called the paratenon; sometimes the site of tenosynovitis (see p. 147).

The Deep Layer of Muscles. In order to increase their mechanical advantage, the digitorum and hallucis longus muscles arise from what appear to be the wrong bones, but the force of pull from the fibula to the big toe is stronger than it would be from the tibia to the big toe and vice versa. Accordingly, the flexor hallucis longus arises from the fibula and the digitorum from the tibia. They give rise to tendons which cross one another in the sole of the foot as they pass to their respective insertions. Deeper to these two muscles, and arising from both bones and the interosseous membrane, is the tibialis posterior, which passes inferiorly and peripherally, crossing deep to the digitorum longus tendon behind the tibial malleolus to its major insertion into the tuberosity of the navicular bone, and all the bones of the tarsus, except the talus.

THE MOVEMENTS OF THE FOOT AND ANKLE

Inversion and Eversion

What is meant by inversion is the turning of the sole of the foot to face inward. Eversion is the opposite. This movement cannot take place at the ankle joint, which is almost a pure hinge; rather, it takes place at the subtalar level, the talus remaining fixed and the other bones of the foot moving in relationship to the talus. Most of the movement takes place at the talocalcaneonavicular joint; the calcaneocuboid joint moves only slightly. The joints between the tarsal and metatarsal bones present a somewhat irregular, horizontal line, owing to the proximal projection of the second metatarsal. Little movement takes place at these tarsometatarsal joints.

It will be seen that all muscles lying on the lateral aspect of the leg are evertors. Their tendons lie peripherally and laterally. They are the three peronei: the tertius in front of the malleoli, and the other two behind.

Those tendons lying medially, and peripheral

to the deep layer of posterior tendons at the back of the calf, are invertors. This group consists of the tibialis anterior and posterior.

Dorsiflexion and Plantar Flexion

It is quite clear that all structures passing in front of the ankle joint are dorsiflexors and all those passing behind the ankle joint are plantar flexors.

Dorsiflexors. The extensor hallucis and digitorum longus muscles are major dorsiflexors, as well as extensors of the toes, whereas the tibialis anterior and peroneus tertius, while mainly inverting or everting, are minor dorsiflexors as well.

Plantar Flexors. Of the deep muscles passing from calf to foot, the hallucis and digitorum, while being flexors of the toes, also flex the ankle joint. The tibialis posterior will do this, but it expends its energy mainly on producing inversion. The most powerful plantar flexors are the gastrocnemius and soleus, acting through the tendo calcaneus.

Additional Bonuses

All muscles with tendons passing behind the joint are additional plantar flexors, and all those with tendons passing in front of the joint are dorsiflexors. The tendons also play a very important part in maintaining the arches of the foot. The tendon of the peroneus longus, by running from the lateral aspect of the leg across the inferior aspect of the tarsus to its medial side, acts as a strong pulley lifting up the lateral longitudinal arch as well as turning the sole of the foot outward. The tibialis anterior and posterior are both inserted into the middle of the tarsus and assist in its elevation. The long flexors of the calf, particularly the flexor hallucis longus running behind the medial malleolus and beneath the sustentaculum tali to the big toe, are also major supports of the arch.

THE RETINACULA

The peroneal retinacula maintain the position of the peroneus longus and brevis, while the superior and inferior extensor retinacula control the tendons crossing the anterior aspect of the ankle joint. Finally, and of major importance, is the thickest retinaculum of all, the flexor retinaculum, running from the medial malleolus to the calcaneus, which holds the tendons passing from calf to foot in position, as well as protecting the underlying vessels.

Tendon Sheaths

Where the tendons lie between the overlying retinacula and the underlying bone, the synovial sheaths enclose both surfaces of the tendon to allay friction. The sheaths of all tendons not reaching the sole of the foot start and stop short distances above and below the retinacula. These include the anterolateral muscles, with separate sheaths for the tibialis anterior and extensor hallucis longus, and the common sheath for the extensor digitorum and the peroneus tertius; the tibialis posterior medially, and the peroneus brevis laterally, which leaves its common sheath with the longus as it runs to its insertion. Those tendons reaching and traversing the sole, pass through fibro-osseous tunnels, where synovial sheaths greatly assist their gliding motion. Thus the peroneus longus, between the long plantar ligament and the cuboid and cuneiform bones, and the flexors hallucis- and digitorum longus, passing over the plantar aspects of the calcaneus and navicular and into the fibrous flexor sheaths of the digits, have sheaths which enclose the tendons almost to their insertion points. The sheath of the digitorum for the middle digits is interrupted for a short distance, as in the hand.

NERVE SUPPLY

The Anterior Tibial Nerve

The anterior tibial nerve enters the anterolateral compartment, and having supplied all the muscles of that compartment, appears on the dorsum of the foot, supplying only the skin of the first web space (that is, it expends most of its energy in supplying muscles).

The Superficial Peroneal Nerve

The superficial peroneal nerve runs between the two peronei and leaves them at a point about two-thirds of the way down the lateral side of the leg, where it pierces the fascia to supply all of the dorsum of the foot, except for the first web space (anterior tibial) and the two borders, which are supplied by the sural and saphenous nerves. The musculocutaneous nerve can actually be rolled on the underlying fibula after it pierces the fascia and is a simple nerve to block should one wish to carry out any surgery on the dorsum of the foot.

The Saphenous Nerve

The saphenous nerve, having started just below the inguinal ligament, accompanies the saphenous vein and ends by supplying the skin of the foot as far as the ball of the big toe, while the sural nerve, accompanying the short saphenous vein, supplies the skin on the lateral side of the foot to the side of the little toe.

ARTERIAL SUPPLY

The Posterior Tibial Artery

The posterior tibial artery runs inferiorly, together with the nerve, behind the deep fascia covering the deep muscles of the leg. It surfaces behind the medial malleolus where, with its accompanying veins, it lies behind the tibialis posterior and digitorum longus tendons. Beneath the flexor retinaculum, it divides into terminal, medial and lateral plantar arteries. This artery is important in determining the blood supply of the leg as it can be palpated two-tendons-breadth behind the medial malleolus. It is important that the flexor retinaculum be relaxed during palpation by inverting the foot.

The Peroneal Artery

The peroneal artery runs inferiorly in the substance of the flexor hallucis longus in very close relationship to the fibula and eventually passes beyond its lower extremity to supply the heel as the lateral calcaneal artery. It gives off a large, perforating branch which, as the name indicates, passes through the interosseous membrane to the anterior compartment of the leg. This is a fairly constant vessel and should be sought in clinical examination. These two arteries supply all the muscles, bones, and joints of the posterior part of the leg.

The Anterior Tibial Artery

The anterior tibial artery, having entered the anterolateral compartment of the leg, runs inferiorly, at first deeply amongst the muscles. It surfaces in front of the ankle joint and is crossed by the extensor hallucis longus tendon on its way to the big toe. This artery, now called the *dorsalis pedis*, usually disappears at the proximal end of the first intermetatarsal space, where it passes deeply to join the deep plantar arch. It supplies branches to the dorsum of the foot and the ankle region. A branch anastomoses with the perforating branch of the peroneal artery as it passes anteriorly.

It should be stated that, in general, one artery is sufficient to supply the foot and, therefore, it is important to be able to determine the patency of the arteries to the foot; the posterior tibial artery, two tendons in breadth behind the medial malleolus, with the ankle inverted to relax the thick retinaculum; the perforating peroneal artery in front of the lower third of the fibula, and also the dorsalis pedis just proximal to the first intermetatarsal space.

THE SOLE OF THE FOOT

The Skin

On the sole, as on the palm of the hand, both the epidermis and dermis are thick, even in the newborn child.

The skin of the sole of the foot becomes even thicker and, on an unshod foot, almost horny. The skin, as in the hand, is attached to the underlying deep fascia by fibrous bands. This divides the subcutaneous fat into numerous small cushions for weight bearing, particularly in the heel region. The presence of these compartments, while very comfortable, makes it difficult to find a foreign body in the sole of the foot. The deep fascia of the sole of the foot is also markedly thickened, especially centrally, where it is called the plantar aponeurosis and extends from both calcaneal tubercles, splitting into five bands, one for each digit. (In the hand it splits into four, as nothing is allowed to interfere with the mobility of the thumb.) Each band bifurcates distally to allow for the passage of the flexor tendons, and the

divisions are attached to the sides of the phalanges, as in the hand. The fascia over the medial and lateral borders of the foot is much thinner. The attachment of the skin to the underlying aponeurosis gives some degree of fixation. The plantar aponeurosis is one of the main struts maintaining the longitudinal arch of the foot.

The Muscles of the Sole

Traditionally, these have always been described as being in four layers, but it is easier to divide them into medial, lateral, and central. The peripheral muscles, one long and one short on each side, reach the proximal phalanges of the digits only. The central muscles are more numerous as they fill the spaces formed by the longitudinal and transverse arches. Except for one muscle running obliquely and transversely to support the transverse arch, all the muscles run longitudinally and are placed one on top of another, the superficial muscles reaching the intermediate phalanges and the deeper muscles, the distal phalanges.

Medial Muscles. The most superficial muscle, called the abductor hallucis, is rather large. Lying deep to it, and more anteriorly, is the short flexor of the big toe; the flexor hallucis brevis. The latter muscle is in two portions: its medial belly is inserted, in common with the abductor, into the medial side of the proximal phalanx, while its lateral head is inserted into the lateral side of the proximal phalanx, in common with another muscle. It is worth knowing that the flexor hallucis brevis has sesamoids, which articulate with the plantar aspect of the head of the first metatarsal bone. Perhaps there was a time when the big toe could be abducted, but now these muscles act as springs for the arches of the foot.

Lateral Muscles. On the lateral side we have the abductor digiti minimi and, deep to that, the flexor digiti minimi brevis. These are inserted into the lateral aspect of the proximal phalanx of the fifth toe. Their function is the same as that of the medial muscles.

Central Muscles. Deep to the plantar aponeurosis is the flexor digitorum brevis, going to the middle phalanx of each toe and, deep to this, the flexor digitorum longus and -hallucis tendons running to the terminal phalanges. Here, an interesting anatomical rearrangement allows these tendons to pull both in straight lines and on more than one phalanx. For example, the flexor digitorum longus, after entering the medial side of the foot and running laterally, at an angle, to allow its tendons to reach the lateral toes, has its pull straightened out by a muscle, the flexor accesorius (quadratus plantae) which arises from the calcaneus and is attached to the tendon to help it to pull in a straight line. The hallucis longus runs in a straight line and does not need any assistance; moreover, as it crosses deep to the digitorum, it gives slips to the tendons to the second and third toes, thereby extending its pull on the whole medial longitudinal arch, which is one of its main functions. Arising from the flexor digitorum longus are four lumbricals which, as in the hand, pass on the thumb—or big toe—side of the digitorum tendons. That being so, the first lumbrical can arise from only one side of the tendon, but the other three lumbricals arise from both tendons, between which they lie. As in the fingers, they pass dorsally to the extensor expansions on the dorsum of the toes and to the distal two phalanges. Deeper, we find the adductor hallucis, which has oblique and transverse heads that are inserted in common with the lateral head of the flexor hallucis brevis into the proximal phalanx of the big toe. They may help in maintaining the transverse arch formed by the metatarsal bones. Finally, deep to this muscle lie the interossei, which, as the name indicates, are between the bones. They have the same function as in the hand, in that they pass across the metatarsophalangeal joints to the dorsal expansion and then to both phalanges (that is, they are flexors of the metatarsophalangeal, and extensors of the interphalangeal joints, as are the lumbricals). They also, however, act as abductors and adductors: they separate and oppose. The difference between the foot and the hand is that the axis of movement occurs through the *second* toe but to the *third* finger. The plan, however, is the same. The *d*orsally placed interossei *ab*duct (mnemonic: dab) and the *p*lantar interossei *ad*duct (pad).

Abduction and Adduction. ABDUCTION OR SEPARATION. The big and middle toes have their own abductors and do not need the aid of the interossei. The abductors are therefore on either side of the second toe, abducting it away from the imaginary line passing through the second toe. The third and fourth toes have interossei inserted into the lateral portions of each proximal phalanx, moving the third and fourth toes away from the second toe.

ADDUCTION OR OPPOSITION. The big toe has its own adductor. The second toe cannot, of course, be adducted to itself, so there remain only three plantar interossei, which are inserted into the medial aspect of the third, fourth, and fifth toes, swinging these toes toward the second toe. Dorsal interossei arise from both bones, and the plantar interossei, from a single bone.

The Functional Anatomy of the Muscles of the Sole. EXTRINSIC MUSCLES. The long flexors of the toes (hallucis and digitorum) are concerned mainly with flexing the terminal phalanges and digging them into the ground to provide a push-off in walking. The hallucis, as it runs under the sustentaculum tali beneath the spring ligament, is a powerful supporter of the medial longitudinal arch and, in fact, as it passes deep to the digitorum to reach the big toe, it gives off slips to the latter muscle which are expended in the second and third toes, thereby emphasizing its importance in maintaining the medial longitudinal arch. The tibialis posterior, like the tibialis anterior, is inserted into the mid-tarsus on the medial side and plays an important part in supporting the arch.

THE PERONEI. The peroneus brevis, passing to the outer part of the mid-tarsus, is a strong evertor, as is the peroneus longus. The latter, however, acts as a pulley, in that it runs across the sole of the foot from the lateral to the medial side and both supports the arch and everts the foot.

INTRINSIC MUSCLES. Many of the intrinsic muscles, as they run posteroanteriorly, approximate the two pillars of the arch on con-

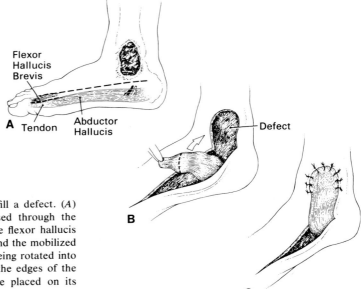

Fig. 3-15. Transposition of muscle to fill a defect. (*A*) The abductor hallucis muscle is exposed through the outlined incision and separated from the flexor hallucis brevis. (*B*) The ulcer has been excised and the mobilized muscle, after division of its tendon, is being rotated into the defect. (*C*) The muscle is sewn to the edges of the defect, after which a skin graft will be placed on its surface.

traction and are therefore very important members in maintaining the mobile arch. The abductors of the big and little toes act mainly as springs and do very little in the way of abduction. The adductor hallucis, as it runs across the sole of the foot, plays a part in maintaining the transverse arch of the metatarsal bones. The lumbricals and interossei, as in the hand, are flexors of the metatarsophalangeal, and extensors of the interphalangeal joints. They are actually very important in that they straighten the toes. Their failure to do so will result in clawing, which means that the interphalangeal joints are flexed and the metatarsophalangeal are extended. This leads to protuberance of the interphalangeal joints, resulting in dorsal corns. The extension of the metatarsophalangeal joints leaves the heads of the metatarsal bones exposed and, so, subjected to increased weight bearing. One needs straight toes and somewhat protected metatarsal heads to provide a satisfactory weight-bearing platform. Clawfeet and -toes tend to occur in diabetics, when neurologic lesions lead to atrophy of the intrinsic muscles of the foot.

Applied Anatomy of the Muscles of the Sole. Recently, muscles of the sole of the foot have been used to close defects of the malleolar region, heel, and dorsum of the foot. The principle underlying the procedure is to transpose the muscles with their neurovascular supply intact, onto or into the defect, and to apply skin grafts to the muscle to complete the closure.

The muscles used are those that lend themselves to easy mobilization near the borders of the foot. The abductors of the big and little toes are the most versatile muscles and can be used to surface the proximal dorsum heel, and malleolar regions. The flexor digitorum brevis and flexor hallucis brevis are less useful but are available for certain types of transpositions.

The principle of the operative approach is to use an incision along the border of the foot (Fig. 3-15), so as to avoid a plantar scar, and to mobilize the muscle by severance of its distal musculotendinous junction until the neurovascular pedicle is reached (Fig. 3-16). Full mobilization is secured by detaching the muscles from their bony origins (Fig. 3-17).

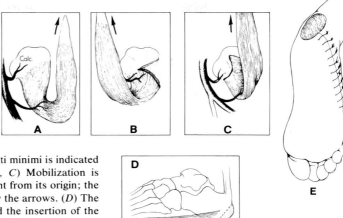

Fig. 3-16. (*A*) The mobilized abductor digiti minimi is indicated before disturbance of its bony origin. (*B*, *C*) Mobilization is increased by partial or complete detachment from its origin; the direction of the mobilization is indicated by the arrows. (*D*) The bone between the origin of the muscle and the insertion of the tendo calcaneus is removed to facilitate implantation of the muscle. (*E*) The muscle occupies the defect, and the incision is sutured.

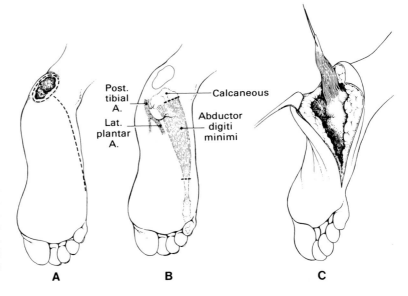

Fig. 3-17. (*A*) The line of excision of the ulcer and the skin incision is demonstrated. (*B*) The blood supply of the muscle is indicated, with the incisions necessary to mobilize the muscle. (*C*) The mobilized muscle is demonstrated prior to its being placed in the defect.

Vessels of the Sole

The sole of the foot has a profuse blood supply, as it is one of the sites from which one loses heat. The *posterior tibial artery* divides into the medial and lateral plantar arteries and gives off the calcaneal branches to the heel, whilst deep to the retinaculum the plantar vessels pass, deep to the superficial muscles of the sole, and run forward to supply digital arteries to the toes. Most of these arise from the medial plantar artery, while the larger, lateral artery expends itself mainly in forming a plantar arch, lying across the bases of the metatarsals, where it meets the termination of the dorsalis pedis as the latter passes deeply through the proximal end of the intermetatarsal space. The deep plantar arch gives off meta-tarsal arteries, which anastomose with the digital arteries.

Nerves of the Sole

The medial and lateral plantar nerves, like-wise, arise from the posterior tibial nerve beneath the flexor retinaculum, after it has given off its calcaneal branches to the heel. The nerves accompany the arteries, and the medial plantar nerve is the larger, behaving exactly as the medial nerve does in the hand. It supplies the skin of the medial three-and-a-half toes, including the dorsal part, and the muscles on the medial aspect of the foot. It supplies the abductor hallucis, flexor hallucis brevis, the first lumbrical, and the flexor digitorum brevis. The lateral plantar nerve runs to the lateral border of the foot to supply the skin of the lateral one-and-a-half toes and then supplies all the remaining muscles of the sole of the foot; in this, it resembles the ulnar nerve in the hand.

4 Biomechanics of the Foot

MICHAEL T. MANLEY

The foot is a complex mechanical structure of 26 bones braced by associated muscles and ligaments. It can carry the full body weight and bear the dynamic forces imposed by gait, yet adapt its contour to all types of terrain.

Although studies of the biomechanics of locomotion can be traced back as far as Aristotle and Leonardo da Vinci, the foot has been traditionally viewed as a static tripod or, at best, a semirigid support for body weight. The three weight-bearing legs of the tripod were assumed to contact the ground at the heel and the first and fifth metatarsal heads, while the integrity of the tripod was supposedly maintained by the longitudinal and lateral arches of the foot. The shape of these arches was assumed to be of the utmost importance, and the excellence (or otherwise) of the foot was often correlated with the height of the arch. To view it in this way is to lose sight of the fact that the foot has evolved primarily for walking and must be studied as a dynamic mechanism which forms an integral part of the locomotor system. The body requires a flexible foot to accommodate the variations in the external environment, a semirigid foot which can act as a spring and lever arm for the push-off during gait, and a rigid foot to enable body weight to be carried with reasonable stability. The biomechanics of the unique structure which forms the foot and which allows it to perform successfully all of these roles can,

therefore, only be understood when studied in relation to the biomechanics of the walking lower limb.

THE ROTATIONAL AXES OF THE FOOT

The major axis of free foot motion is the ankle joint, formed by the articulation of the talus with the tibial and fibular malleoli. In the frontal plane the ankle axis is not horizontal but is inclined away from the ground on the medial border of the foot at a mean angle of about 80 degrees (± 10°) to the long axis of the tibia (Fig. 4-1A). In the transverse plane the axis of the ankle is rotated internally some 84 degrees to the long axis of the foot (Fig. 4-1B).[1] The obliquity of the ankle axis has this effect: if the foot is raised from the floor with the leg fixed, plantar flexion will cause the forefoot to move laterally. Conversely, when the foot is bearing weight, plantar flexion and dorsiflexion can only be achieved if there is associated rotation of the tibia and fibula about the long axis of the leg (Fig. 4-1C). The normal range of motion of the foot about the ankle joint, from the right angle position, is approximately 20 degrees of extension (dorsiflexion) and 50 degrees of flexion (plantar flexion).[2]

The second critical degree of freedom of the foot occurs at the subtalar joint, which is the articulation between the talus and the calcaneus. The axis of the subtalar joint is also

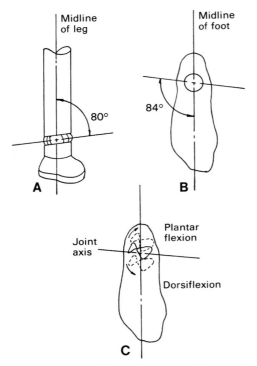

Fig. 4-1.   Geometry of the ankle joint. (*A*) Frontal plane. (*B*) Transverse plane. (*C*) The rotations imposed upon the tibia and fibula during ankle flexion and extension if the foot is fixed to the floor.

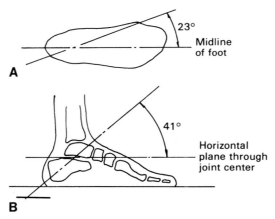

Fig. 4-2.   The geometry of the subtalar joint. (*A*) The transverse plane. (*B*) The anterior/posterior plane.

oblique, but here the obliquity is at an angle of about 23 degrees to the midline of the foot and 41 degrees to a horizontal plane through the joint center (Fig. 4-2).

Because of the obliquity of the axis of the subtalar joint to the normally accepted coordinate system used to describe motions of the lower limb, the subtalar joint allows both a degree of abduction–adduction and dorsiflexion–plantar flexion of the foot. In addition, the calcaneus can rotate on the talus about the foot's midline to produce inversion (elevation of the medial border) or eversion (elevation of the lateral border). When all of these subtalar movements occur simultaneously (i.e., when the foot freely rotates about the subtalar axis) they produce supination, which is a combination of inversion, adduction and plantar flexion, and pronation; a combination of eversion, abduction, and dorsiflexion.

The third significant rotational axis in the hindfoot is the transverse tarsal joint, which is formed by the articulation of the talus on the navicular and the calcaneus on the cuboid. The relatively large talar surface which articulates with the adjacent surface of the navicular allows inversion and eversion of the foot to occur at the talonavicular joint, while the free motion available at the calcaneocuboid is limited, in the main, to abduction and adduction. Since the transverse tarsal joint comprises these two minor joints, any movement in the talus or calcaneus will affect the transverse tarsal axis. In fact, in the pronated foot the axes of the talonavicular and calcaneocuboid are parallel to one another, allowing relatively free transverse tarsal motion. By comparison, in the supinated foot the two axes are divergent, transverse tarsal motion is restricted, and the foot is stable.

Finally, one forefoot 'joint' deserves brief consideration. The so-called metatarsal break is the oblique axis that overlies the metatarsophalangeal joints and runs from the second to the fifth metatarsal head at an angle of about 50 degrees to the long axis of the foot. The metatarsal break interacts with the plantar aponeurosis, which runs from the inferior tubercle of the calcaneus to the base of each proximal phalanx, to stabilize the foot significantly, prior to toe-off. As the metatarsophalangeal joints extend (i.e., as the toes are dorsiflexed), the plantar aponeurosis is

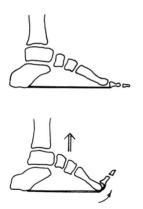

Fig. 4-3. The windlass effect of the plantar aponeurosis, with dorsiflexion of the toes causing elevation of the longitudinal arch of the foot.

wrapped around the metatarsal heads, causing a "windlass action" and increasing tension across the longitudinal arch of the foot. This increased tension across the arch causes its span to shorten, and the complete arch is forced into an elevated and more stable position (Fig. 4-3).

THE MECHANICS OF LOCOMOTION

The normal gait or walking cycle can conveniently be divided into two distinct phases: the stance phase, during which the foot is bearing weight, and the swing phase, during which the limb is swinging forward. The swing phase is concerned with preparing and aligning the swinging foot for heel-strike and also ensuring that the swinging foot clears the floor. The stance phase, which occupies some 60 per cent of the total gait cycle is concerned with weight bearing and body stability.

Five distinct events occur during the stance phase: heel-strike, when the swinging foot first contacts the floor; foot-flat, the instant when the forefoot touches the floor; mid-stance, when the intact lower limb is vertical; heel-rise, which occurs as the body drives onward and the heel leaves the floor; and finally, toe-off. The mechanisms that control gait and foot function will be described in relation to one or more of these events.

Locomotion is the translation of the body in space from one point to another. It has been said that human locomotion can be compared to a wheel rolling over the ground with the legs being two of the spokes; the spoke that touches the ground representing the stance phase and the spoke moving about its center of rotation representing the swing phase.[2] However, this analogy is somewhat misleading, as two rigid spokes undergoing a pendulumlike motion would cause the center of mass of the body to rise and fall during gait, thus wastefully expending energy. The locomotor system attempts to minimize such wasteful energy expenditure by a number of subtle movements which minimize vertical motion of the center of mass as the legs propel the body forward. For example, during the swing phase the pelvis tilts toward the swinging leg, which is, in turn, slightly abducted with knee and hip flexed to allow the foot to clear the floor. In addition, the pelvis rotates forward with the swinging leg and shifts laterally over the weight-bearing leg to maintain body balance as the swinging leg is lifted from the ground. The knee, which is fully extended at heel-strike, flexes until the foot is flat upon the ground and then extends again, so that at toe-off the joint is fully extended. At heel-strike the ankle joint is in an approximately neutral position. Simultaneously with knee movement, it undergoes plantar flexion to become flat upon the ground as the weight-bearing limb becomes vertical, and then dorsiflexes once again until toe-off occurs.

These so-called gait determinants smooth the otherwise undulant course of the body's center of mass as well as increasing gait efficiency and decreasing energy expenditure. However, the forward rotation of the pelvis with the swinging leg mentioned above is transmitted as an inward rotation about the longitudinal axis of the entire lower segment and, as will be shown, is used as a mechanism for stabilizing and destabilizing the weight-bearing foot.

THE MECHANICS OF FOOT FUNCTION

During normal locomotion the inward and outward rotation of the pelvis causes the femur, fibula, and tibia to rotate about the long axis of the limb. The magnitude of this rotational motion increases progressively from pelvis to tibia; for example, during normal walking on level ground the pelvis undergoes a maximum rotation in each gait cycle of about 6 degrees, while the tibia undergoes a rotation of about 18 degrees in the same period. In general terms the intact limb rotates medially during the swing phase and early stance phase and then laterally until the stance phase is complete and toe-off has occurred. The typical rotational motion of the pelvis, femur, and tibia during gait is shown in Fig. 4-4.

At the beginning of the stance phase (heel-strike) the tibia is rotated internally about 5 degrees from its neutral position, and the ankle joint is either in its neutral position or in slight plantar flexion. Immediately after heel-strike, the foot flexes toward the floor, the dorsiflexors controlling this plantar motion to prevent the foot slapping down to the foot-flat position. From heel-strike to just before foot-flat, the increasing inward rotation of the tibia and fibula is transmitted through the ankle mortise to the talus. The inward rotation of the mortise,

combined with the plantar flexion position of the ankle, tends to shift the forefoot medially from its neutral, toe-out position. Additionally, the talus rotates medially on the calcaneus about the subtalar axis, forcing the calcaneus into eversion and causing pronation of the foot. In this condition free motion is available at the transverse tarsal joint, so that, distal to the navicular and cuboid the foot remains supple and is allowed to bend into intimate contact with the supporting surface.

As the foot moves into the foot-flat position, the direction of rotation of the lower limb is reversed and the leg begins to rotate externally (Fig. 4-4). The forefoot is now fixed on the floor and the entire external rotation of the ankle mortise is passed to the talus. As the magnitude of external rotation increases, the subtalar joint forces the calcaneus into increasing inversion, causing supination of the foot and increased stability at the transverse tarsal joint. This, in turn, produces a more stable longitudinal arch of the foot. In addition, the foot is now carrying an increasing proportion of the body weight, and stability of the transverse tarsal joint is further improved by the convex head of the talus seating more firmly into the concave face of the navicular.

Once the leg has passed over the (by now) weight-bearing foot, the ankle begins dorsiflexion, and there is increasing activity of the intrinsic muscles. Soon after heel-rise the ankle joint moves back into plantar flexion, and the metatarsophalangeal joints are forced to extend. The windlass effect of the plantar aponeurosis running over the metatarsal heads further elevates the longitudinal arch, increasing foot stability. Just before toe-off, the talus has reached its maximum degree of external rotation, and the foot is solidly locked in the supinated position. At this instant the combination of weight bearing, windlass effect, supination, and intrinsic- and posterior calf muscle activity ensures that the foot is in a maximally stable position for lift-off.

As toe-off is completed, the leg begins to rotate inward, once again everting the foot and unlocking the transverse tarsal joint. The ac-

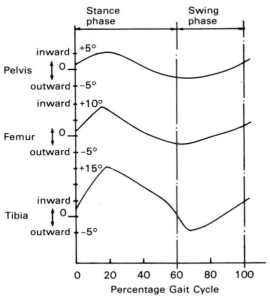

Fig. 4-4. Rotation of the lower body segment during one gait cycle.

tivity of the intrinsic- and the posterior calf muscles also ceases, and the foot returns to its flexible state for the swing phase of gait.

A schematic of a typical gait cycle, showing joint rotations and muscle activity, is shown in Fig. 4-5.

FUNCTIONAL ASSESSMENT OF THE WEIGHT-BEARING FOOT DURING LOCOMOTION

Clinical assessment and analysis of the weight-bearing foot in abnormality and disease is most often based on the subjective judgment of a physician. Although anatomical abnormalities are often apparent at examination, the accurate assessment of an abnormality of function is more difficult, particularly if the malfunction is apparent only under dynamic loading conditions.

The numerous studies into the biomechanics of locomotion reported in the literature have tended to concentrate on the lower limb (particularly the resolution of gait forces through the hip and knee), and the foot has been rather ignored. The monitoring systems used in most studies of this type consist of floor-mounted force plates together with high-speed movie-

or television cameras. Synchronous recordings of the forces applied by the foot to the plate, and high-speed film records of the position of the limb in space allow the forces acting through the segment of interest to be computed at any instant in the stance phase. As a result the biomechanics of limb motion is now well understood. However, an analysis of the biomechanics of foot (as opposed to lower limb) function is almost impossible with systems of this type. It is difficult to see the subtle movements occurring in the foot during the stance phase and therefore difficult to relate the gross reaction forces measured by the plate to specific anatomical sites on the foot. A better approach would be to record the changing localized forces or interface pressures across the plantar surface, and then relate the plantar loading pattern to an image of the foot's plantar surface.

Attempts to measure pressures at the foot-ground interface for diagnostic purposes stretch back as far as the nineteenth century. An early researcher in this field was Beely[3] who in 1882 attempted to relate interface pressures to the depth of a foot impression in a thin bag filled with plaster-of-Paris. Later researchers, such as Elftman[4] and Morton[5]

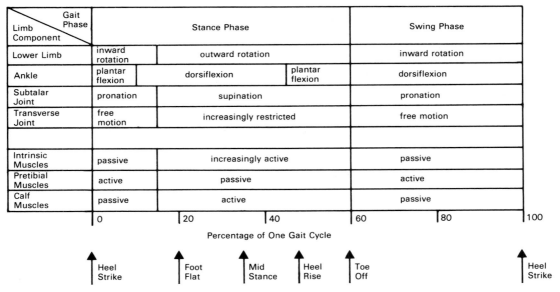

Limb Component \ Gait Phase	Stance Phase			Swing Phase
Lower Limb	inward rotation	outward rotation		inward rotation
Ankle	plantar flexion	dorsiflexion	plantar flexion	dorsiflexion
Subtalar Joint	pronation	supination		pronation
Transverse Joint	free motion	increasingly restricted		free motion
Intrinsic Muscles	passive	increasingly active		passive
Pretibial Muscles	active	passive		active
Calf Muscles	passive	active		passive

| 0 | 20 | 40 | 60 | 80 | 100 |

Percentage of One Gait Cycle

Heel Strike   Foot Flat   Mid Stance   Heel Rise   Toe Off   Heel Strike

Fig. 4-5. Summary of the biomechanics of one gait cycle.

used the deformability of rubber projections on a walkpath mat to measure localized loads. A similar method has been proposed recently, in which an optical technique is used to display the localized loads as a set of circular interference fringes.[6]

All these methods allow an easily assimilated visualization of the loading patterns of the standing foot to be displayed, but the rapidly changing loading patterns developed during gait make the recording and interpretation of data very difficult. In order to simplify the data-handling problem, some investigators have fixed flexible pressure transducers over selected anatomical sites by inserting them into specially constructed shoes or attaching them to the sole of the bare foot.[7-9] Discrete pressure transducers have the attraction of simple calibration, but they must be extremely carefully located on the foot, as discrepancies in transducer placement on subsequent occasions can make follow-up studies almost meaningless.

The increasing professionalism in sport and the growth of running or jogging in the wider population has caused a dramatic increase in sport-related injuries to the foot in recent years. Many of these injuries are intrinsic in that they are self-inflicted or caused by overuse, and the special care required has stimulated greater interest in the analysis of foot function. Current diagnostic studies of the walking or running foot use high-speed motion picture techniques to achieve close-up shots of ankle and subtalar joint motion. Unfortunately, the assessment of function or injury depends upon the skill of the observer, and there is still a need for a simple method of quantitatively assessing the function of the weight-bearing foot.

A new technique that has been described recently may well fill this need.[10] The system consists of a segmented force plate, two television cameras, and a signal processing and display unit. The force plate is constructed of 16 narrow transparent beams mounted at right angles to the direction of walking in a walkway. When the foot touches the plate, its plantar surface is photographed through the plate by one camera while its lateral aspect is photographed by the second camera mounted adjacent to the walkway. The signal-processing unit immediately generates a video display which shows a close-up lateral view of the foot, a view of the plantar surface, and a histogram-type display of the load applied to each beam by the foot. Additionally, the processing unit calculates the position of the center of pressure on each beam and electronically superimposes center-of-pressure lines on the image of the plantar surface. By using this system it is possible to see at a glance, not only the magnitude of the load carried by different sections of the foot throughout the stance phase but also the patterns of loading applied to the plantar surface together with the position that the foot has reached in the stance phase.

Figure 4-6 shows a series of still photographs which illustrate the stance phase of normal gait as seen by this system. The instants in the stance phase depicted here are heel-strike, the approach to foot-flat, foot-flat, mid-stance, heel-rise, and the approach to toe-off. The upper third of each photograph shows the lateral aspect of the foot, the middle third shows the plantar surface with center-of-pressure lines superimposed, and the histogram in the lower third displays the total load carried on each segment of the foot.

The series of photographs clearly show that, as predicted by traditional gait studies, the heel is subjected to an impact load of considerable magnitude at heel-strike. The lateral view shows that at this instant the ankle joint is in slight plantar flexion, and the position of the center-of-pressure lines shows that the calcaneus is slightly everted. As the forefoot descends toward the plate and the lower leg moves towards the vertical, the heel still carries the majority of the applied load, but the increasing loading of the mid- and forefoot is carried somewhat laterally to the longitudinal midline. The longitudinal arch remains the major weight-bearing area from foot-flat to mid-stance, but although the loading is reasonably evenly distributed along the arch at foot-flat, by mid-stance increasing load is

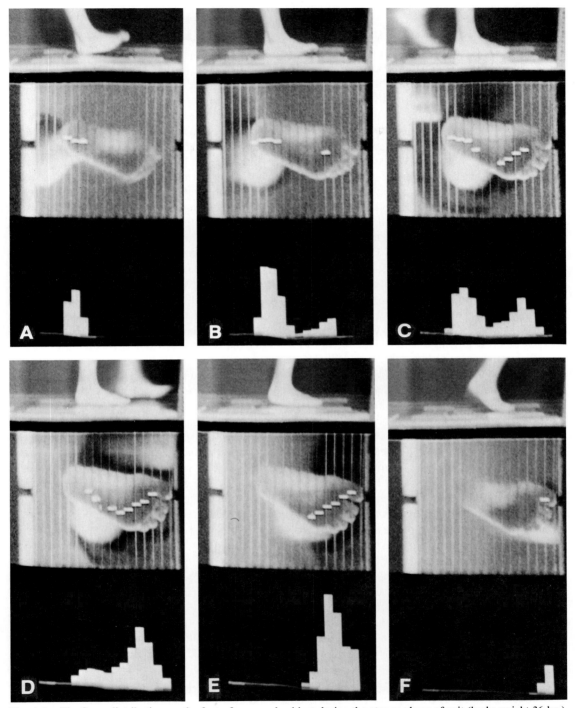

Fig. 4-6. The force distribution on the foot of a normal subject during the stance phase of gait (body weight 36 kg.).

(A) Heel strike	(D) Mid-stance
(B) Approaching foot flat	(E) Heel rise
(C) Foot flat	(F) Approaching toe off

Full-scale deflection on the bar chart represents 160 newtons.

27

building on the forefoot. When heel-rise occurs, the foot is fully supinated, and the loading moves medially across the metatarsal heads, along the line of the metatarsal break, toward the big toe. The center of the forefoot is now carrying the large, impulsive load generated by the lower segment, which drives the body forward. The approach to toe-off shows further medial movement of the weight-bearing area with rapid decrease in applied loading, until the final contact occurs between the plate and the big toe.

By comparison, a series of photographs taken at similar instants in the stance phase of the right foot of a 10-year-old patient with arthogryposis is shown in Fig. 4-7. This recording was made 4 months after lower tibial and fibular osteotomies had been performed. Recordings taken before surgery show that the untreated patient was only able to bear weight on the forefoot during gait because his arthogrypotic ankles prevented sufficient dorsiflexion to allow the heel and hindfoot to contact the plate. This postoperative series of photographs shows that the osteotomies now allow the patient to exhibit a reasonably normal heel-strike and early stance phase. However, later in the stance phase the stiffness inherent in this foot does not allow a normal loading progression across the line of the metatarsal break from fifth to first metatarsal head as the heel leaves the floor. Surgical treatment has thus made a significant improvement to the weight-bearing function of this arthogrypotic foot. However, this postoperative recording of the forces acting during the patient's stance phase can still not be mistaken for the smooth progression of plantar loading (i.e., from heel, along the lateral border and then across the metatarsal break) which is seen in the normal foot.

It can be seen from these two series of photographs that this technique of imaging and assessing the foot clearly shows the difference between normal and abnormal foot function. The sequence depicting the normal foot shows that the movement of the foot and the way in which load is transferred between the foot and ground is not compatible with the tripodlike behavior that the traditional view would have us believe. Pronation and supination provide flexibility and then stability of the mechanical structure of the foot, and the loading patterns between foot and ground move from the midline of the heel, along the lateral border of the flexible foot, and then across the metatarsal break of the stabilized foot as the stance phase progresses.

It is unfortunate that prostheses currently available for ankle or whole-foot replacement are usually based on simple hinge mechanisms and constrain the normal plantar loading pattern with consequent adverse effects on foot function and the patient's gait pattern. Studies of both the normal and abnormal foot now show that a better approach to the prosthetic ankle may be to replace the traditional hinge with a spiral or a pseudo-helix, as the range of movement available at this type of joint will allow the natural lateral to medial shift of the forces between foot and ground during the stance phase of the gait cycle. The design and development of suitable prostheses, however, and a full understanding of the role of the foot in creating locomotor disorders, can only be achieved if proper methods for analyzing the walking foot find a regular place in clinical practice. It is to be hoped that this hitherto rather neglected but vital component of the locomotor system will receive the attention that has been lacking to date.

REFERENCES

1. Mann, R. A.: Biomechanics of the foot. *In* Atlas of Orthotics. St. Louis, C. V. Mosby, 1973.
2. Cailliet, R.: Foot and Ankle Pain. Philadelphia, F. A. Davis, 1968.
3. Beely, F.: Zur Mechanik des Stehers. Langenbecks Archiv fur klinische chirurgie, *27:*457, 1882.
4. Elftman, H.: A cinematic study of the distribution of pressure in the human foot. Anat. Rec., *59:*481, 1934.
5. Morton, D. J.: The Human Foot. New York, Columbia University Press, 1935.
6. Arcan, M., and Brull, M. A.: A fundamental characteristic of the human body and foot—the foot ground pressure pattern. J. Biomechanics, *9:*453, 1976.

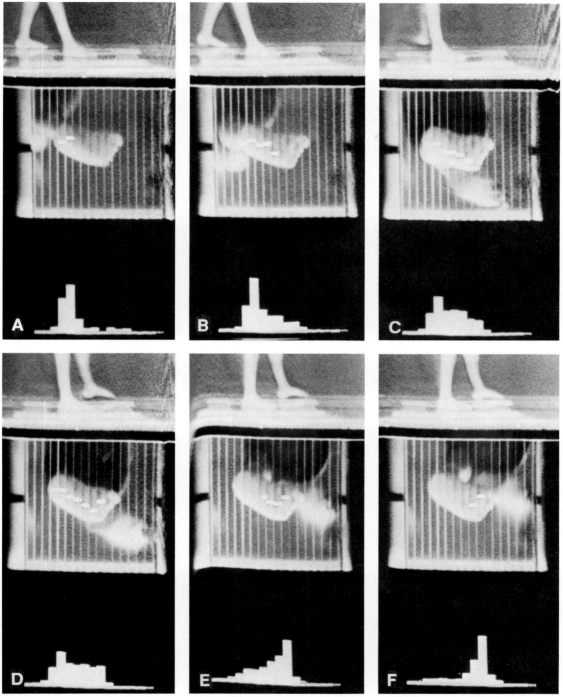

Fig. 4-7. The force distribution on the foot of a patient with arthogryposis after tibial and fibial osteotomies (body weight 19 kg.).

(A) Heel strike	(D) Mid-stance
(B) Approaching foot flat	(E) Heel rise
(C) Foot flat	(F) Approaching toe off

Full-scale deflection on the bar chart represents 125 newtons.

29

7. Holden, T. S., and Muncey, R. W.: Pressure on the human foot during walking. Aust. J. Appl. Sci., *4:*405, 1953.

8. Schwartz, R. P., and Heath, A. L.: The oscillographic recording and quantitative definition of functional disabilities of human locomotion. Arch. Phys. Med., *30:*568, 1949.

9. Bauman, J. H., and Brand, P. W.: Measurement of pressure between foot and shoe. Lancet, *1:* 629, 1963.

10. Manley, M. T., and Solomon, E.: The functional assessment of the weight-bearing foot. in Proc. of Engineering for Health, 7 CMBEC, Vancouver, Canada 1978.

5 Dysfunction of the Foot

FATIGUE AND ACUTE FOOT STRAIN

We all know what is meant by a tired foot. Everyone has heard someone say, "My feet are killing me," and, "I must get off my feet"; equally descriptive of suffering and of the natural remedy.

Tiredness may be considered the reaction of muscles to an activity that is normally comfortable but has been prolonged or increased unduly. The stamina of the muscles is exhausted, and they protest their willingness or ability to continue. We have, as yet, no definition that accurately defines the clinical or pathological state.

Symptoms of tiredness develop earlier in the weak and elderly, with pain mainly in the arch, the ball of the foot, and under the heel. Pain is accompanied by swelling, which is always present to some degree. Swelling, for example after prolonged sitting, especially in an aircraft, or as a complication of varicose veins, cardiovascular failure, or malnutrition, produces a feeling of heaviness, of tiredness.

Profound fatigue may reach the point of near paralysis or collapse of the affected muscles. Toward the end of a forced march the tibialis posterior may give way, with dramatic collapse of the longitudinal arch, or the peronei may weaken until the ankle gives way into inversion. The latter condition must be differentiated from instability secondary to disruption of the ligaments (see Chap. 12, Sprain of the Lateral Ligaments), for in the former condition rehabilitation of the muscles with temporary bracing is necessary, *not* surgical reconstruction of the ligaments.

Other consequences of severe fatigue are muscle spasm, myositis, and ischaemia, but they are related to the severity of the strain and respond to a more protracted course of the same treatment. Muscle inhibition may also occur as a reaction to pain. A sudden strain, stenosing tenovaginitis, or a loose body in one of the joints may cause a sudden pain, leading to muscle inhibition and the giving way of the joint.

Accurate diagnosis will point the way to correct treatment. In the initial stages, rest brings relief, but the more severe the symptoms, the longer it may take.

CHRONIC FOOT STRAIN

Swelling causes stiffness. In due course the swelling and stiffness become persistent and may not disappear without treatment.

Chronic foot strain is a term which defies precise definition. *Foot strain* is related to stress and excessive fatigue of the muscles and tendons, the working, moving tissues of the foot. *Sprain* of joints describes injury to the capsule and ligaments, the fixed soft tissue structures which encompass and reinforce, but also limit the excursion of, the joint. The sprain may be limited to a minor distraction of intramural fibers or, more severely, a partial or complete rupture or avulsion of the ligament from its bony attachments, with or without a fragment of bone. Evidence of strain is manifest when the swelling becomes organized to form fibrous adhesions. These limit the free play of the muscles and movement of the joints. What Burrows and Coltart described as "scar tissue which interferes with the free play between the parts of the motor system" occurs at the junction of tissues of differing elasticity, for example, where muscle fibers or ligaments are attached to bone or tendon. The fine, fibrous adhesions are responsible for pain on movement as they are subjected to tension.

In our well-shod and motorized age, foot strain is a common phenomenon that occurs most frequently in the middle-aged and elderly and in those whose occupations are relatively sedentary or demand much standing, such as housewives, shop assistants, and policemen. Feet that are not exercised sufficiently weaken.

When the muscles are too feeble, or when they tire, the toes do not straighten during walking and the weight is borne on the heads of the metatarsals and the tips of the curled toes, areas not designed for weight bearing. Pain and tenderness result. At the same time, the curled toes rub against the uppers of the shoes, which produces painful corns. In time, friction from the shoes over the flexed, proximal, interphalangeal joints causes similar inflammation and pain.

Prolonged fatigue and swelling may reach a chronic state, so that the supple foot becomes semirigid and, eventually, quite stiff. With stiffening, weight bearing is increasingly concentrated on the bony prominences. Calluses develop. At first they are protective in nature and not necessarily painful or tender. The development of adventitious bursae changes this. As the feet stiffen and become painful, walking is more tiring. The calves take abnormal strain and ache in their turn. In the end, degenerative joint changes occur with enlarging osteophytes, beneath which secondary adventitious bursae develop.

Treatment of Foot Strain

The treatment of foot strain is the treatment of the symptoms. These frequently follow in sequence: aching with fatigue; metatarsalgia; corns; aching under the longitudinal arches and aching in the calves on walking. All are aggravated by swelling and stiffness. The approach to treatment depends on the stage that has been reached, and particularly on whether the feet are supple, mildly stiff, painful on forced movements, or quite stiff.

A mobile or supple foot is one that can be moved through a full range of movements in all directions. This includes straightening and plantar flexion of the toes. The mildly stiff, or semirigid, foot has a range of comfortable movement, but, when the limit is reached, further movement, whether active or passive, causes increasing discomfort or pain.

Supple feet can be restored to comfort and vigor by the correct application of rest, local heat, and exercise. In severe cases, rest should consist of a few days spent in bed. In less severe cases it may be achieved by limiting activity, with or without foot supports. In the early stages, the usual longitudinal arch supports are rarely required. All that the patient needs is a metatarsal pad or platform, which relieves the heads of the metatarsals from full weight bearing and helps to straighten the toes (Fig. 5-1). By holding the heel vertical, a Helfet heel seat takes the stress off the arch and often provides relief within a short time. Longitudinal arch supports, which convert the arch into a weight-bearing surface, weaken the foot and, in many instances, the patient cannot again do without them. Their use is not advised.

Initially, exercise should be "non-weight-bearing" and should be directed toward strengthening the short muscles that straighten and separate the toes. The patient is instructed to do the exercises for short periods, two or three times a day, while seated. The traditional instructions to walk on the outer borders of the feet serve no purpose, since only the muscles of the calf are exercised by this means.

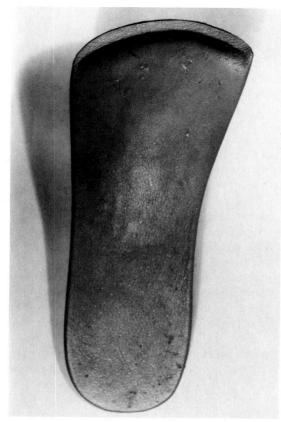

Fig. 5-1. A transverse metatarsal pad fitted within a leather sole.

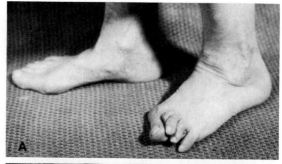

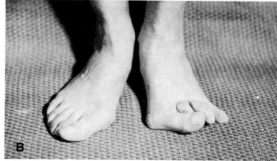

Fig. 5-2. A typical rigid flat foot with marked secondary collapse of the toes on the left side; (*A*) lateral view, (*B*) anterior view.

The patient is instructed in the foot regimen described below. When the patient can straighten and separate the toes actively, good progress has been made. Longitudinal arch supports are prescribed only when the condition is of long standing and marked by weakness or wasting. The supports should be made-to-measure of a resilient, nonrigid material.

Rigid Feet. In comfortable shoes, rigid feet (Fig. 5-2), though weak, are often painless. If not, the prime requisite is a pair of firm, custom-built supports, made from plaster-of-Paris casts. Stock sizes are seldom adequate. If standard shoes do not fit, special shoes must be made, or surgery will be necessary to reshape the foot. Physiotherapy should aim only at reducing swelling and improving the circulation.

Semirigid Feet. When the patient complains of pain on forced, passive movements, a clinical decision must be made. Either the feet must be mobilized by physiotherapy and manipulation and then treated as a supple, strained foot, or we must accept the disability and treat it as a rigid foot. The judicious use of manipulation under general anesthesia, adequate rehabilitation, and appropriate support is usually effective in relieving symptoms.

Manipulation is a passive, yet gentle, stretching of the foot through a full range of motion, including inversion and eversion of the subtalar joints; flexion, extension and rotation of the midtarsal region; and distraction, flexion, and extension of all the metatarsophalangeal and interphalangeal joints of the toes.

The Foot Regimen[1]

Contrast Bathing. Take two buckets of water; one as hot and the other as cold as the feet can stand. The feet are immersed in the hot water for 1 minute and then in the cold for a half minute. This is repeated five times. The feet are then dried vigorously with a rough towel, after which the exercises are performed.

"Non-Weight-Bearing" Exercises. Each exercise should be performed six times at first, working up to twelve.

1. FOOT SHORTENING. Sit with the feet on a towel. Keep the toes straight by pressing them against the towel with the fingers. Then attempt to bring the heels toward the toes, so that the longitudinal arch lifts slowly. Keep the knees firmly in position and do not allow them to separate.

2. TOE RAISING. Raise the toes, keeping the ball and the rest of the foot firmly on the floor.

3. FOOT INVERSION. Keeping the knees together and the outer borders of the feet on the ground throughout the whole exercise, arch and invert until the big toes and balls of the feet touch at the midline.

4. TOE-CLAWING. Using the toes, claw the towel into a ball under the foot. Pick up a pencil, a ball of wool, or some similar object, with the toes.

5. TOE MOVEMENTS. Put the foot on a chair so that the ball of the foot and the toes extend just over the edge. Flex and extend the toes, resisting these movements with the fingers. Spread out the toes as much as possible without flexing or extending them. If the big toe will not abduct, hold it in abduction with the fingers and try and maintain it in this position.

6. HEEL RAISING. Keeping the toes straight and the ball of the foot on the ground, raise the heels as high as possible.

Weight-Bearing Exercises. After the above exercises have been performed two or three times a day for a fortnight, Exercises 1, 2, 3 and 6 should be carried out while standing. Again, the patient should start with six and work up to twelve repeats.

METATARSALGIA

Metatarsalgia is the term usually employed to denote pain in the forefoot, and especially under the ball of the foot. It often presents problems in diagnosis. The pain may originate locally in muscles, ligaments, joints, or nerves, or it may be a manifestation of a disorder of circulation, systemic disease, or infection. It occurs most frequently in the everted foot, the high-arched clawfoot, and in feet with limited dorsiflexion due to short Achilles tendons. The pain may be a result of foot strain. It may be associated with hallux valgus and bunions, with fatigue fractures of the metatarsals, in adolescents with Freiberg's infraction of the head of the second metatarsal, or with entrapment or damage to the interdigital nerves.

Metatarsalgia occurs most frequently in adults over 30 years of age, and more often in women than in men (especially those who wear tight, high-heeled shoes). The first symptom is often an aching sensation, followed by burning or cramp in the ball of the foot. The patient may describe the sensation of a bone slipping out of place. The symptoms, on occasion, are so severe as to be disabling. The pain may be referred into the toes or up the leg. Symptoms are usually relieved by rest and by removing the shoe.

Examination reveals tenderness of the heads of the affected metatarsals. A callosity may be present. The toes are curled in some cases. At first they are mobile but later become fixed due to contractures.

To relieve the condition, the particular cause of pain must be diagnosed and treated; be it flat, everted feet, high-arched feet with clawed toes, or chronic foot strain. Metatarsal platforms, Haig forefoot suspensions (Fig. 5-3), or corrective heel seats may be appropriate to relieve the pressure on the heads of the metatarsals (see Chap. 11, Claw Toes). A metatarsal- or roller bar is suitable in some cases (Fig. 5-4). The foot should be strengthened by contrast bathing and "non-weight-bearing" exercises (see above).

Calluses, once the pressure is removed, are not usually painful, in contradistinction to plantar warts, which are acutely sensitive and need determined treatment (see Chap. 12).

Fig. 5-3. Haig forefoot suspension for the treatment of clawed toes, especially following chronic foot strain. (*A*) The apparatus itself consists of a proximal loop to fit around the heel, and two distal loops for the second and fourth toes. It can be seen that the sides of the proximal loop are elastic. (*B*) The Haig suspensions on a foot, showing that the toes are held straight when the foot is relaxed. (*C*) When weight is borne on the toes, the suspension apparatus prevents clawing because of its elasticity.

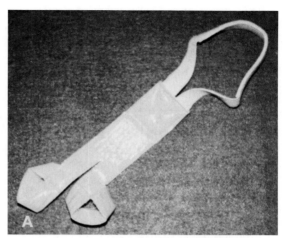

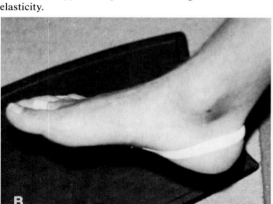

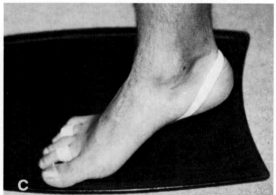

Fig. 5-4. A shoe in which a roller bar has been inserted onto the leather sole beneath the metatarsal heads. By extending the toes the patient is able to adopt a normal gait without causing metatarsalgia.

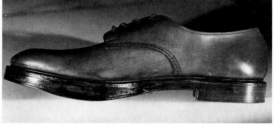

DIFFERENTIAL DIAGNOSIS OF THE CAUSES OF METATARSALGIA

Several specific causes of metatarsalgia will be described in detail because accurate diagnosis is required for their treatment.

Metatarsophalangeal Synovitis

Occasionally, a young adult, or even a patient in late adolescence whose epiphyses are not yet fused, develops persistent pain in the second metatarsophalangeal joint. In rare instances the third joint may be the one that is affected.

The condition is usually associated with a long second toe, often longer than the hallux, that habitually adopts a clawed position, with hyperextension of the metatarsophalangeal joint. Examination reveals swelling and thickening of the joint lining itself, with marked local tenderness as the troublesome symptom. Movements of the joint elicit characteristic pain.

The condition usually settles within 2 to 3 weeks after the injection of 40 mg. of intraarticular corticosteroid and 1 ml. of 2-per-cent lidocaine (Lignocaine), provided the patient performs toe exercises to overcome the residual stiffness and wears shoes that do not cause repetition of the abnormal posture.

In the uncommon event of pain and swelling persisting after treatment, the joint is exposed via a short vertical incision in the ball of the foot over the area of greatest swelling. A florid, inflammatory synovitis is present in the second metatarsophalangeal joint. In chronic cases, it may appear almost villonodular in type, with excessive pouching of the synovium beneath the metatarsal head. Since the abnormal hyperextension of the joint has pressed the metatarsal head firmly downward and set up the synovitis, synovectomy is not curative. The toe must be shortened, either by excision of the metatarsal head or, preferably, by excision of the base of the proximal phalanx, to form a flaccid, fibrous joint. Excision of the metatarsal head interferes with the normal weight-bearing function of the metatarsal arch and is likely, in young patients, to cause trouble in the adjacent joints later in life.

"Clicking" Metatarsalgia

In some young patients with normal feet and toes metatarsalgia may be accompanied by a painful "clicking" sensation. Sometimes the feeling is one of pain on bearing weight on the transverse arch that continues until the condition is relieved suddenly by a click, only to recur hours or days later. It may follow prolonged sporting activity. The pain stops the patient in his tracks. Walking is impossible until relief is obtained by removing the shoe and squeezing the foot, when another click may herald sudden comfort.

On examination, there is no stiffness or swelling of the joints, nor is there any tenderness of the metatarsal heads. Tenderness of one of the transverse intermetatarsal ligaments, usually that between the third and fourth metatarsal heads, can be elicited, however. The pathognomonic sign is reproduction of the painful click. This is performed by grasping one of the metatarsal heads between the finger and thumb of one hand, and the adjacent head between the finger and thumb of the other. If the heads are then moved up and down in opposing directions, the click, sometimes associated with pain, may be elicited by the examiner. Similarly, compression of the whole transverse arch by the examining hand causes the metatarsal heads to roll on each other, reproducing the click. If the ligament ruptures with use, abnormal, vertical movement may be present, or a chronic sprain of the ligament may result in a small, bony spike in one or the other of its attachments, visible on suitable radiographs.

Treatment consists of rest, steroid infiltration, and, when indicated, the use of a metatarsal bar. Occasionally, symptoms persist, and excision of one of the metatarsal heads is the cure.

Freiberg's Disease

Freiberg and Kohler described a condition of damage to the second metatarsal head in adolescence (Fig. 5-5A).[2-4] It has also been called epiphyseal ischemic necrosis, epiphyseal osteochondritis, and infraction of the head of the second metatarsal.

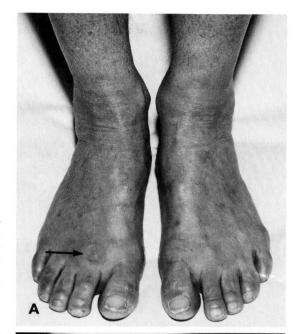

Fig. 5-5. (*A*) The feet of a young adult. The arrow points to a callosity overlying a bony lump in the second metatarsal head. (*B*) A radiograph shows typical fragmentation with early degenerative changes in the second metatarsal head. (*C*) This radiograph shows Freiberg's disease in the third metatarsal head. Early osteoarthritic changes are present. While most cases of Freiberg's disease occur in the second metatarsal head, the third may be affected.

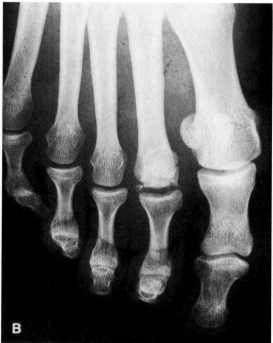

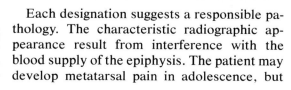

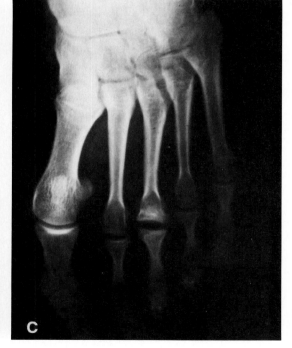

Each designation suggests a responsible pathology. The characteristic radiographic appearance result from interference with the blood supply of the epiphysis. The patient may develop metatarsal pain in adolescence, but not necessarily; sometimes the symptoms are not troublesome until middle age, when the forefoot has weakened and splayed. The pain is felt on walking and is relieved by rest. The head of the metatarsal, invariably the second, is tender and can be felt to be enlarged. The fact that the second joint is involved may be due to a long second toe, subjecting the epiphysis to unacceptable pressure.

Radiographs show the typical changes of avascular necrosis, with rarefaction and patchy areas of increased density so typical of other forms of epiphyseal osteochondritis, such as Perthe's disease in the upper femoral epiphysis. Lateral views of the metatarsal head reveal the earliest changes to be in the dorsal metaphyseal bone. As this crumbles, the epiphysis slips and tilts dorsally. The condition, in some, if not all, cases, is equivalent to slipping of the upper femoral epiphysis.

Later, after epiphyseal fusion is complete, radiographs show a distorted, flattened, and enlarged head (Fig. 5-5B). This is a typical end result after osteochondritis in other epiphyses. Finally, some 10 years or more later, secondary osteoarthritis occurs (Fig. 5-5C), with loss of articular cartilage, sclerosis, capsular fibrosis, and peripheral osteophyte formation.

A metatarsal platform, contrast baths, and exercise often relieve the symptoms, but this program of treatment must be continued; if not, the patient will require surgery. *A prolonged trial of conservative treatment is always merited,* for it is surprising how often normal, comfortable function is possible in spite of a poor radiograph. Metatarsal platforms, of the type described, are preferred to metatarsal bars on the soles of the shoes. Carefully measured, they are more effective, more comfortable, and less obvious, especially in women's shoes. Most last about a year before they must be replaced.

Young patients with marked dorsal collapse are treated, occasionally, by reduction of the epiphysis (by an operation equivalent to Dunn's procedure for the slipped, upper, femoral epiphysis[5]). The procedure is performed through a dorsal incision, which extends to the neck of the metatarsal. The joint is opened longitudinally, when the dorsally tilted epiphysis is found. It is usually loose and can be tilted downward into its normal position by a blunt lever. The gap left by the crushed, posterior, metaphyseal cancellous bone is packed with cancellous chips from the shaft. The wound is closed in layers.

If reduction proves impossible, and certainly if the epiphysis has fused, as well as in patients who later suffer osteoarthritic changes, the metatarsal head must be exercised. Retraction of the toe, which is cosmetically unattractive, may follow. The appearance is improved by syndactilizing the second toe. The operation, however, is not simple, for technical skill is required to fashion adequate skin flaps to accomplish syndactyly without breakdown of the flaps.

"Sesamoiditis"

Apley has shown that the sesamoids under the first metatarsal head do, on occasion, show radiographic changes similar to those seen in the patella, including chondromalacia, osteochondritis dissecans, osteoarthritis, and even osteomyelitis, which may lead to transverse rupture of the bone.[6]

In rare instances, such pathological changes may cause persistent metatarsalgia.[7] It usually responds to relief of pressure by an excavated metatarsal pad, but if not, excision of the sesamoid bone is indicated. Sesamoidectomy leads to a surprising amount of pain and disability; recovery may take months, or even years.

Neural Pain Beneath the First Metatarsal Head

Pain beneath the first metatarsal head that is frequently diagnosed as a traumatic lesion of a sesamoid is often, and perhaps usually, due to injury to the medial, digital nerve of the big toe. Fibrosis around the nerve causes the symptoms.

Shortly after the medial plantar nerve enters the sole of the foot it gives off the medial digital nerve to the big toe, which runs obliquely forward and medially, in line with, but superficial to, the flexor hallucis longus. At the place where the tendon reaches the fibrous mass which contains the two sesamoids, the nerve crosses the medial half of the medial sesamoid.

In 1954 the following cases were reported:[8]

CASE 1: In April, 1952, a staff nurse bruised the soft tissues under the head of the metatarsal bone of the right great toe. The resultant swelling and broad tenderness resolved in 6 weeks, but severe local tenderness persisted over the lateral sesamoid bone of the long flexor tendon. Insoles, metatarsal bars, and physiotherapy did not relieve the pain she endured when walking.

In September, an operation for removal of the sesamoid bone was arranged. When the tendon was exposed, it was noticed that the digital nerve to the medial border of the great toe crossed the lateral sesamoid bone and the long flexor tendon. At the crossing, the nerve was embedded in scar, and both nerve and scar were adherent to the tendon sheath. The nerve was freed from adhesions and realigned away from the weight-bearing surface. The scarred portion of the tendon sheath was excised. The longitudinal skin incision in the line of the long flexor tendon healed perfectly. The patient soon recovered and suffered no discomfort thereafter.

CASE 2: In August, 1953, a man, aged 21, described similar symptoms, which he had had for 3 years, since he first injured his foot. There was a small area of reduced sensitivity over the medial border of the big toe. Radiographs showed multiple centers of ossification in the sesamoids. His doctor had tried all forms of conservative treatment and suggested removal of the sesamoid bone.

At operation, exactly the same conditions were present as were found in the foot of the staff nurse (Case 1). Again, freeing and transfer of the nerve and excision of the adjacent portion of the tendon sheath led to complete relief of pain. Sensation on the medial surface of the toe was also recovered.

It is possible that, on occasion, the sesamoid bones of the great toe have been removed when neurolysis and transposition of the digital nerve is all that is required.

The operation is performed through a slightly curved incision in the sole, edging the medial, "non-weight-bearing" border of the ball of the big toe. The branch of the medial digital nerve is found, usually thickened by scar tissue and adherent where it crosses the sesamoid and the sheath of the long flexor tendon. The nerve is carefully mobilized and transposed medially, away from the sesamoid. The skin is sutured and a padded, elasticized bandage is applied, "Non-weight-bearing" movements of the big toe commence next day.

After this simple operation there is no loss of function, whereas after removal of a sesamoid there is residual disability. Two famous cricketers, both fast bowlers, retired after excision of the sesamoid bone. They could no longer slap the foot down while bowling, which is necessary at the moment of delivery of a fast ball in both cricket and baseball.

The results of the operation have been almost uniformly good. Pain is relieved and sensation is restored to the medial surface of the big toe. During rehabilitation, a metatarsal platform should be worn.

Morton's Metatarsalgia

Morton, of Philadelphia, originated the term in 1876 to describe an acute, painful affliction of the forepart of the foot, a condition which has since had the eponym, Morton's metatarsalgia.[9] He considered that pain was due to compression of a digital nerve as it passed between the heads of the metatarsal bones; usually that between the third and fourth. Betts attributed the symptoms to a fibroneuroma of the fourth interdigital nerve resulting from traumatic neuritis.[10] Nissen ascribed them to ischemia of an interdigital neuroma.[11]

The condition occurs at any age and follows chronic compression of the nerve on bearing weight, either because of clawing of the toes or constant wearing of high-heeled shoes.

The patient suffers from typical pain on walking. It is burning in nature and referred to the interdigital cleft between the third and fourth toes. Paresthesia in the same distribution soon occurs. There is local tenderness of the nerve, and the symptoms are reproduced. These can be relieved temporarily by wearing an insole suitably excavated to prevent bearing weight on the nerve.

Operation is usually required to cure the condition. An incision is made over the nerve, extending from the ball of the foot into the skin of the digital cleft. The nerve is dissected and found to be thickened and fibrous—to the extent of having a fusiform swelling, or even a fibrous nodule, just proximal to its bifurcation. The thickened area is usually so large that the nerve cannot be transposed from the vulnerable area. It must, therefore, be transected proximal to the swelling. The nerve is then dissected distally and its two branches divided as they enter the adjacent toes. The whole segment is removed and sent for histological section. After suture of the skin, a firm dressing is applied. At least a half inch of the nerve above and below the neuroma should be excised.

The operation is curative, but at a price. The patient is left with permanent loss of sensation in the digital cleft and the adjacent sides of the affected toes. It is important to warn the patient of this effect of the operation, lest the surgeon be vulnerable to medicolegal attack. Interdigital neuromas, while most common beneath the third and fourth metatarsal heads, may occur beneath any of the metatarsals. Symptoms are similar to those in Morton's metatarsalgia. At operation, the nerve is found to be thickened at the point where it passes over the intermetatarsal ligament. The thickening has been called a neuroma, but is due to interstitial fibrosis and sometimes to proliferation of the neurolemma. Sometimes a small bursa is found, which should also be removed. It is wise to divide the intermetatarsal ligament in most cases.

Joplin's Neuroma

Joplin described perineural fibrosis of the plantar proper digital nerve, a terminal branch of the medial plantar nerve.[12] It is probably due to repeated trauma, as are other neuromas, or to involvement of the nerve in scar tissue after operation on the metatarsophalangeal joint. Hallus valgus and bunions characteristically cause severe pain on the plantar medial aspect of the joint, even in young people. This may be due to the outward rotation of the valgus toe on walking until weight bearing affects the digital nerve. Local tenderness and paresthesia are typical of a neuroma.

Joplin recommends excision of the nerve from the middle of the metatarsal shaft. Pain is relieved, but the area remains numb and, in contrast to what happens in Morton's metatarsalgia, the affected area of skin is not opposed to another protecting surface. It is on the medial side of the great toe, and for the rest of the patient's life it is vulnerable, like all insensitive areas of skin, to pressure necrosis.

We consider, therefore, that mobilization of the nerve and transfer to the medial side of the metatarsophalangeal joint, which usually relieves the pain, is the preferred procedure.

TARSAL TUNNEL SYNDROME[13]

The deep fascia around the ankle is strengthened posteriorly by the flexor retinaculum. The medial ligament of the ankle stretches from the lower border of the medial malleolus to the calcaneus. With the flexor retinaculum, it forms a tunnel which conducts the posterior tibial nerve, vessels, and tendons from the back of the ankle into the sole of the foot.

While less common than median neuropathy in the hand, posterior tibial neuropathy due to tarsal tunnel compression is the result of tenosynovitis of the flexor tendon sheaths or edema within the tunnel following trauma or thyroid dysfunction. Occasionally the nerve is compressed by collapse of the longitudinal arch, usually owing to intrinsic muscle atrophy and mid-tarsal degenerative joint changes in late middle age.

The condition affects men and women equally. The early and main complaint is of a burning pain and disordered sensibility in the toes and the soles of the feet. Sometimes the pain is referred up the leg, as in the carpal tunnel syndrome. It may be worse at night; exercise or hanging the leg out of bed may bring some relief.

Examination may reveal a fusiform swelling of the soft tissues behind the medial malleolus. The posterior tibial nerve is usually tender. Venous engorgement, by the use of a sphygmomanometer cuff inflated above the diastolic blood pressure, may reproduce the symptoms. Sensory impairment may be demonstrated in the skin supplied by the affected nerve.

The condition must be differentiated from pain due to peripheral vascular disease and the occasional posttraumatic, stenosing tenovaginitis of a posterior tendon sheath. In the early stages, physical therapy, including the intraarticular injection of steroid and a local anesthetic agent, may be helpful. In the older patient with fixed planovalgus deformity, a molded insole sometimes brings relief. More often, division of the roof of the tarsal tunnel is required. It may not always overcome sensory loss, but usually cures the pain.

THE FOOT IN OLD AGE

The strains and stresses of weight bearing take their inevitable toll of the feet. Even where there is no vascular disease or neurological damage, pathological changes take place.

Gradual relaxation of the ligaments leads to progressive collapse of the bony structure of the longitudinal and transverse arches. With sagging, abnormal weight bearing occurs.

Atrophy of the intrinsic muscles of the sole causes further collapse of the transverse arch, increasing the abnormal pressure on the skin beneath the heels and metatarsal heads. Intrinsic muscle atrophy leads to gradual stiffening of the toes. If they adopt a stiff, clawed position, the tips develop callosities. Hammer deformities, with a different pattern of callosities, may also develop.

Weakening of the calf muscles, so-called extrinsic muscle collapse, causes sagging of the longitudinal arch. Abnormal weight bearing at the center of the bony arch (i.e., at the talonavicular and mid-tarsal joints) leads to osteoarthritis. As these joints, by degrees, lose articular cartilage and develop peripheral osteophytes, subluxation of the mid-tarsal joints occurs.

The combination of loss of muscle control, relaxation of the ligaments, and osteoarthritis leads to increasing stiffness. Nothing is more conducive to pain in the feet than the combination of stiffness and callosities. Pain arises both in the joints of the feet and in the skin beneath the bony prominences.

Unprotected callosities may lead to pressure sores, in which case the patient is vulnerable to infected ulcers. Since such ulcers usually communicate with the metatarsal and pha-langeal joints, septic arthritis inevitably results. The danger of spreading infection, requiring local amputation, looms in the background. Reduced sensation, or vascular insufficiency, may precipitate a major catastrophe.

To pay careful attention to the feet in old people is essential, not only for their comfort, but to prevent major problems. Hygiene is important: dirt embedded in epidermal folds can lead to desquamation and even dermatitis, which may become infected. The toenails should be trimmed adequately, especially if onychogryphosis is present. Since few old people can reach their toenails with ease, and many suffer from defects of eyesight, it is often necessary that they obtain help from family members or friends, or arrange regular visits from the district nurse. Ingrowing toenails can cause severe pain and even ulceration.

Callosities are a common source of pain. Although thickening of the horny layer of the epidermis is the result of abnormal pressure, nodules within the cornified layer exacerbate the condition. Regular attendance at the surgery of a competent chiropodist is recommended.

The feet of old people should be kept warm, both in bed and outdoors in cold weather. To this end, old-fashioned bedsocks and lined slippers are useful, while great care must be taken to keep the feet dry. Footwear is a significant factor. Shoes (or boots, if weakness of the ankles is a problem) must be properly fitted for the shape of the individual foot, well-padded, and with no abnormal pressure points in either the sole or the uppers. Molded insoles may be required to spread the load of standing and walking.

There are occasions when surgery is required for deformities, especially of the toes, that cannot be controlled adequately by shoes. The surgeon should approach such operations with extreme caution, since he can easily precipitate necrosis of skin flaps, leading to spreading gangrene. General anesthesia is indicated, unless the patient's cardiac or pulmonary condition prevents it absolutely. Local anesthetic infiltration can become infected. A bloodless field should never be used. Surgery must be performed gently, since traumatized tissue may not survive. In the author's experience a condition of the feet in old age that frequently requires surgery to allow a comfortable shoe to be worn is complete dislocation of the second toe. It results from fixed hallux valgus. The consequent bunching of the toes may lead to dislocation of the second metatarsophalangeal joint. A totally useless, deformed, second toe is usually displaced dorsally to such an extent that it cannot be fitted even into a surgical shoe. Amputation, if carefully performed, is usually highly successful, as the incision, placed vertically between the first and third toes, is usually made through skin that is eminently viable, unless there is obstruction to a major artery in the leg.

REFERENCES

1. Helfet, A. J.: The treatment of the soldier's foot. Roy. Army Med. Corps J., May, 1941.
2. Freiberg, A. H.: Intraction of the second metatarsal bone. Surg., Gynecol. Obstet., *19:*191, 1914.
3. Freiberg, A. H.: The so-called infraction of the second metatarsal bone. J. Bone Joint Surg., *8:*257, 1926.
4. Kohler, A.: Typical disease of the second metatarsophalangeal joint. Am. J. Roentgenol., *10:*705, 1923.
5. Dunn, D. M.: The treatment of adolescent slipping of the upper femoral epiphysis. J. Bone Joint Surg., *46B:*621, 1964.
6. Apley, A. G.: A System of Orthopaedics and Fractures. ed. 5. London, Butterworths, 1977.
7. Inge, G. A. L., and Ferguson, A. B.: Surgery of the sesamoid bones of the great toe. Arch. Surg., *27:*466, 1933.
8. Helfet, A. J.: Neurological cause of pain under head of metatarsal bone of big toe. Lancet, *2:* 846, 1954.
9. Morton, T. G.: A peculiar and painful affection of the fourth metatarsophalangeal articulation. Am. J. Med. Sci., *71:*35, 1876.
10. Betts, L. O.: Morton's metatarsalgia: neuritis of fourth digital nerve. Med. J. Austral., *1:*514, 1940.
11. Nissen, K. J.: Plantar digital neuritis: Morton's metatarsalgia. J. Bone Joint Surg., *30B:*84, 1948.
12. Joplin, R. J.: Some common foot disorders amenable to surgery. A.A.O.S. Instructional Course Lectures, *15:*144, 1958.
13. Lam, S. J. S.: The tarsal tunnel syndrome. Lancet, *2:*1354, 1962.

6 Flatfoot

MOBILE FLATFOOT

The term *flatfoot* is generally used to describe a condition in which the longitudinal arch is lower than normal when bearing the weight of the body (Fig. 6-1). About one third of all adults have such feet, although not always bilaterally equal. Like the rest of their primate cousins, most children have this characteristic at birth, and even when they begin to walk, flat feet are the rule (Fig. 6-2). Over the succeeding 4 or 5 years a muscular support to the arch is created by the development of involuntary reflexes that brace the bone and the ligamentous bridge of the longitudinal arch.

The normal infant's foot, with its tendency to calcaneovalgus, differs from true talipes calcaneovalgus in that it is fully mobile. A pad of fat under the arch emphasizes this appearance. It is unlike the thick pad of fibrofatty tissue, obviously protective in character, in the soles of many barefoot, African tribes. The pad is not obvious in those who grow up with what may be considered the handicap of shoes.

The feet of most children are everted and bear weight along the inner borders, which are not designed or suitable for weight bearing. Until a sense of balance is acquired, gait is awkward (Fig. 6-3). The infant learns to walk on a wide base with the feet splayed outward; the typical "Charlie Chaplin" gait. Some try to compensate by walking pigeon-toed. This stance inverts the heels and lifts the inner borders of the feet—a sounder and stronger posture. Those who walk in this manner usually develop a well-shaped arch. Walking on tiptoe also forms the arch and is to be encouraged as a means of strengthening feet: in this way the development of the reflex support of the arch is stimulated. There is probably a critical stage in the growth of the child for the development of such reflexes. Children older than 5 or 6 years who have not developed reflex support seldom do so later. However hard they exercise to strengthen the intrinsic muscles of the foot, they merely increase the bulk of the muscle and improve the voluntary support of the longitudinal arch, but not the effortlessness of involuntary reflex control (Fig. 6-4). This is not as simple as one might think: some 20 per cent of adults never develop the reflex pattern, even in countries where shoes are not worn habitually. A genetic aspect may be responsible for this lack, for it often occurs in families whose members have similarly shaped feet (Fig. 6-5) and who may fail to establish the reflexes.[1] Also, some foot shapes naturally stimulate the growth of the necessary synapses: feet of other shapes do so only if stimulated by suitable exercises at the appropriate time.

In rare examples, young children, usually between the ages of 18 months and 3 years, seem to develop an abnormal variation of intrinsic reflexes and are able to walk only on

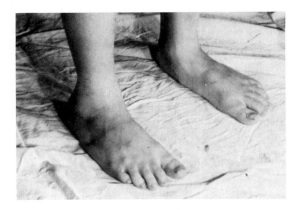

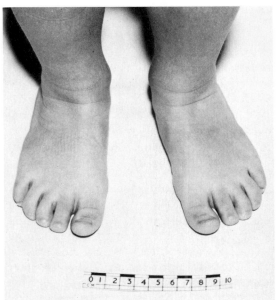

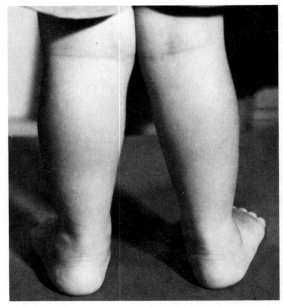

Fig. 6-1. An example of flat feet in which the longitudinal arch is lower than normal. In this case the patient is bearing weight upon the arch.

Fig. 6-2. In children under age five, as in this example, flatfoot should be regarded as normal.

Fig. 6-3. Until the intrinsic reflexes have developed, walking is awkward; the typical "Charlie Chaplin" gait.

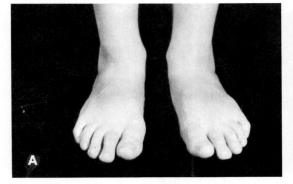

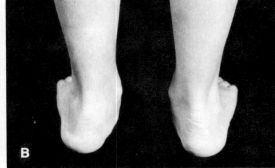

Fig. 6-4. (*A*) An anterior view of the feet of an older child shows persistent dropping of the longitudinal arch. (*B*) A posterior view shows persistent valgus position of the heels.

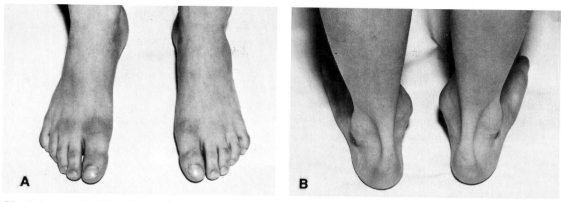

Fig. 6-5. Anterior (*A*) and posterior (*B*) photographs of the long, thin, planovalgus feet that occur in some families.

tiptoe. The resulting fixed, equinus gait distresses the parents, and they seek orthopaedic advice. One of the authors has seen two such cases in 8 years of practice in a community of 252,000 people. Both were healthy children with normally developed and -shaped feet. The calf muscles were not unduly tight, nor, when the patients were at rest, was any deformity discernible; yet, as soon as they stood up, they rose naturally to stand on the metatarsal heads with the feet in full equinus. Their gait was not ungainly. They were able to run. Both overcame the strange manner of walking within a few months; both reverted to normal movement suddenly, suggesting that the pattern of reflexes had adapted to a more adult type.

A third child, who seemed on superficial examination to have the same condition, showed slight, fixed equinus. The tightness did not disappear, however, and some months later minimal spastic paraparesis was obvious, with increased reflexes and a persistent, positive Babinski plantar response.

There is a widespread belief that flatfoot in children corrects spontaneously; that treatment is unnecessary. A visit to a foot clinic in any orthopaedic department dealing with adults or, more especially, to a military recruiting depot, will dispel any such illusion.

The late Dr. Goldman of the Poriah Hospital, near Tiberius, in Israel, told one of the authors that he had examined the feet of 3000 3-year-old children in kibbutzim in the Galilee. Ap-

proximately 80 per cent had flat feet. They were not treated. More often than not, many walked barefoot. At the age of sixteen, some 21 per cent of the boys and 19 per cent of the girls still had flat feet. Dr. Goldman found no way of determining which feet would reform and which would not.

Anatomical Factors that Predispose to Persistent, Mobile Flatfoot:

Pronation of the Forefoot (Fig. 6-6). Intrauterine development of the hind limb is not only axial but includes repeated folding of the

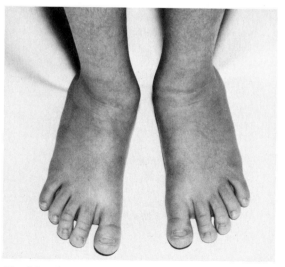

Fig. 6-6. Apparent pronation of the foot causes the child to stand on the medial border. There is gross valgus distortion of the heel, and if the heel were held vertically, the forefoot would be supinated.

limb bud; for example, the angle between the neck and shaft of the femur may be considered an internal, rotational fold, while that of the lower end of the femur would be external.

Inspection of the weight-bearing foot reveals that the forefoot has folded into a position equivalent, in the hand, to a palm-down posture; that is, the forefoot is pronated on the heel. At birth the human foot is fixed in a pronated position by the shape of its constituent bones. This adaptation has led to the characteristic plantigrade human posture.

Many children, when they first start to walk, have incomplete pronation (a relative *supination*) of the forefoot. The consequence is that the child finds it difficult to bring the head of the first metatarsal to the ground. He manages to do so by further pronational development of the bone structures, or he may compensate for the supination by tilting the heel into valgus or eversion. This brings the medial border of the foot to the ground, and the child walks with a seemingly flat foot. Examination, however, reveals a normal arch (Fig. 6-7).

The apparent flattening may be corrected by rolling the heel into a vertical position during standing, so forcing the completion of forefoot pronation by further growth. The condition causes awkwardness in the child but distress chiefly to the parents.

Congenital Pes Planus (Fig. 6-8). True, mobile, flatfoot is usually the result of ligamentous laxity. This may be a manifestation of one of the rare, hereditary diseases of ligamentous elasticity, such as the Ehlers-Danlos syndrome, or congenital hypermobility. The latter is not a disease but merely a variant of human type. It may be generalized, with abnormal hyperextensibility of elbows, wrists, thumbs, knees, and metatarsophalangeal and interphalangeal joints, or it may manifest only distally, affecting the hands and feet. Severe types cause pes planus, multiple joint pains, and premature degenerative changes in major weight-bearing joints. (A surprising finding is that persons so affected tend to enjoy longevity.) Mobile pes planus, seen in childhood, persists to an advanced age. Stiffness occurs only when degenerative osteoarthritis supervenes, usually in the midtarsal region. This type of pes planus is a handicap to both the child and to the adult.

Pes Planovalgus. A more complex deformity of the foot at birth may be the congenital planovalgus type. Because of the valgus shape there is a true, flatfoot, despite its mobility. The intrinsic muscles do not develop, and the foot remains flat, with the heel in valgus.

The Tight Achilles Tendon (Fig. 6-9). Whatever the original cause of valgus heel, if the position is maintained, the heel cord is kept continually in a lateral, "bow-string" position. As a result the calf muscle never grows to its full length in relation to the length of the limb. The Achilles tendon has become a cause of continuous valgus deformity of the heel and, consequently, of persistent flatfoot. If the heel is held in a vertical position for a sufficient

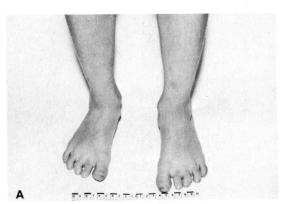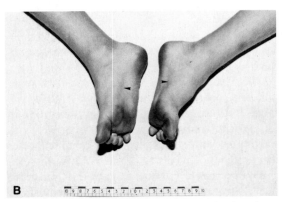

Fig. 6-7. (*A*) Another example of planovalgus feet due to relative supination of the forefoot. (*B*) Examination shows that a normal arch is present (*arrows*).

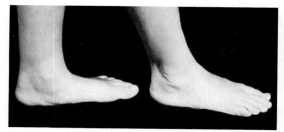

Fig. 6-8. True pes planus associated with congenital hypermobility.

length of time, the calf muscle will grow to its correct length and the valgus will be overcome. The flatfoot improves with the stretching of the heel cord. It is possible to dorsiflex the ankle further when the foot is everted. This explains the frequent association of a short Achilles tendon and feet apparently flat.

Occasionally the Achilles tendon is so tight that a raised heel is required for normal walking. A planned regimen for gradual lowering of the heel leads to stretching of the muscle. Only in very rare cases is lengthening of the tendon required. It is an effective method of overcoming the deformity, but it weakens the calf muscles and they may never recover fully.

Flatfoot as a Response to Postural Variation Elsewhere. A child with a normal arch at rest may adopt a flatfooted stance in order to compensate for postural variation elsewhere (Fig. 6-10). Planovalgus feet, and any of the other variations that lead to such a stance, may be reinforced by the posture of the rest of the limb.

Anteversion or retroversion of the femoral neck, knock knees, internal or external tibial torsion (Fig. 6-11)—all combine in differing patterns of rotation with flatfoot. The knock knees usually straighten, and normal alignment of the hip develops with further growth of the limb, especially after correction of the everted feet.

In other words, the normal activities of childhood may lead to the correction of these variations, but correction is more certain if measures are taken to ensure that the child stands and walks as often as possible with the foot in its desired position; that is, with a normal arch. A child's limbs and back grow

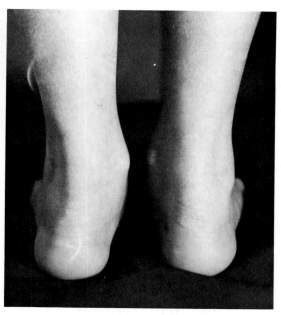

Fig. 6-9. In this posterior view of the heels, valgus deformity is present. The tight heel cord can be seen.

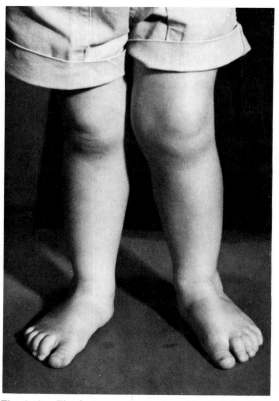

Fig. 6-10. Flat feet secondary to knockknee deformity.

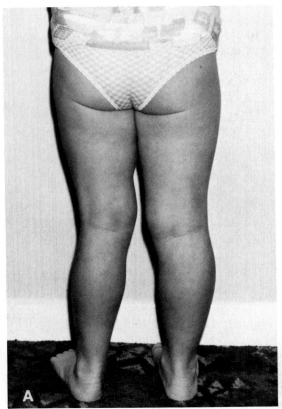 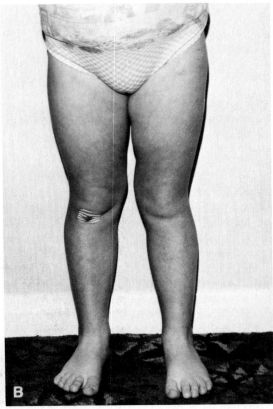

Fig. 6-11. (*A*) A back view of a standing child. The left foot seems flatter than the right. It can be seen that although the leg lengths are equal there are rotational differences between the two. The left buttocks is not as well developed as the right, a condition usually associated with retroversion. The left foot is rotated outward compared with the left knee owing to external tibial torsion. (*B*) Anterior view of the same child. The rotational deformities are well hidden. However, the bandage below the right knee is indicative of the child's ungainly gait and tendency to fall.

in the position in which they are used. If he walks and stands constantly with an elevated, longitudinal arch, the foot will grow in that shape and will be strong and stable; to attain this is the main object of the heel seat.

Although many feet correct spontaneously, this is not always the case. The child with grossly everted feet; the fat or sluggish child, whose activities are not sufficient for the development of strong feet; those suffering from Ehlers-Danlos syndrome or other causes of slack ligaments; may become flatfooted adults and therefore require treatment as early as possible.

Treatment of Flatfoot

The authors consider that the normal arch for a supple foot is formed when the heel is vertical. We know that dorsiflexion of the big toe, and walking or standing on tiptoe, tighten the plantar fascia and contract the plantar muscles, so correcting the eversion of the heel and restoring the arch. Exercises based on these movements correct the eversion and, by strengthening the muscles, ease walking with a vertical heel and raised longitudinal arch, even if the reflex support never develops. Active exercise may stimulate adequate growth of the bone of the arch.

We have been discussing the mobile, painless flat foot. The symptoms are mainly awkwardness of gait, early fatigue, and a tendency to develop strain. Such patients may go through life comfortably enough, with reasonable function except for a tendency to wear out their shoes quickly. Not all, however, are free of pain in adult life, and some suffer quite severe fatigue; many have problems with footwear. For these reasons, as well as for the parents' sake, an attempt at active correction is worthwhile, provided the cure is not worse than the disease. In the growing child, correction can be achieved in a simple way by using the heel seat described later.

Arch Supports. Most European specialists, as well as many in other parts of the world, traditionally prescribe rigid arch supports. These do raise and hold the arch, but work only by persisting with a forced and unnatural weight-bearing area. The muscles of the arch are not exercised and consequently do not strengthen. The foot lapses when the support is removed.

This method of treating flatfoot in children led to many adults having to wear rigid arch supports. These, for example, were standard issue in the German army during the 1939–1945 war. They were carried routinely in the quartermaster's stores. In other words, once a child becomes used to arch supports, they cannot be abandoned. The support has replaced the action of the muscles which have not had the exercise necessary for strength and stability. The feet are weak and lazy. The ordering of arch supports for a child is more than a prescription: it may be a life sentence.

The Elongated Heel Wedge. The second method, devised by Hugh Owen Thomas a century ago, was used almost universally in English-speaking countries. Correction of the eversion of the heel was attempted by tilting and elongating the heel of the shoe by means of a medial wedge on the inner side. If the back of the shoe fits snugly, the tilt does counter eversion.

The elongation of the heel on the medial side of the sole is necessary to protect the welt of the shoe on its inner side, but it also inverts the forefoot. Consequently, however long the child wears these altered shoes, the foot and heel relapse, to some degree, afterward.

In an attempt to supinate the forefoot, some surgeons prescribe a lateral, tilting wedge on the sole of the shoe to balance the medial heel tilt. In theory, this combination should hold the heel vertical while pronating the transverse

arch. It does not work, even in the best-made leather shoes. The upper soon loosens, and the twist breaks the sole of the shoe or loosens the heel. The combination is unsatisfactory (Fig. 6-12).

With a Thomas' heel wedge it is difficult to preserve the snug fit of the shoe around the child's heel, since the foot tends to slip down the sloping sole, deforming the outer wall of the upper and causing increased wear on the outer border of the heel.

Once the grip on the heel is lost it is necessary to repair or renew the shoes, otherwise the method is inefficient. In the case of hard-playing little boys, the heels have to be repaired at least every 2 to 3 weeks, and the shoes themselves do not long retain their shape. Repairs and replacements become expensive and irksome.

To be effective, the shoes with tilted, elongated heels must be worn constantly. The child must not walk barefoot, and he should also refrain from wearing slippers, sandals, rubber boots, and football boots, because it is impracticable to alter these types of footwear.

So many shoes with tilted heels, with or without a molded insole as a support for the arch, are manufactured and sold commercially, that it is worth reiterating their disadvantages:

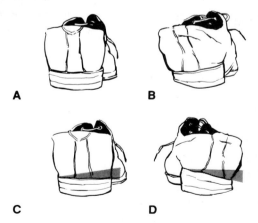

Fig. 6-12. The tilting heel wedge. (*A*) The back of a child's shoe. (*B*) The everted or flat foot tends to deform the outer stiffening of the back of the shoe and wears down the heel on the inner side. (*C*) A heel wedge within the shoe is intended to prevent eversion tilting, but (*D*) this merely transfers the wedge to the outer side of the heel, and the upper is distorted in the opposite direction.

although suitable for treating knock knees in young children, they are not wholly effective in forming or reforming the arch of the foot. To be so at all, there must be continuity of treatment, which prevents the child from walking barefoot or wearing other forms of footwear. To remain effective, the shape of the shoe and the tilt of the heel need conscientious and constant supervision, frequent repair, and renewal. This is expensive.

The Corrective Heel Seat. The heel seat described here is useful in correcting the flat, everted feet of growing children.[2] It does not suffer from the disadvantages of the tilted, elongated heel wedge. It is a method which forms and develops a normally arched foot in a positive manner.

The idea for the corrective heel seat is based on two premises:

When the forefoot is held flat on the floor, inversion of the heel produces a longitudinal arch, and the greater the inversion, the higher the arch. In other words, with the heads of the first and fifth metatarsals bearing weight normally in the shoe, correction of the eversion of the heel corrects the flatfoot. A vertical heel gives the flatfoot its normal arch (Fig. 6-13).

The growing foot develops and functions in the shape in which it is held; if the growing foot is held and allowed to function in the normal shape, it will "set" in that shape. An extreme contrast is provided by the ancient Chinese custom of constant binding of the feet of baby girls into a "club" shape. With growth, they developed fixed clubfeet. Not only does the child develop normally-shaped feet, if we allow them to function with a normal arch, but if the arch is not supported, it will develop strong muscles. The result will be a strong foot.

The heel seat shown in Fig. 6-14A and B is so constructed that it fits snugly into the back of a shoe, sandal with heel, or even slipper, so long as the stiffening of the upper is strong enough to maintain it in position (Fig. 6-14C). When so fitted, the inner surface of the heel seat is the shape of the normal heel in the vertical position. As soon as the child puts on a shoe containing the heel seat, any eversion

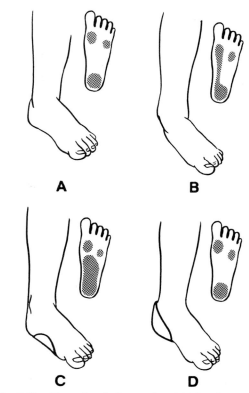

Fig. 6-13. Normal and abnormal weight bearing on the arches of the foot. (*A*) The diagram shows that, with normal longitudinal and transverse arches, weight is borne on the "tripod" consisting of the heel and the first and fifth metatarsal heads. (*B*) In the flat foot, weight is borne along the medial longitudinal arch. (*C*) The use of an insole merely spreads the weight bearing further to the longitudinal arch. (*D*) A heel seat, by keeping the heel vertical, restores the "tripod."

is corrected. It is a virtue of the appliance that the child does not experience any discomfort. If socks are worn, the heel seats fit into the shoe outside them, so the plastic does not stick to sweating skin.

The weight of the body on the base of the heel seat levers the inner wall to an upright position and so corrects pronation of the heel, or prevents its occurrence. The inner wall is shaped to the curves of the normal heel. Tilting the base of the heel seat, as is sometimes done to simulate the tilted heel wedge, is wrong, because it reduces the corrective effect.

Heel seats, based on the principle of correcting the valgus heel, have been used since 1956 for children with mobile, flat feet; for

Fig. 6-14. (*A*) The Helfet heel seat. (*B*) A diagram, drawn in cross section, of the heel seat applied to the valgus heel before weight bearing commences. (*C*) The heel seat when weight is borne. The vertical arrow represents body weight. It can be seen that the curved inferior surface of the heel seat forces the heel to adopt a vertical position by transferring the body weight as a corrective force to the heel. This is represented by the horizontal arrow. (*D*) A different diagrammatic representation of the heel cup. In this drawing, the horizontal corrective force is represented in the opposite direction to indicate that the appliance depends upon the strength of the upper of the shoe.

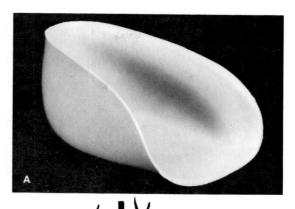

A

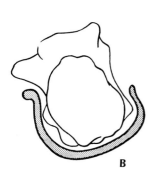

B

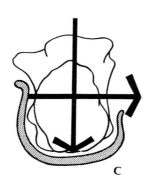

C

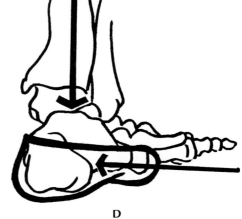

D

children and adults with footstrain; and in the rehabilitation of convalescent patients recovering from confinement to bed for long periods through illness or injury.

After heel seats have been prescribed, the child's gait is improved almost immediately. Pigeon-toed or splayfoot gaits are corrected, and the child is more agile and less awkward. The effect on gait can be assessed by the way in which the shoes wear down. Whereas, previously, the heels of the shoes wore down quickly on the outer side and the upper became deformed, with the properly fitted corrective heel seat the heel wears evenly and the shoe maintains its shape. Moreover, shoes last twice as long before they need repair.

PIGEON TOES AND FEMORAL AND TIBIAL TORSION

Children with toe-in gait seldom suffer pain in the feet, but the condition worries the parents, who seek medical advice. It is common before the age of 5 years, occurring equally in boys and girls, and is often familial: grandparents will say that one or the other of the parents had similar trouble in childhood.

Children with such feet walk in an ungainly way and, if the condition is severe enough, there is a tendency to fall repeatedly when the toes of one foot catch against the heel of the other. Healed abrasions of the knees or face may be visible. The feet alone may be affected, but knock knee deformity, bow legs and anteversion or retroversion of the femoral necks are often present in some combination.

It is obvious that the deformity, if deformity it is, is rotational in nature. What is not always realized is that it is not the foot that is rotated. Examination of the feet show that they are normal in shape for a child of that age. Since toe-in gait is most common in young children, especially soon after they have learned to walk, development of the arch is incomplete, and the foot may well be everted.

The rotational deformity is in the leg, and the foot merely draws attention to the position of the leg. Furthermore, the internal rotation is complex, the sum of all the rotations of the leg being internal. Where do the rotational deformities occur?

The Femoral Neck

Rotation in the femur does not take place throughout the shaft of the bone. It is confined mainly to the angle that the femoral neck makes with the shaft. At birth the femoral neck is anteverted 40 degrees, and in the adult this is reduced to 20 degrees, on the average. The angle of 40 degrees is usually described as the fetal position of the femoral neck. Any angle greater than 40 degrees is defined as increased anteversion; if the rotation does not "unwind" in due time, the position is termed *persistent fetal alignment.*

Persistent fetal alignment implies that, when the child is standing or walking and the hips are fully extended, there is a greater range of internal- than of external rotation. The insertions of the muscles around the hip tend to pull the limbs into an internal rotational posture during walking. This posture causes a toe-in gait, but it is not the only factor.

Internal Tibial Torsion

Rotational deformity can also occur in the tibia, but, unlike the femur, the rotation is present throughout the shaft. In many instances the condition is diagnosed as bow legs. The legs are bowed, but examination shows them to be internally rotated as well. Tibial torsion plays a large part in the appearance of the toe-in gait.

The condition may be inherited or associated with the position of the legs in utero, especially in the last trimester, when the increasing size of the fetus causes it to be packed tighter and tighter. The final factor in the development of the combination of bow legs and internal tibial torsion may well be the onset of walking. The strength of the tibias may not be sufficient to support the weight of the body, and the deformity occurs. At the same time the wearing of diapers causes the child to walk on a wide base, increasing the deformity.

The toe-in gait is the sum of the rotational deformities, controlled by the action of the muscles. In most children the condition improves gradually with further growth, but it may not be maximal when the child first learns to walk. Sometimes the pigeon toes are most severe 18 months to 2 years later. Repeated examination of such children shows that it is the femoral component that unwinds before the tibial. It may be that unwinding of tibial torsion is due to the change of forces on the tibia that takes place after the femoral rotation unwinds. In effect, femoral rotation is "the conductor of the orchestra."

Children in whom toeing-in increases after walking has begun usually have extreme internal tibial torsion combined with retroversion of the femoral neck. The sum of opposing rotations is toeing-in. As the retroversion is overcome by growth of the femur, internal tibial torsion remains and the toe-in gait increases. Later, the tibial torsion unwinds as well and the position of the foot gradually improves.

The rotational deformities of the legs are not necessarily symmetrical. Differences between the two sides are commonly present in children, with or without toeing-in or clinically obvious bow legs or knock knees. Examination of many adults shows that such rotational differences are present in many people throughout life but that a balance exists in the rotations, so that the feet point more or less in the right direction. For example, increased rotation of one femur may well be balanced by increased rotation of the tibia in the same leg, but in the opposite direction. In other cases, increased rotation of one femur may be accompanied by increased tibial torsion in the other leg in the *same* direction. Such differences are seldom noticed, because the precise angle of rotation of femur or tibia is difficult to measure accurately. They may account for the advent of unilateral osteoarthritis of one joint or another later in life.

Treatment. Little treatment is required, apart from reassuring the parents that the condition will gradually improve.

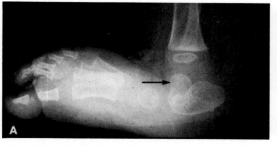
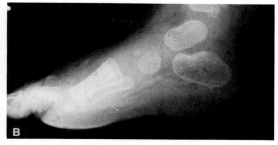

Fig. 6-15. (*A*) Radiographs of the foot of an infant with congenital vertical talus (*arrow*). The soft tissue shadow reveals the true shape of the foot, which is completely flattened. (*B*) The opposite foot is normal, both in the shape of bones and the soft tissues.

Heel wedges may improve the gait in some instances, as may heel seats. Severe anteversion of the femoral heads may be overcome by the use of Denis-Browne night splints, with the shoes locked onto the bar in extreme external rotation. The authors do not recommend such therapy, since it may cause inadvertent retroversion of the femoral necks. In particular, all such medieval paraphernalia as leather night splints with buckles and straps are contraindicated. They do not treat the rotational distortions, since they are based on a two-dimensional assessment of the deformities. They are inadequate and unnecessary, and the effect of the treatment is less therapeutic than punishing to the child.

STIFF FLATFOOT

Vertical Talus

This rare condition is present at birth.[3-5] It is also, and perhaps more properly, known as rocker-bottom foot, from the shape of the deformity.

The name *vertical talus* derives from the position of the ossification center visible on radiographs (Fig. 6-15), but careful examination reveals a more complex deformity.

Essentially the condition is one of dorsal dislocation of the forefoot, the dislocation occurring through the mid-tarsal region and, in particular, the talonavicular joint. As a result, the neck (and head) of the talus, normally approximately horizontal, is pushed downward until it is almost vertical. The dorsally dislocated navicular bone comes to lie anterior to the neck of the talus (Fig. 6-16).

Since the elements of the foot are well-formed, it is obvious that the dislocation occurs late in fetal development, from abnormal intrauterine pressure. There are two reasons why, in rare cases, intrauterine pressure causes dislocation of the forefoot, when usually it results in the more common calcaneovalgus deformity.

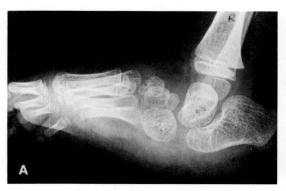
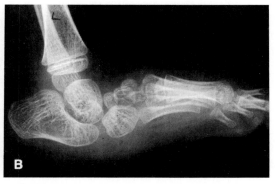

Fig. 6-16. Radiographs of both feet of an older child. The vertical talus can be seen in each foot, together with the dorsal dislocation of both forefeet. The navicular bones can be seen to be lying dorsal to the neck of each talus.

Abnormal laxity in the mid-tarsal region is one cause. Harrold described a case in which at operation it was discovered that there was no tendon of the tibialis posterior.[6] This abnormality has not been recorded elsewhere; it resulted in sufficient laxity to allow dislocation. More commonly, the hindfoot is seen to be abnormal. A fixed equinovarus is present. Presumably, a clubfoot deformity has been converted into vertical talus by compression of the forefoot.

Congenital vertical talus is a severe deformity which, unless corrected, leaves the growing foot stiff and in an abnormal shape that will not fit into a conventional shoe. The head of the talus projects into the sole, giving rise to intense pain from abnormal weight bearing. Treatment is essential—and *before* the child begins to walk. Surgery offers the only hope of changing the shape of the foot. Open reduction of the dislocated talonavicular and mid-tarsal joints must be performed and, if necessary, stainless steel Kirschner wires inserted across the joints to maintain reduction. The shape and position of the hindfoot is assessed to determine whether a residual equinus or equinovarus deformity needs to be corrected by further dividing the constricting soft tissues (see Chap. 8).

Spasmodic Flatfoot

The term *spasmodic, flatfoot* describes a painful foot in marked eversion, due to peroneal muscle spasm.[7] The spasm is caused, not by any neurologic lesion but by the reflex contraction of the peroneal muscles, which, in turn, is caused by irritation of tarsal joints.

The condition usually starts in adolescence. Since most cases are associated with a congenital abnormality of the tarsal bones, an interesting feature is that symptoms are not present when the child begins to walk.[8,9] It is the rare patient in whom no abnormality is present. Such patients are usually adolescents of lanky and indolent type, or thin adults whose occupations require long periods of standing. This rare, idiopathic variety is not seen as frequently as it was before World War II.

The pain and spasm may start suddenly, or they may develop insidiously over a few months. Symptoms usually develop at, or shortly before, puberty.[10] Pain is usually felt on the lateral side of the tarsus, and local tenderness with involuntary peroneal muscle spasm is present. Any attempt to overcome the eversion spasm causes pain. There may be local swelling on the lateral border of the foot.

The reflex eversion may be regarded as protective in nature, since it is movement of the affected tarsal joints that gives rise to the pain. The patient is able to walk with fixed eversion, although in the acute stage every step is painful, and the patient walks with an awkward, shuffling gait. Later, secondary changes in the tarsal joints lead to bony rigidity, and the pain may subside.

The cause of spasmodic flatfoot is a congenital synostosis or synchrondrosis between two of the bones of the hindfoot. Usually it consists of a calcaneonavicular bar (Fig. 6-17),[11] although there may be a calcaneotalar bridge behind the sustentaculum tali. These abnormalities can be demonstrated by appropriate oblique radiographs, which are not easy to obtain because the position of the foot is critical if the bone images are not to overlap on the film.

The hindfoot cannot be normal in childhood if a bony or cartilaginous bar is present. There is always some degree of stiffness in the talar joints, leading to a limitation of inversion and eversion. The pain is usually caused by a stress fracture of the bar, resulting in delayed union and pseudarthrosis, with consequent inflammation and reflex spasm (Fig. 6-18).

Injection of a local anesthetic agent into the tender area relieves the spasm and overcomes the symptoms temporarily. In the absence of a bony abnormality, the deformity may be corrected by manipulation under general anesthesia, followed by immobilization in a walking plaster cast for 4 to 6 weeks. Thereafter, foot exercises and physical treatment, such as ultrasound or local heat, accompanied by the use of a heel seat, can help to maintain normal foot posture and a mobile foot.

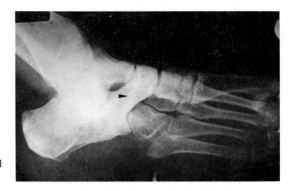

Fig. 6-17. Spasmodic flatfoot. A very broad congenital calcaneonavicular synostosis is present (*arrow*).

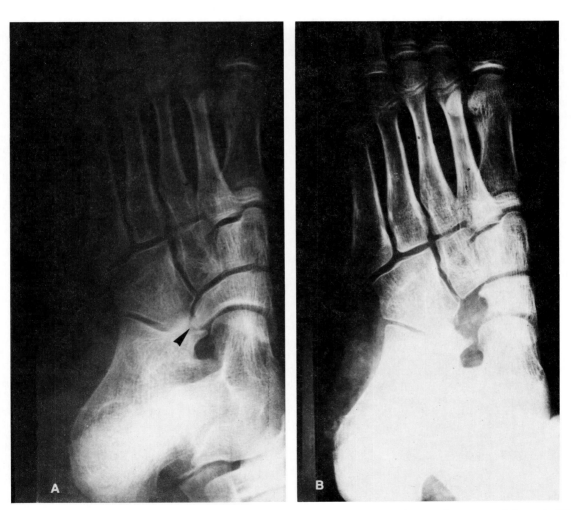

Fig. 6-18. (A) Radiograph of a calcaneonavicular synostosis in which a stress fracture has occurred (*arrow*). (b) Radiograph of the same patient after surgical excision of the calcaneonavicular bar.

Immobilization relieves the pain and, in rare instances, leads to fusion of the pseudoarthrosis and recovery; but in the great majority of cases in which a congenital bar is present, such conservative therapy is unavailing. Surgery offers the only opportunity of overcoming the symptoms. Sometimes excision of the congenital bar cures the condition, but the operation is difficult and the results may be disappointing.[12] Despite apparently adequate excision, reflex spasm occasionally persists. In most cases, combined subtalar and midtarsal arthrodesis (so-called triple arthrodesis) is necessary for a cure.

Posttraumatic Stiff Flatfoot

Many injuries to the bones and joints of the foot result in stiffness (Fig. 6-19), but in one particular type of injury (namely fracture of the calcaneus) it is the usual outcome. The heel is commonly fractured in a fall from a height in which the patient lands on his feet. Minor fractures, in which there has been no displacement of fragments or avulsion injury of parts of the calcaneus, unite well, and, if exercises are undertaken, a mobile, comfortable foot will be regained. The result in the

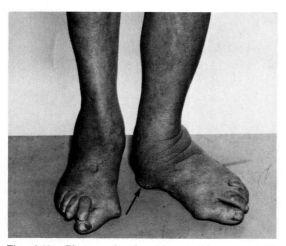

Fig. 6-19. Photograph of a 51-year-old woman with severe rigid flatfoot. A large bony lump can be seen projecting from the medial border of the foot (*arrow*). This patient was suffering from severe erosive rheumatoid arthritis, and complete lateral dislocation of the forefoot had occurred. The bony lump is the head of the talus projecting subcutaneously.

severely crushed heel is very different. The calcaneus is broken into small fragments, and the posterior and anterior subtalar joints are disrupted. The angle between the two parts of the calcaneus is lost, with consequent flattening of the heel. At the same time the distal fragment is displaced laterally. The result is flatfoot with a thickened, widened heel and stiffness of the subtalar joints amounting, in many cases, to fibrous ankylosis.

The resulting foot is poorly adapted to walking because of the crushed shape, the abnormally stiff joints, and the fact that it will no longer fit into a normal shoe. The lateral tilt of the heel may cause direct impingement of the distal tip of the lateral malleolus against the surface of the calcaneus, causing local pain.[13]

Other less common crush injuries may result in a stiff flatfoot. Direct crush injuries of the midtarsal region caused, for example, by a heavy vehicle passing over the top of the foot, may collapse the longitudinal arch, with multiple fragments of the tarsus eventually uniting by fibrous, or even bony, ankylosis. Where indicated, excision of the bony lumps, or fusion after realignment of the joints, may bring some alleviation of the pain, stiffness and awkwardness of this disability.

Paralytic Flatfoot

Spastic Paralysis. Paralysis may be associated with increased or decreased tone, that is, with an upper- or lower motor neuron lesion. Spastic paralysis due to upper motor neuron lesions manifests with increased tone in the leg. By far the most common cause of spastic paralysis is a stroke, in which all the muscles of the limb are affected. The paralyzed foot is usually pulled into a position of fixed equinovarus, since the flexor and invertor muscles prove to be stronger than the evertors. The patient walks with a "dropped" foot. Occasionally, the balance of paralyzed muscles results in the opposite deformity: spastic calcaneovalgus flatfoot.[14] This outcome is fortunate for the patient, since walking is easier than with the "dropped" foot.

As a rule, the only treatment needed is

careful attention to the fitting of shoes. In rare instances orthotic splinting may be required, especially if the calcaneovalgus spasticity is severe.

Flaccid Paralysis. Whatever the cause, paralyzed flat feet with decreased muscle tone may well require stabilization for effective walking. This usually entails specialized orthotic splinting.

REFERENCES

1. Griffiths, R. K.: The evolution of the foot. *In* Klenerman, L.: The Foot and Its Disorders. London, Blackwell Scientific Publications, 1976.
2. Helfet, A. J.: A new way of treating flat feet in children. Lancet, *T:*262, 1956.
3. Osmond-Clarke, H.: Congenital vertical talus. J. Bone Joint Surg., *38B:*334, 1956.
4. Colton, C. L.: The surgical management of congenital vertical talus. J. Bone Joint Surg., *55B:*566, 1973.
5. Eyre Brook, A. L.: Congenital vertical talus. J. Bone Joint Surg., *49B:*618, 1967.
6. Harrold, A. J.: Congenital vertical talus in infancy. J. Bone Joint Surg., *49B:*634, 1967.
7. Braddock, G. T. F.: A prolonged follow-up of peroneal spastic flat foot. J. Bone Joint Surg., *43B:*734, 1961.
8. Challis, J.: Hereditary transmission of talonavicular coalition in association with anomaly of the little finger. J. Bone Joint Surg., *56A:*1273, 1974.
9. Bersani, F. A., and Samilson, R. L.: Massive familial tarsal synostosis. J. Bone Joint Surg., *39A:*1187, 1957.
10. Leonard, M. A.: The inheritance of tarsal coalition and its relationship to spastic flat foot. J. Bone Joint Surg., *56B:*521, 1974.
11. Lapidus, P. W.: Congenital fusion of the bones of the foot. (Report of a case of congenital astragaloscaphoid fusion.) J. Bone Joint Surg., *14:*888, 1932.
12. Mitchell, G. P., and Gibson, J. M. C.: Excision of calcaneo-navicular bar for painful spasmodic flat foot. J. Bone Joint Surg., *49B:*281, 1967.
13. Isbister, J. F., St. C.: Calcaneofibular abutment following crush fracture of the calcaneus. J. Bone Joint Surg., *56B:*274, 1974.
14. Duckworth, T., and Smith, T. W. D.: Treatment of paralytic convex pes valgus. J. Bone Joint Surg., *56B:*305, 1974.

7 The Foot in Athletics

DANIEL N. KULAND

People of all ages, shapes, and sizes now participate in athletics. Running is the primary activity: some run marathons of 26 miles and 385 yards, while others run or jog shorter distances, in an unprecedented movement toward fitness. Primitive man possessed very heavy limbs, so running would have been an unusual activity, designed for extreme situations such as fleeing from danger. The robust bone structure of the distal phalanx of the great toe, which bears the thrust during push-off, is evidence of a striding, rather than a shuffling, gait.[1]

THE FOOT AND KNEE CONNECTION

Many conditions of the knee, such as chondromalacia patella, sprains, and bursitis, are primarily the result of foot imbalance. A linkage system extends up the limb from the foot, and that is the source, in running athletes, of most knee problems that may be alleviated or avoided by attention to the foot.[2,3]

Medial pain in the knee can be caused by excessive pronation of the foot, resulting in valgus strain of the knee; lateral pain, by a rigid foot with varus jamming; and patellofemoral pain, by tight heel cords and resulting deep knee flexion during mid-support.

Female athletes have additional problems. Their wider hips and the more angled course of the quadriceps mechanism to the kneecap and insertion into the tibial tubercle (the Q angle) result in a tendency of the kneecap to slide laterally. The increased angle, combined with flat kneecaps, shallow femoral grooves, and ligamentous laxity with recurvation, results in subluxation or dislocation of the patellas, and chondromalacia. This may be accentuated if the quadriceps have not been strengthened by training. The movement of the patella is exaggerated by pronation of the foot, with consequent valgus strain at the knee, an increase in the Q angle and lateral slide. Subluxation of the kneecap can be limited or, in some cases, avoided by using an orthosis which limits pronation. An elastic rubber knee strap with controlling pad may help to hold the kneecap in the groove.

In 1976, 89 participants in the United States Bike-centennial Tour were examined. They cycled from Reedsport, Oregon to Yorktown, Virginia: a distance of 4500 miles. Orthopaedic and fitness studies were done in Eugene, Oregon and again at the University of Virginia.[4] Very few knee problems arose and most occurred in the first few days, as the riders traversed the Cascade Mountains. The pain behind the kneecap ceased as soon as the riders learned that intermittent changes in saddle height would eliminate it by changing the point of contact between patella and femur. This simple expedient eliminated the trouble during a trip involving 2 million pedal strokes.

Some participants over 60 years of age had some degenerative changes in the knee, but they reported that their knees had never felt better than they did after the completion of the tour. This may have been due to the flexibility exercise of cycling and the nutritive milking of the articular cartilage. In comparison to cycling, the jamming of the knees in running can cause subchondral microfractures and loss of the shock-absorbing capacity of trabecular bone. The overlying articular cartilage must then absorb the shocks and can break down.[5]

Osgood-Schlatter's disease, or apophysitis of the tibial tubercle, is seen in some fast-growing, active youths. The tibial tubercle is part of the epiphysis of the knee, and microtears in the insertion of the patellar tendon with flaking of cartilage results in a painful, swollen tubercle region.[6] Treatment includes a knee-resting program followed by daily quadriceps stretching. A youngster's quadriceps are usually strong, but these young athletes do not often work on stretching of the quadriceps as a means of preventing Osgood-Schlatter's syndrome. The appropriate exercises should therefore be added to the young runner's warm-up (Fig. 7-1).

INJURIES OFTEN ASSOCIATED WITH ATHLETICS

Shin Splints

In the United States, the term *shin splints* is used to describe a feeling of pain and tightness in the shin. There are two types: anterior shin splints, due to microtears at the origin of the tibialis anterior from the tibia; and posterior shin splints, involving the posterior tibial muscle.[7]

The anterior shin splints are most prevalent when the person begins a program of running, or when he runs on hard surfaces, downhill, or in shoes that have a sharply-angled heel. Under all these conditions, the runner's foot slaps down after heel-strike. In order to slow

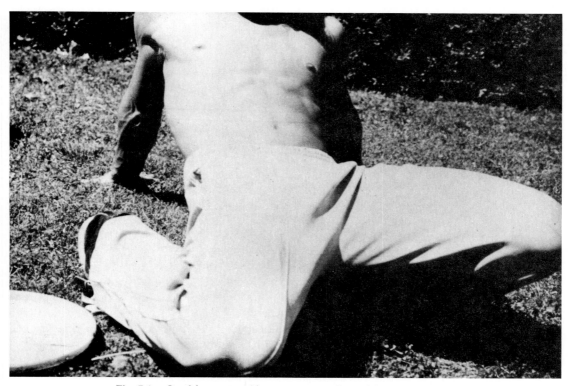

Fig. 7-1. Quadriceps stretching can prevent Osgood-Schlatters disease.

down a fast slap, the tibialis anterior contracts eccentrically, and small tears can arise at its origin. Such shin splints can be avoided by running on softer surfaces, such as grass or wood chips; also, the runner should wear, as a buffer, shoes with rounded and absorptive heels. He should avoid downhill runs, which accentuate the slap, and he must strengthen his tibialis anterior and stretch the antagonistic heel cord.

Posterior shin splints occurs in athletes with pronated feet and those who run in sand or on humped roads. The pronated foot stretches out and irritates the posterior tibial muscle and tendon, causing posteromedial tibial pain. Running on a beach causes the foot to pronate through the sand. The athlete who constantly runs along the edge of a canted road has to pronate the higher foot more than the lower one, and this pronation also stretches the posterior tibial muscle and tendon. Treatment of posterior shin splints consists in avoiding running on surfaces such as those described above, which force pronation, and by using orthoses to limit pronation.

Rupture of the Heel Cord

Although an athlete can suffer a ruptured heel cord at any time, there are two circumstances and times when it is especially likely.[8] The first is during the young, competitive years, in events such as the long jump. The ankles are dorsiflexed during landing and then quickly converted to plantar flexion by contraction of the calf muscle. This combination of forced dorsiflexion and dynamic plantar flexion may result in rupture of the heel cord. The plantaris tendon usually remains intact and can be used in the repair of these ruptures. If the patient is treated nonoperatively, with an equinus cast, healing occurs, but the tendon junction is weak and heel cord pain often persists. Rupture should therefore be repaired surgically, using the plantaris tendon as a "living weave." The tendon should not be fanned out and used as a sheath for the heel cord, since it can strangle the tendon tissue. After repair, the ankle is held in equinus until the limb is ready to bear weight, followed by

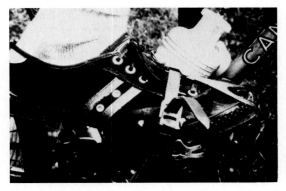

Fig. 7-2.   These cycling shoes have a thin counter and can irritate the subcutaneous bursa.

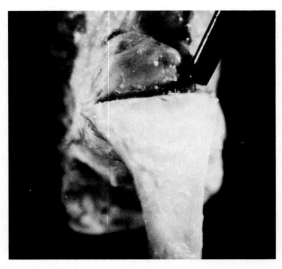

Fig. 7-3.   The heel cord inserts into the calcaneus, leaving room for the retrocalcaneal bursa.

an equinus walking cast and then a shoe with a built-up heel. A systematic program of stretching and flexibility exercises, together with muscle strengthening, is vital for the best results.

Conditions of the Heel Region

The heel is a complex structure.[9] Behind it are the subcutaneous bursa, the heel cord, and the retrocalcaneal bursa. Beneath the heel are the impact point of the calcaneus, the fat pad with its septa, and the plantar fascia.

The subcutaneous bursa can be irritated by shoes with a thin, unpadded counter, like those in some cycling and running shoes (Fig. 7-2).

The insertion of the heel cord begins ¾ inch distal to the uppermost posterior part of the calcaneus (Fig. 7-3) and extends onto the plantar surface. The proximal area between the calcaneus and the heel cord is occupied by the retrocalcaneal bursa. Prolonged irritation of the retrocalcaneal region (e.g., by women's high-heeled shoes) may cause an exostosis to develop on either side of the heel cord insertion. This "pump bump" can be seen on radiographs as a prominent roundness of the posterosuperior aspect of the calcaneus which may cause Achilles tendinitis due to friction. Flared-heel training shoes may alleviate this by diminishing rocking at heel strike. An oblique osteotomy may eventually be needed to remove the bump.

Irritation of the heel cord occurs when a cyclist "ankles" too much. This happened to many on the Bikecentennial Tour as they crossed the Cascade Mountains. They soon found that by reducing ankle motion they eliminated the heel cord irritation.

During running, Achilles' tendon pull can cause avulsion of pieces of calcanal bone, leading to "runners' bumps" (Fig. 7-4). Achilles tendinitis and bump pain is treated by putting a lift under the heel and starting stretching exercises, since a tight heel cord is the primary cause of the problem. The wider heel is also helpful in limiting rocking.

Because of the close juxtaposition of structures in this region, a combined diagnosis of "pump bump," retrocalcaneal bursitis, Achilles tendinitis, and subcutaneous bursitis is sometimes made. The athlete may thus need a soft counter, a heel lift, flared-heel shoes, stretching exercises, and perhaps an oblique, calcaneal osteotomy.

Ankle Sprains

Prolonged disability can result when lateral ankle sprains are undertreated.[10,11] Treatment with ice, followed by an elastic wrap, is not optimal. The tear is usually in the anterior talofibular ligament and results in a puffiness in this area. The ankle sometimes swells like a balloon, and it is important to use a bulky dressing and elevation to reduce swelling.

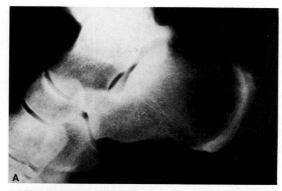
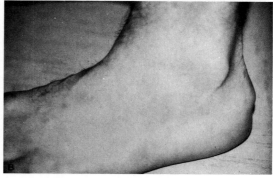

Fig. 7-4. (*A*) The Achilles tendon can avulse pieces of calcaneal bone. (*B*) These avulsed pieces of bone cause a "runner's bump."

More severe tears extend through the calcaneofibular ligament.

An injection of lidocaine into the hematoma allows stress testing for evaluation of stability. In minor ankle sprains I use a compression dressing and contrast baths to allow rapid return to competition. The contrast baths are done in a warm whirlpool bath and a cool tub, the contrasting temperatures inducing a pumping action that reduces swelling. The athlete then works on flexibility, so that his heel cord does not tighten up, and he uses isometric exercises to maintain the strength of all muscle groups. For moderate sprains, a foam pad is placed over the swollen area, sheet wadding is wrapped around the limb, and a stirrup splint and posterior plaster splint are applied and held in place by a snug, elastic wrap. The limb is elevated, and crutches are used for walking. The swelling has usually resolved after 5 days, and then either a stretching and strengthening program or a walking cast is used, depending on the symptoms at the time of removal of the splint.

In complete tears, some surgeons use casts and others operate.[12,13] A lateral heel wedge is used in the shoes after all sprains to reduce inversion stress on the lateral side of the ankle joint and a U-shaped pad is wrapped in place, distal to the malleolus, to massage out any swelling. In late cases with chronic instability, a reconstructive procedure is needed to restore stability.[14,15]

There are various kinds of sneaker uppers, including high-top, medium-height, and low-quarter shoes. The high-top canvas shoe may give more support to the ankle than the others, but there is controversy about the effectiveness of ankle taping, since the tape tends to loosen after a few minutes of play.[16,17] Ankles that have never been sprained are generally wrapped, while ankles that have been sprained in the past are taped, although the effectiveness of taping is debated. Rounded heels and soles

help to prevent injury caused by a quick turning of the ankle.

Peroneal Tendon Problems

The great mimic of ankle sprain is dislocation of the peroneal tendons. These tendons run behind the lateral malleolus. Forceful ankle dorsiflexion with peroneal contraction ruptures the overlying retinaculum and frees the tendons (Fig. 7-5). If this is misdiagnosed as ankle sprain, and the retinaculum does not resume its place over the tendons, recurrent dislocation of the peroneal tendons will occur.[18] The diagnosis can be made by reproducing the tendon dislocations and finding tenderness behind the lateral malleolus.

Early diagnosis permits repair of the retinaculum, but in late cases it may be so atrophied that it cannot be reattached over the tendons.[19] Pain, snapping, and instability result. Where treatment has been delayed, the tendons are restrained by swinging the outer part of the fibula backward using an osteoperiosteal flap, an Achilles tendon strip, or the plantaris ten-

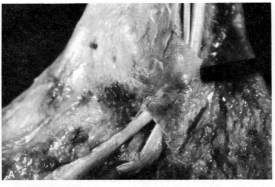

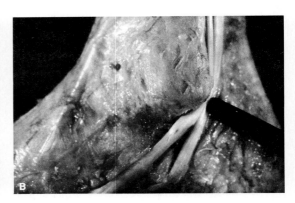

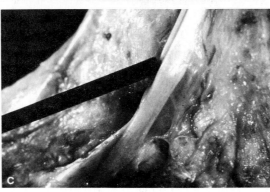

Fig. 7-5. (*A*) The peroneal retinaculum covers the peroneal tendons. (*B*) The tendons run in a groove behind the lateral malleolus. (*C*) The peroneal tendons dislocate over the lateral malleolus when the retinaculum is removed.

don.[20-23] Another method is to reroute the peroneal tendons deep to the strong calcaneofibular ligament.[24]

The peroneus brevis tendon passes behind the lateral malleolus and inserts into the tubercle of the fifth metatarsal. Jumping rope has become a popular fitness activity, but tears of the insertion of the peroneus brevis tendon or fractures of the metatarsal metaphyses are common. These metaphyseal fractures heal quickly, but stress fractures of the fifth metatarsal proximal diaphysis (the Jones fracture) may not unite.[25] Intramedullary screw fixation through the prominent base of the fifth metatarsal was successful in promoting healing of this fracture in one group of athletes.[26]

Problems in the Toes

An intermetatarsal neuroma can form when a digital nerve is pinched between the metatarsals. Pain occurs during weight bearing and is referred along the opposing surfaces of the third and fourth toes when the metatarsals are squeezed together. The neuroma occurs most commonly between the third and fourth metatarsal heads. A soft insert in a shoe with a proper forefoot fit usually relieves the pain. If pain persists, the neuroma should be excised.

Ganglion Cyst. Sometimes, during activity, a firm mass appears dorsally in the web space between the toes (Fig. 7-6A); it spreads the toes apart but recedes with rest. At operation a ganglion cyst can be traced to the flexor sheath (Fig. 7-6B). The ganglion, forced from the plantar surface by the rough, tight, and moving structures, follows the path of least resistance between the toes to the dorsum. The ganglion can be removed completely by tracing it down to the flexor sheath.

"Turf toe" is a metatarsophalangeal plantar capsule sprain in the great toe.[27,28] It occurs in players who wear flexible, soccer-style shoes on artificial turf and is often caused by hypertension of the metatarsophalangeal joint during push-off. If a player is down on his knees and another player lands on his heel, the metatarsophalangeal joint can be violently hyperextended, spraining the capsule or frac-

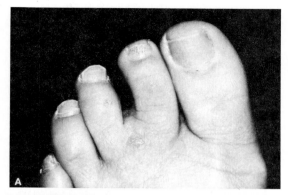

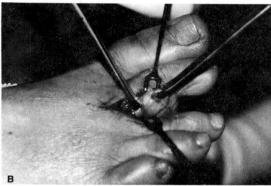

Fig. 7-6. (*A*) The second and third toes are pressed apart by a mass in the web space. (*B*) The mass is a ganglion containing jellylike fluid.

turing a sesamoid bone.[29] Rest is needed after these injuries, the great toe is taped, and a firmer shoe with a spring steel or Orthoplast forefoot splint is worn for protection.[30]

Subunqual hematoma of the great toe, or the toe that projects farthest forward, occurs in tennis ("tennis toe") and other sports where there are sudden stops (Fig. 7-7).[31] The excellent traction of modern-day shoes on nonskid surfaces stops the shoe, but the foot continues to move forward. The toe jams against the toe box and a subungual hematoma can result. Tennis toe is painful, and sometimes the subungual blood must be drained (e.g. by the physician using a flame-sterilized paper clip to puncture the nail). A properly fitted shoe with a large toe box can prevent tennis toe (Fig. 7-8).

Hammer Toes. Athletes often have hammer toes caused by ill-fitting shoes worn in childhood. Painful corns form over the dorsum of

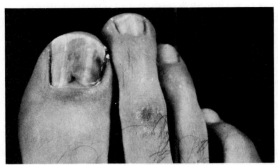

Fig. 7-7. Subungual hematoma of the great toe ("tennis toe") is painful and can result in a lost nail.

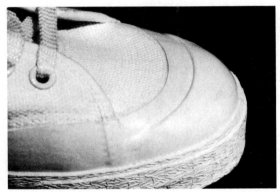

Fig. 7-8. Roomy toe boxes free the toes.

the flexed, proximal, interphalangeal joints. A shoe with a large toe box frees the toes, or a simple diaphysectomy of the proximal phalanx can relieve the pressure. The bone heals with some shortening of the toe, but the phalanges line up well and cease to be a problem.

Athlete's Foot. Tinea pedis is usually caused by the fungus, *Tricophyton rubrum* or *T. mentagrophytes.*[32] Team shower rooms, humid locker rooms, and sweaty socks provide an environment for the spread of the fungi. Some athletes are more susceptible than others to these organisms. *T. rubrum* infection causes scaley soles and web areas and *T. mentagrophytes* gives itchy vesicles and pustules. A potassium hydroxide examination is used to diagnose fungal infections, and most cases can be cured with the new topical antifungal agents. These medications are also active against *Candida* species. Athletes should dry their feet well, especially between the smaller

toes, since bacteria can invade these regions. Cotton placed between the toes keeps these areas dry. Some athletes are sensitive to the rubber of athletic shoes or to their socks and develop a contact dermatitis. A fungal infection can become much worse if it is mistaken for contact dermatitis and treated with a steroid cream.

RUNNING—ITS MECHANICS AND ITS EFFECTS ON THE FEET

Running is essentially a series of bounds or smoothly coordinated jumps rather than accelerated walking. The double-support phase of walking is absent in running.[33] A running cycle consists of two steps, with a support and a recovery phase. The support phase includes heel-strike, mid-support (pronation), heel-rise (supination), and toe-off. The recovery phase has a follow-through stage from toe-off to forward-swing. At the end of the forward swing the foot reverses direction and quickly descends to heel-strike.[34-36]

Running Surfaces

The best surfaces for running are grass and wood chips. Next come the composite tracks. Last on the list would be the beach, because the soft sand causes pronation, while the firmer sand near the water is canted; or hard surfaces, such as asphalt and banked, wooden running tracks.

The hardest track surfaces are not the fastest. A pliant surface acts like a spring and can be tuned to the mechanics of running, so that the runners' times should improve. A "tuned" indoor track with a surface of optimal compliance has been constructed at Harvard University.[37] It has a polyurethane surface and a wooden substructure that gives two to three times the stiffness of an average runner. The usual jolt of vertical force as the heel strikes the ground is absent; the length of stride is increased; and contact time is shortened. On this track runners have fewer injuries and better times than they do on other tracks.

The galloping racehorse supports itself on one finger that has evolved into the hoof. Hard training before the growth plates are closed may lead to breakdown of bones and joints in a 1200-pound thoroughbred. Many horses are thus rendered unsound for later competition in events such as jumping or dressage. Similarly, young people can train too hard. High-school cross-country runners used to average 3 miles a day; now it is not unusual for them to average 6 miles daily, and some run more than 100 miles a week. Although we have shock-absorbing mechanisms in the foot, ankle, leg, and knee, the forces applied are considerable and can cause early breakdowns and traumatic arthritis. Most running injuries occur in long-distance runners rather than in sprinters.[38]

Problems in Running

Heel-Strike. At heel-strike only a small portion of the calcaneus contacts the ground. The hip is adducted, and the leg rotates internally. The fat pad acts as a cushion at heel-strike, and in young persons strong septa encase the fat lobules. As the athlete ages, the septa become flimsy, and the fat becomes more liquefied and amorphous; this cushion is not as effective, and the heel can be more easily bruised. The *stone bruise* is due to a concussion to the calcaneal impact point that results in subperiosteal bleeding. Scar tissue forms, and the heel can remain permanently painful. One form of treatment is to use a doughnut-shaped foam pad (Fig. 7-9). A hole in the central impact area of the foam pad allows the irritated region to float freely and avoid contact with the shoe during heel strike. Another device is the molded plastic heel cup, which holds the heel snugly, compacts the heel pad, and has shock-absorptive properties of its own. The foam heel cup is compressed to a very thin cup that is, however, extra-thick in the heel contact area. This material has good, shock-absorbing properties and wears well, since it is precompressed.

The Support Phase of Running. The leg continues to rotate inward after heel-strike, and the foot must pronate to achieve a plantigrade position (Fig. 7-10A,B). *Pronation* refers to dorsiflexion, eversion and abduction at

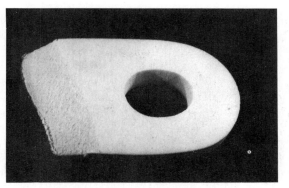

Fig. 7-9.   The foam doughnut heel pad protects the heel.

the subtalar joint (Fig. 7-10C). Excessive pronation causes many runners' problems, ranging from knee pain and shin splints to plantar fasciitis. It is also a cause of medial knee pain due to sprain of the tibial collateral ligament from valgus knee stress. Lateral knee pain results from jamming, if the foot is rigid and supinated.

A runner's center of gravity reaches its lowest point during mid-stance—knee flexion and ankle dorsiflexion. *A tight heel cord* is the major cause of runner's knee, or chondromalacia of the patella, since more knee flexion is needed to cushion the shock normally absorbed by ankle dorsiflexion. Pain behind the kneecap is commonly noted when running down hills or walking down stairs, when the knee is held in a flexed position to shift the center of gravity behind, so that the athlete does not fall forward. The knee flexion results in increased patello-femoral contact and pressure.

Tight heel cords are responsible for a running style of flexed knees and increased patellofemoral contact and pressure, as well as foot pronation to increase ankle dorsiflexion. Eversion allows more dorsiflexion than an inverted or neutral position. A heel-cord stretching regimen can often slowly, but surely, eliminate retropatellar pain.

Pronation of the foot causes a chronic tugging on the plantar fascia, resulting in *plantar fasciitis*. This tugging irritates the origin of the plantar fascia at the medial tuberosity of the calcaneus. The periosteum forms a heel spur

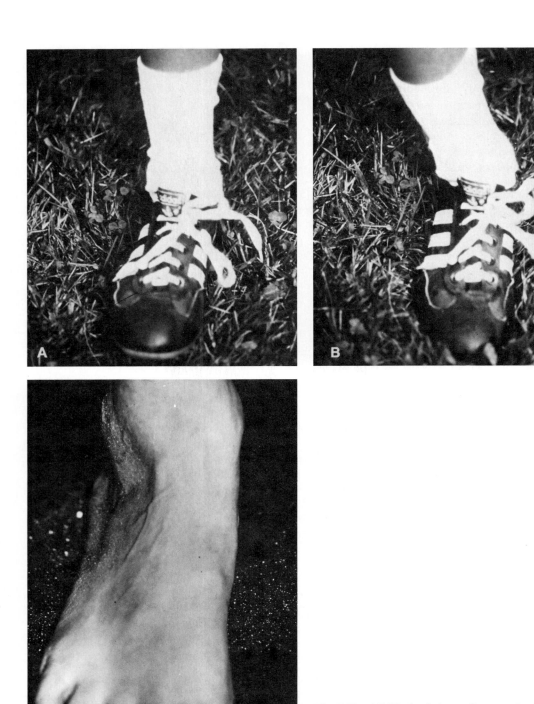

Fig. 7-10. (*A*) The leg is internally rotated at heel strike. (*B*) During the support phase the leg rotates further internally and the foot pronates. (*C*) Pronation involves dorsiflexion, eversion, and abduction at the subtalar joint.

by laying down reactive bone (Fig. 7-11). The presence of heel spurs indicates some plantar fascial tension, but the heel spur itself is not the cause of pain; hence doughnut pads or cups, prescribed for pain and tenderness in this region, do not effect a cure. Pronation is the etiology and must be limited in order to reduce the tension. A plantar fascia-stretching regimen, however, is a useful adjunct to treatment (Fig. 7-12). Steroid injections lead to tissue degeneration at the origin of the plantar fascia, and a more intractable problem.[39] The injections treat only the inflammatory effect of the pronation and can result in plantar fascia rupture.[40]

Toe-Off. During the push-off or toe-off phase, the leg rotates externally, and the foot supinates and becomes a rigid lever. During push-off the plantar and great-toe flexors that arise from the fibula draw the bone toward the tibia.[41] This recurrent, rhythmic, to-and-fro movement is pronounced when the athlete runs on his toes on hard surfaces. The point of greatest stress is near the inferior tibiofibular

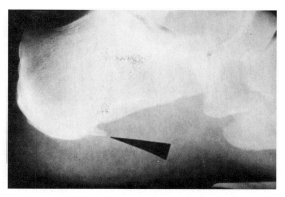

Fig. 7-11. The plantar fascial tug results in a heel spur, but the spur itself it not the cause of pain.

joint: a cortical break usually occurs about 6 cm. above the tip of the lateral malleolus (Fig. 7-13).

Stress fractures through the posteromedial cortex of the lower third of the tibia are also seen in runners.[42] This injury differs from the upper-third fractures of recruits[43] and the middle-third stress fractures of ballet dancers.[44] The stress fracture may, in fact, be a "fracture

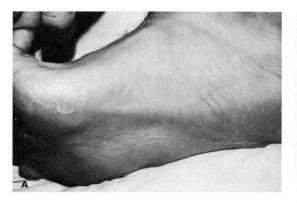

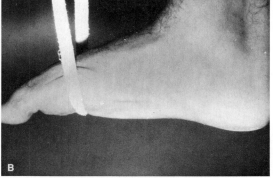

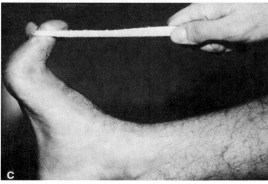

Fig. 7-12. (*A*) The plantar fascia can be stretched by extending the great toe. (*B*) If the great toe is not extended the stretch is not optimal. (*C*) This sling method of stretching is effective.

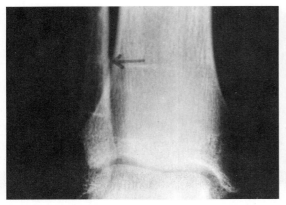

Fig. 7-13. Stress fractures are commonly seen about 6 cm. from the tip of the lateral malleolus.

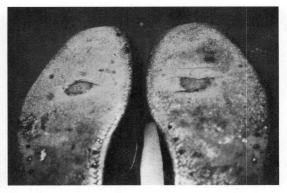

Fig. 7-14. The maximum force during push-off is under the second metatarsal head, and shoes are often worn down in this area.

before a fracture," since osteoclasts are busy remodelling the bone to accommodate stress.[45] Sometimes the osteoclastic action is so rapid that a defect forms, which is essentially a fracture or a loss of continuity of the bone. (This exceptional osteoclastic activity may account for some of the growing pains of children.)

The diagnosis of stress fracture is aided by noting pain at the fracture site when the examiner strikes the heel sharply. Pain is elicited at the tibial fracture site when the examiner uses his own knee as a fulcrum to "spring" the tibia. New bone can sometimes be seen on oblique radiographs at 2 weeks if a bright light is used to view them. Supportive strapping is worn until the soreness is gone; sometimes a cast is needed.

Stress fractures must be differentiated from the more serious *anterior compartment syndrome.* This syndrome involves swelling within the tight fascial compartments of the leg and characteristically fails to improve with rest and ice treatment. There may be numbness between the great and second toe and weakness of the extensor hallucis longus. The numbness and weakness appear in this distribution, since the anterior tibial nerve and extensor hallucis longus are the deepest structures in the anterior compartment and are under the most pressure. Wick catheter determinations of pressure are useful in determining progression and indicating when fasciotomy is necessary.

In the propulsive phase, *the plantar fascia* is again stretched. During walking, the plantar pressure area extends from the heel along the lateral border of the foot and across the metatarsal heads, with the maximum force on the second metatarsal head during push-off.[46] High-heeled shoes cause the metatarsal heads to be jammed against the ground. This area of wear is noted on the soles of old shoes, where a hole may form in the area under the metatarsal heads (Fig. 7-14). In running, the forces also go through the second metatarsal head and are more pronounced than in walking. This causes the second metatarsal bone of marathon runners to hypertrophy and sometimes become broader than the first metatarsal.[47] The distribution of force can result in stress fractures of the second, third, and fourth metatarsals of runners. Radiographs may show a normal foot in the early stages. Forefoot pain and swelling that are relieved by rest and then recur with weight bearing are features in the early stages of stress fracture.

ATHLETES' SHOES

Design Problems

The sole of the training shoe should be flexible and of soft rubber. The thickness of the rubber does not necessarily correlate with the shock-absorptive capacity, since this depends on the hardness of the material used. A useful improvement in tennis shoe design places extra rubber under the pivot point (Fig.

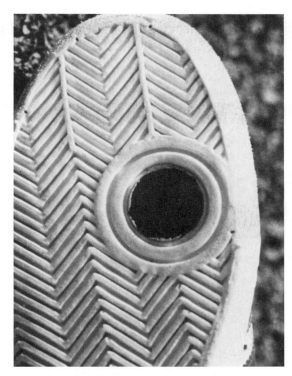

Fig. 7-15. These tennis shoes have a reinforced pivot point.

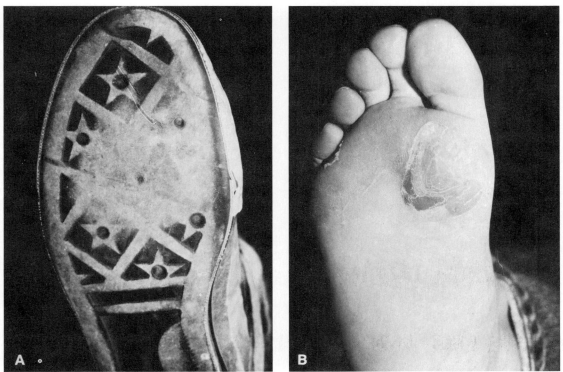

Fig. 7-16. (*A*) Wear is pronounced in tennis shoes at the pivot point. (*B*) Blisters and calluses form at the pivot point, owing to shifting skin.

7-15). This is the area where pivoting occurs, and it is also the region where painful callosities are apt to develop (Fig. 7-16).

Some *training shoes* have been advertised as "made for your knees." These shoes have a very wide heel and are supposed to set the heel down without any side-to-side rocking, hence eliminating a need for the knee to compensate. However, some runners who have used these shoes complain that they cause, rather than eliminate, knee pain. The use of a slightly widened heel seems to be a good compromise.

Eighty Super Senior tennis players were evaluated at the National Clay Court Championships.[48] The Super Seniors are men over 70 years of age who have averaged more than 50 years of competitive tennis. They had minimal foot and knee problems, which might be attributable to their having played mostly on clay courts (Fig. 7-17). Currently, most tennis players use hard courts, and it is important that their shoes cushion the shocks. In future, senior tennis players will surely have many foot and knee problems if flimsy shoes are worn.

The insole in athletic footwear has not kept up with the overall improvements in shoe design. Athletes are susceptible to callus de-velopment, and this can be prevented by using custom-made plastazote inserts (Fig. 7-18). Sheets of this nitrogen-blown foam of medium hardness are heated in an oven so that they become workable. The material is then allowed to cool down somewhat, so that it can come in contact with the skin. The athlete steps on the foam, and it is molded to his foot. The foot outline is traced, and the insert is cut out and smoothed. The foam is sometimes backed with neoprene for extra wear. These inserts are especially effective in football cleats and baseball spikes, which have notoriously poor insoles. Basketball players now are bigger, jump higher, and land harder, and the blown-foam inserts help to protect against long arch tears, calluses and foot fatigue.[49]

The popular game of soccer involves a great deal of running and kicking. The forward cleats on soccer shoes, which are stubby, do not catch during kicking. Youngsters should use soccer balls that are the proper size for their feet. The youngest should use a No. 3 ball, the middle group a No. 4, and older children can move on to the regulation No. 5 (Fig. 7-19). Otherwise, foot sprains and exostoses may occur and lead to pains and arthritis in later life.

Tennis shoes should have a reinforced toe bumper, so that the toe-plate rubber does not wear away during serving (Fig. 7-20). If a runner has a toe problem, it is important to check the contour of his training shoe toe box. Reinforcing material may be rubbing the toes, and a change to another shoe brand with a different style of toe box might eliminate the problem (Fig. 7-21). Runners now have many styles of training and competition shoes to choose from, and some athletic shoe stores have repair shops where soles, heels, toe bumpers, arch cookies, and insoles are replaced.

In reaching for a tennis ball, heel impact is accentuated by shoes with sharp-edged heels that act like a wedge and drive into the foot. Some of the better tennis shoes have a slight roll to the heel, allowing absorption of force and avoidance of jamming (Fig. 7-22A). Training shoes with softer rounded heels also

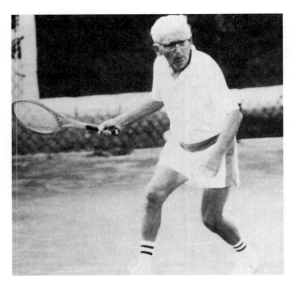

Fig. 7-17. This Super Senior, 80-year-old national tennis champion is playing on shock-absorbing clay courts.

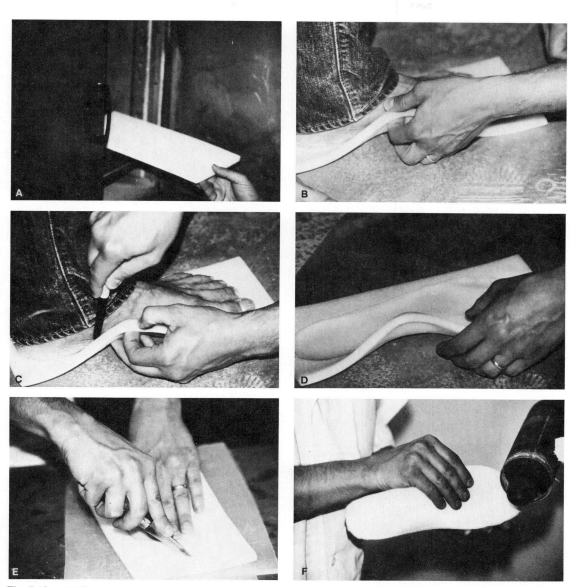

Fig. 7-18. (*A*) To make a custom-fitted shoe insert, plastazote material is heated so that it becomes workable. (*B*) The material is pressed under the arch as the athlete stands on it and the outline of the athlete's foot is traced (*C*). The shaped insert is now ready for trimming (*D*). (*E*) Trimming is accomplished using a knife and, (*F*) the insert is smoothed and inserted into the shoes.

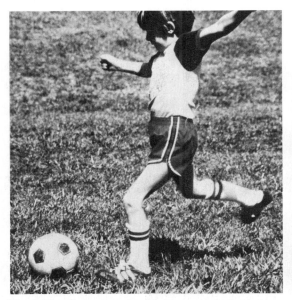

Fig. 7-19. Youngsters should use soccer balls that are the proper size for their small feet.

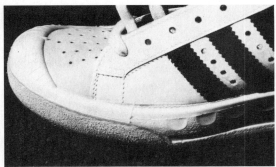

Fig. 7-20. The reinforced toe bumper in tennis shoes preserves this area during the tennis serve.

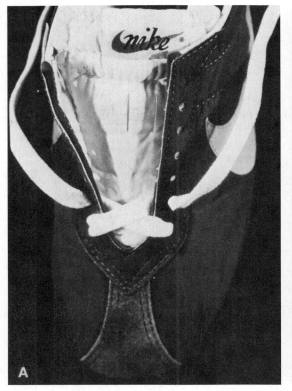

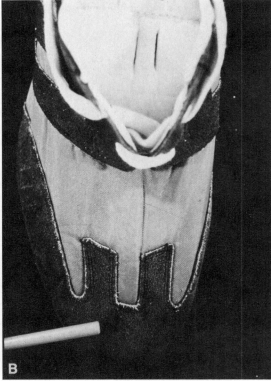

Fig. 7-21. Toe boxes can take various shapes and may be responsible for toe problems.

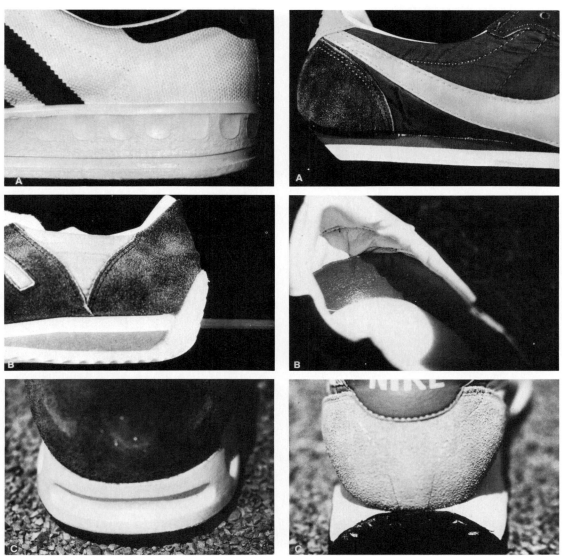

Fig. 7-22. (*A*) The rolled heel of tennis shoes absorbs force and avoids jamming. (*B*) The rounded heel of training shoes dampens impact. (*C*) The carved-out wedges in this heel permit reproduction of subtalar motion.

Fig. 7-23. (*A*) This foam counter holds the heel and keeps it from shifting. (*B*) This foam material snugly holds the heel and prevents shifting. (*C*) The mildly widened heel dissipates impact forces and limits locking.

dampen impact during running (Fig. 7-22B). Another training shoe modification is a wedge carved out posteriorly, laterally, and medially on the heel (Fig. 7-22C). This permits some subtalar motion.

The heel of a good training shoe has a firm, supportive counter that keeps the heel from shifting (Fig. 7-23A). Some have an added foam material that conforms to the runner's heel (Fig. 7-23B). The mildly widened heel also seems effective in controlling heel-strike and dissipates the impact force over a broader area (Fig. 7-23C). Athletes should periodically check their shoes and reinforce worn areas of the heel, to prevent imbalances from asymmetrical wear.

The ripple sole was developed for soldiers in World War II. Each successive wave dis-

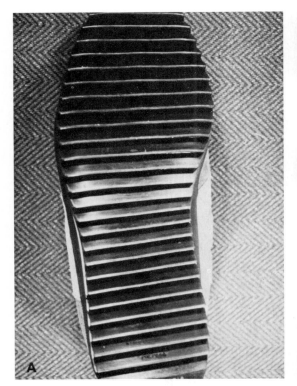

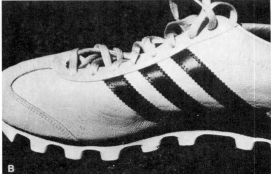

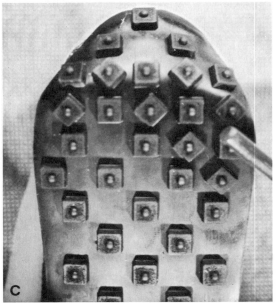

Fig. 7-24. (*A*) Each ripple-sole wave dissipates some shock. (*B*) These large ripples absorb shock on hard surfaces. (*C*) Each protruding waffle absorbs some shock.

sipates some shock. Training shoes that have adopted the ripple sole take up the shock on hard surfaces (Fig. 7-24A,B). The waffle sole, so-called since it resembles the batter cake of that name, has protuberances that protect against shock (Fig. 7-24C).

Both the posterior part and the underside of the heel have problem areas, and changes following overuse can be a summation of many of these. A given person might have a weak heel-pad with flimsy septa, a heel bruise or subperiosteal bleed and scarring, a heel spur and plantar fasciitis. He may thus need a foam pad and an orthosis.

The midfoot support given by shoes varies. Stripes are not merely for ornamentation; they

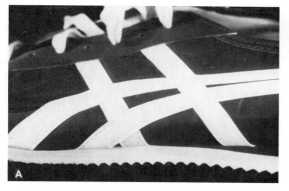

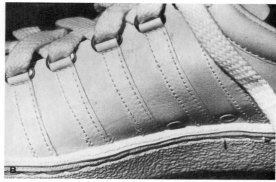

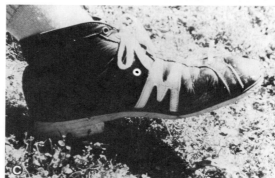

Fig. 7-25. (*A*) The stripes are an integral supportive aspect of the shoe. (*B*) The stripes extend to the eyelets, and when the laces are tied the stripes give good mid-foot support. (*C*) The weight lifter's shoe is a sturdy one, and the heel helps stablilize the lifter.

are an integral part of the supportive structure of the shoe, and in some shoes the stripes extend from the undersurface to the eyelet area (Fig. 7-25A,B). When the laces are snug, the whole midfoot portion of the shoe is appropriately snug.

The weight lifter's shoe is sturdily built, with good support in the mid-tarsal region (Fig. 7-25C). The heel helps stabilize the lifter in the clean and jerk, especially in the snatch move.

Pronation Supports

Many devices have been used in an attempt to limit pronation. The small, longitudinal arch cookie that comes in most training shoes does not contribute much to the support of the long arch, let alone control pronation. Sometimes these cookies are badly located and may cause blistering of the arch. If an athlete has a new cookie put in his shoe, it must be placed in such a position that it will not cause irritation. Long arch cork-leather supports can be worn in the athlete's every-day walking shoes, but they are too bulky for training shoes. Usually the walking shoes have very firm insoles, and the addition of a plastazote insert or cork-leather arch support helps cushion the foot.

The *subtalar, talonavicular, and calcaneocuboid* joint regions are complex. When the foot is dissected and opened like a book, the multiple articulations are striking. A foot orthosis to limit pronation is constructed with the foot in neutral position.[50] This is the position where the talonavicular joint is congruent. To ascertain the neutral position, the foot is allowed to dangle off the examining table and the talar head is grasped in one hand while the forefoot is held in the other (Fig. 7-26). As the forefoot is rocked medially and

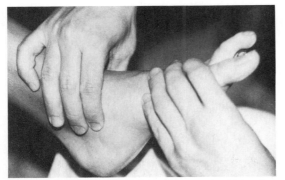

Fig. 7-26. The neutral position is ascertained by palpation.

laterally the congruency of the talus and navicular changes. If the talus protrudes medially, the navicular must be moved medially to restore congruency. If the talus is prominent laterally, then the navicular must be shifted laterally. When the neutral position is achieved, the necks of the fourth and fifth metatarsals are then pushed up, and when resistance is felt, the foot is "locked" and ready for casting in this neutral position. A plaster slipper is made by placing plaster splints over the plantar surface of the foot and wrapping them over the dorsum (Fig. 7-27A).[51]

The plaster is smoothed out to conform to the foot, and after it has set, it is peeled off and allowed to dry (Fig. 7-27B). Baby powder is sprinkled into the slipper, plaster-of-Paris is poured in, and the mold is placed in a sand bin to dry and set (Fig. 7-27C,D), after which the polypropylene is pulled over the positive mold and is then trimmed and smoothed (Fig. 7-27E–G). Neoprene bumpers are glued to the orthosis if they are needed, and a protective plastic plate is glued to the neoprene (Fig. 7-27H). The orthosis is then ready to wear but should be "broken in" gradually, otherwise

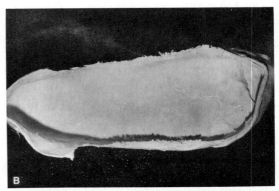

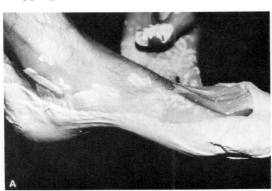

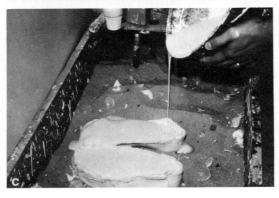

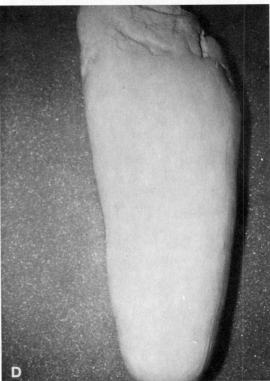

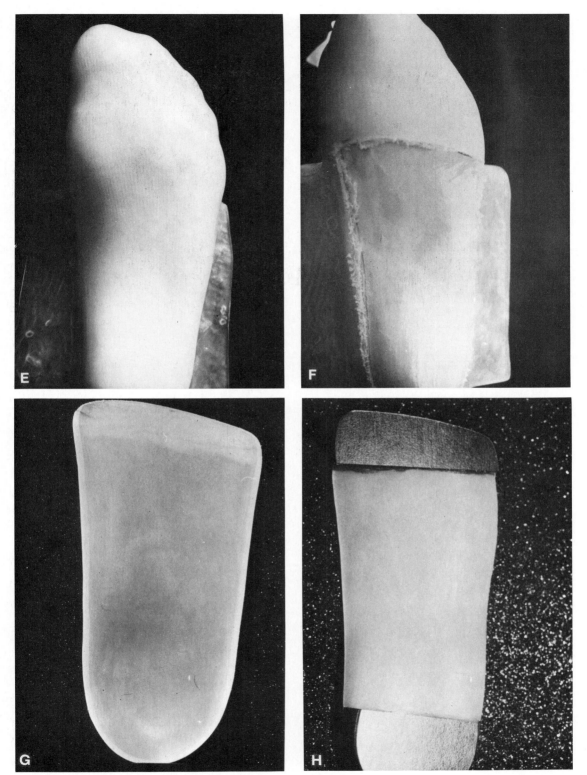

Fig. 7-27. (*Facing Page*) (*A*) A plaster slipper is applied while the foot is held in neutral position. (*B*) The slipper cast is removed and reinforced. (*C*) Plaster is poured into the slippers and allowed to set. (*D*) The plaster positive is smoothed and ready for the orthotic material. (*This Page*) (*E*) Polypropylene is pulled over the positive of the foot. (*F*) The orthotic device is cut out. (*G*) The orthosis is smoothed. (*H*) Neoprene posts are glued in place and covered with plastic plates.

painful pinch calluses can develop. Sometimes the orthosis needs trimming or other small revisions. The cost is raised if the doctor has to send them away for these adjustments, and "tune-ups" at a distance are unsatisfactory. A pair of orthotic devices can cost from $70 to $100, but they are necessary to treat certain difficult pronatory foot problems that have not responded to other methods. The devices also lessen—and in some cases eliminate—knee pains, especially medial pain due to valgus stress caused by excessive pronation. These orthoses are particularly effective in dealing with pain at the origin of the plantar fascia caused by overpronation.[52,53]

Some athletes have a short, *hypermobile first metatarsal*. This type of foot has to pronate excessively to achieve a plantigrade first ray, and pinch calluses of the great toe and under the second metatarsal head, form. The excessive pronation may cause medial knee joint pain secondary to valgus strain. A Morton's extension pad adds bulk under the first ray, so that it need not travel as far to reach the ground; (the ground is "brought up" to the foot).

The Ideal Shoe

When examining a shoe, be certain that the upper, behind the heel, is soft; that the counter is firm and that the heel is rolled and contains a wedge to absorb shock. The upper should be well-built, and the stripes should be a structural element of the shoe rather than being merely decoration, thus giving support to the midtarsal area. Ideally, each athlete should wear shoes with a form-fitting heel seat and a cushioning insole. There should be forefoot flexibility and a toe box that does not jam the toes. For a runner with a foot problem, shoes are required that will help, and not hurt, his feet (Figs. 7-28A,B).

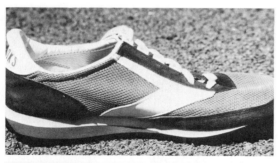

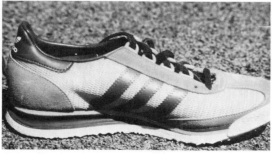

Fig. 7-28. (*A*) This training shoe incorporates excellent features and also has a varus wedge to limit pronation. (*B*) This training shoe has a shock-absorbing cut-out wedge to reproduce some subtalar motion.

REFERENCES

1. Napier, J.: The antiquity of human walking. Sci. Am., *216:*56, 1967.
2. Hlavac, H. F.: The Foot Book: Advice for Athletes. Mountain View, CA, World Publications, 1977.
3. Subotnick, S. I.: The Running Foot Doctor. Mountain View, CA, World Publications, 1977.
4. Kulund, D. N., and Brubaker, C. E., Injuries in the Bikecentennial tour. Phys. Sports Med., *6:*674, 1978.
5. Radin, E. L., and Paul, I. L.: Importance of bone in sparing articular cartilage from impact. Clin. Orthop., *78:*342, 1971.
6. Mital, M. A., and Matza, R. A.: Osgood-Schlatter disease: the painful puzzler. Phys. Sports Med., *5:*60, 1977.
7. Round Table: Leg pains in runners. Phys. Sports Med., *5:*43, 1977.
8. Round Table: Achilles tendon problems increase. Phys. Sports Med., *4:*43, 1976.
9. Seder, J. I.: Heel injuries incurred in running and jumping. Phys. Sports Med., *4:*70, 1976.
10. Bosien, W. R., *et al.*: Residual disability following ankle sprains. J. Bone Joint Surg., *37A:* 1237, 1955.
11. Jackson, D. W., *et al.*:; Ankle sprains in young athletes. Relation of severity and disability. Clin. Orthop., *101:*215, 1974.
12. Staples, O. S.: Ruptures of the fibular collateral ligaments of the ankle: result study of immediate surgical treatment. J. Bone Joint Surg., *57A:* 101, 1975.
13. Woodward, E. P.: Ankle ligament surgery: experience over 18 years. Phys. Sports Med., *5:*49, 1977.

14. Chrisman, O. D., and Snook, G. A.: Reconstruction of lateral ligament tears of the ankle. J. Bone Joint Surg., *51B:*904, 1969.
15. Zenni, E. J., Jr.: Lateral ligamentous instability of the ankle: a method of surgical reconstruction by a modified Watson-Jones technique. Am. J. Sports Med., *5:*78, 1977.
16. Routine ankle taping: benefit or hazard (a panel) Consultant, 188, Oct., 1976.
17. Distefano, V., and Nixon, J. E.: An improved method of taping. Am. J. Sports Med., *2:*209, 1974.
18. Marti, R.: Dislocation of the peroneal tendons. Am. J. Sports Med., *5:*19, 1977.
19. Stover, C. N., and Bryan, D. R.: Traumatic dislocation of the peroneal tendons. Am. J. Surg., *103:*180, 1962.
20. Kelly, R. E.: An operation for the chronic dislocation of the peroneal tendons. Brit. J. Surg., *7:*502, 1926.
21. Watson-Jones, R.: Fractures and Joint Injuries. ed. 4. vol. 2. Baltimore, Williams & Wilkins, 1952.
22. Jones, E.: Operative treatment of chronic dislocations of the peroneal tendons. J. Bone Joint Surg., *14:*574, 1932.
23. Miller, J. W.: Dislocation of peroneal tendons: a new operative procedure. Am. J. Orthop., *9:*136, 1967.
24. Sarmiento, A., and Wolf, M.: Subluxation of peroneal tendons: case treated by rerouting tendons under calcaneofibular ligament. J. Bone Joint Surg., *57A:*115, 1975.
25. Jones, R.: Fracture of the base of the fifth metatarsal bone by indirect violence. Ann. Surg., *35:*697, 1902.
26. Kavanaugh, J. H., *et al.:* The Jones fracture revisited. J. Bone Joint Surg., *60A:*776, 1978.
27. Cooper, D. L.: Turf toe. Phys. Sports Med., *6:*139, 1978.
28. Bowers, K. D., Jr., and Martin, R. B.: Turf-toe: a shoe-surface related football injury. Med. Sci. Sports, *8:*81, 1976.
29. Coker, T. P., *et al.:* Traumatic lesions of the metatarsophalangeal joint of the great toe in athletes. Am. J. Sports Med., 326, Nov.–Dec., 1978.
30. Garrick, J. G.: Artificial turf, pro's and con's. Phys. Sports Med., *3:*41, 1975.
31. Gibbs, R. C.: Tennis toe. J.A.M.A., *228:*24, 1974.
32. Millikan, L. E.: Athlete's foot-scratching beneath surface of fungal ailments. Phys. Sports Med., *3:*51, 1975.
33. Slocum, D. B., and Bowerman, W.: The biomechanics of running. Clin. Orthop., *23:*39, 1962.
34. Nelson, R., and Gregor, R.: Biomechanics of distance running: a longitudinal study. Res. Q., *47:*417, 1976.
35. Slocum, D., and James, S.: Biomechanics of running. J.A.M.A., *205:*721, 1968.
36. James, S., and Brubaker, C. E.: Biomechanical and neuromuscular aspects of running. *In* Wilmore, J. (ed.): Exercise and Sports Sciences Review. New York, Academic Press, 1973.
37. McMahon, T. A., and Greene, P. R.: Fast running tracks. Sci. Am., *239:*148, 1978.
38. Brubaker, C. E., and James, S.: Injuries to runners. J. Sports Med., *2:*189, 1974.
39. Kennedy, J. C., and Willis, R. B.: The effects of local steroid injections in tendons: a biomechanical and microscopic correlative study. Am. J. Sports Med., *4:*11, 1976.
40. Leach, R. *et al.:* Rupture of the plantar fascia in athletes. J. Bone Joint Surg., *60A:*537, 1968.
41. Devas, M. B., and Sweetnam, R.: Stress fractures of the fibula: a review of fifty cases in athletics. J. Bone Joint Surg., *30B:*818, 1956.
42. Devas, M. B.: Stress fractures of the tibia in athletes or "shin soreness." J. Bone Joint Surg., *40B:*227, 1958.
43. Elton, R. C.: Stress reaction of bone in army trainees. J.A.M.A., *204:*314, 1968.
44. Burrows, H. J.: Fatigue infraction of the middle of the tibia in ballet dancers. J. Bone Joint Surg., *38B:*83, 1956.
45. McBryde, A. M., Jr.: Stress fractures in athletes. Am. J. Sports Med., *3:*212, 1975.
46. Collis, W., and Jayson, M.: Measurement of pedal pressures. Ann. Rheum. Dis., *31:*215, 1972.
47. Slocum, D. B.: Overuse syndromes of the lower leg and foot in athletes. A.A.O.S. Instructional Course Lectures, *17:*359, 1960.
48. Rockwell, D. A., and Kulund, D. N.: Super Senior Tennis. Paper Presented at the Annual Meeting of the Virginia Orthopaedic Society. Williamsburg, Virginia, May, 1977.
49. Steingard, P. M.: Foot failures in basketball. Phys. Sports Med., *2:*64, 1974.
50. James, S. L., *et al.:* Injuries to runners. Am. J. Sports Med., *6:*40, 1978.
51. Root, M. L., *et al.:* Neutral Position Casting Techniques. ed. 1. Los Anreles, Clinical Biomechanics Corp., 1971.
52. Subotnick, S. I.: Orthotic foot control and the overuse syndrome. Phys. Sports Med., *3:*75, 1975.
53. Subotnick, S. I.: Podiatric sports medicine. Mount Kisco, N.Y., Futura Publishing, 1975.

8 Congenital Deformities of the Feet

SOME ASPECTS OF THE MANAGEMENT OF THE FAMILY WITH A DEFORMED CHILD

Before entering on any detailed consideration of foot deformity in childhood, some aspects of the management of the children and their families deserve attention. One might think it a simple matter; once the diagnosis has been made, all that the practitioner has to do is to apply the correct principles of management to the limb, and in due time the problem will be solved. This is far from the truth.

In the first place, only a small percentage of children who are brought to the doctor with a problem in one or both feet are suffering from any abnormality at all. Even in a child with a fixed, and therefore uncorrectable, deformity, there are seldom any symptoms from the disease. What turns an apparently simple task of child management into a complex situation is the worry in the mind of the parent or guardian about a possible abnormality in the child.

It is natural for parents to be concerned about a deformed foot in one of their offspring, but there are other, less logical, motives at work in the minds of parents with young children: protective feelings, guilt, transferred ambition, or feelings of personal inadequacy.

It is not difficult to understand the shock and horror that parents must feel when a child is born with or subsequently develops a severe deformity. To see the outcome of so much hope expressed in this way causes a severe, psychic trauma, especially since any abnormality of the limbs is so immediately obvious in the postpartum period.

Klaus and Kennell have described the problem in detail.[1] They have shown that the first few hours after the birth of a child are critical for the development of the parent-child bond. It has both physical and mental components and occurs in an orderly sequence; if this is disturbed, the consequences may be far-reaching, not only on the relationship between parent and child but also upon the physical development of the child itself.

Deformity Present at Birth

Solnit and Stark have likened the crisis of the birth of a child who is found to have a malformation, to the emotional crisis that occurs in parents when a child dies.[2] The mother is forced to abandon her fantasies when faced with the reality. In effect, she first has to mourn the loss of her expected child, and she must then become attached to her actual, damaged infant. This process of reorganization takes time. It has been described in the following way, with each emotional attitude giving way to the next in order: her first reaction is *shock,* followed in short order by *denial* of the situation; gradually this feeling gives way

80

to one of *sadness* mixed with *anger*.[3] She looks for someone to blame, sometimes even herself. In the end *adaptation* occurs, as she has to deal with day-to-day problems.

The unexpected course of events may be complicated if she is in a busy maternity ward. In most such wards, the child will have been taken from her soon after birth. This routine, established many years ago to ease the burdens of busy members of staff, may damage the development of the bond between a mother and her normal child. In a malformed infant the effect can be catastrophic. The mother is forced back upon her fantasies, but now they have become nightmares. Her relief is usually considerable when at last she has the opportunity to see her child's deformities for herself: her imaginings have been worse than any reality.

In the case of deformities of the limbs, the medical and nursing staff often have little specialized experience of the problem as far as management and prognosis is concerned. Because they are largely untrained in coping with the mother's dilemma, they tend to withdraw from her until the arrival of the specialist orthopaedic surgeon. Attempts at cheerfulness magnify her alarm, since she can so easily identify their unease. She has also to deal with the other women in the ward, whose relief at the normality of their own babies is evident.

Any delay in the arrival of the orthopaedic surgeon compounds the injury, and this at a time when she is approaching the normal postpartum depression that so commonly follows the birth of a child. The mother becomes isolated in the midst of a busy ward. Her husband's visits are usually for short periods only, and he is equally at sea, his own state being emotional at a time when his wife needs calm assurance.

Congenital Deformity Presenting Later

At least, the family presented with a child malformed at birth have to come to terms with the facts. Children with congenital or orthopaedic deformities seldom require hospital treatment for long in the first instance. Some abnormalities of the lower limbs, while hered-itary or congenital in origin, are not visible at birth, nor possible to diagnose until months or, in some cases, years have elapsed. The parents do not have the advantage of coming to terms with the problem within a short time. That some of the diseases which occur in this way are not as serious as those discussed above does not minimize the family's anxiety. The opposite may be true.

The problem comes to their attention gradually. Many of the diseases that start in this way are neurologic in origin, showing first as delay in the child's development. Smiling may begin late, and the child may prove difficult to feed. Sitting does not take place at the proper time and the child appears sluggish and slow to react to external stimuli. What begins in an ill-defined way may end some years later as a florid case of spastic paraplegia, accompanied by mental deficiency.

The parents' complacency gives way to doubt; doubt alternates with hope, and gives way, in the end, to a full knowledge of the situation. When the parents have reached this stage, the doctor knows that at least the family has understood the position, and he can build on that. In many ways they have reached the same stage as the parents who are presented with the facts at birth. In time they will come to terms with the problem and react to it, even if, as often happens, they concentrate their attention on a developing abnormality of the feet, which is the least of the child's problems as far as the medical practitioner is concerned. He knows, for example, that the child is developing increasing signs of spasticity and that in due time athetosis, cranial nerve deficiency, and mental deficiency will manifest themselves.

Although the doctor may have difficulty giving a prognosis, he can advise and support the parents in each stage of the developing abnormality. He knows that if the outlook is poor, the parents will be forced to face reality in the end and deal with it as they may. His role, in such cases, is an important one. There is much he can achieve: advising on the day-to-day care of the child; arranging for help that the mother needs to look after the infant;

watching the effect of the situation on the other siblings; and planning and performing the necessary surgical and orthotic procedures.

Most practitioners will confirm that, not only do parents usually come to terms with a permanent problem, but often the afflicted child comes to hold a special place in their affections and may be the most cherished of their offspring. In our unscientific way we can only marvel at the way nature finds compensation for an unsatisfactory "genetic experiment," or a catastrophe of birth.

It is often with children with minor deformities of the feet or those with mild abnormalities that the parents show the least ability to cope. Perhaps self-delusion is easier when the child is so nearly normal. The author has been surprised, on occasion, at the refusal of some parents to accept the presence of a minor deformity.

CASE HISTORY: A middle-aged couple brought, for examination, an only child, aged 4 years. He was suffering from minimal spastic diplegia of both legs, which caused him little trouble apart from weakness and slight uncoordination of both calf muscles, which were underdeveloped. The right leg was more severely affected, with the result that contracture of the right calf was present, and the child had a fixed equinus deformity of the right ankle. The tight heel cord had brought him to the doctor.

The author advised Achilles tendon lengthening, to bring the child's heel to the ground and allow him to walk more normally. The parents refused, the father stating that he himself was quite capable of coping with the problem by stretching the child's calf muscles three times a day. They had merely wanted confirmation that the child's teacher had been wrong advising the boy not to play too much sport.

Feeling that such conscientious parents ought to be encouraged, the author fell in with this plan of management and asked the family to return in 6 months, or earlier, if the deformity became worse. Four years later, the family was still attending the clinic at 6-month intervals. The equinus deformity was the same: it had not become worse, probably because of the constant attention, but was certainly no better. The child still bears no weight upon the right heel, as is shown by the abnormal wear from bearing weight on the front of the shoe. The parents hope the child will be able to play soccer next season. Their unrealistic expectations are characteristic of their problem. They have not faced

reality, and the child is subjected to physical pressures beyond his capacity.

Responses of the Parents

When undertaking the management of children with malformation of one or both lower limbs, the practitioner should bear in mind the psychological components of the family's behavior and prevent these from distorting the treatment.

Parental Guilt. Beneath the logical concern that parents feel, and express, to the doctor when they bring a child to him for examination and diagnosis lies a pervasive and illogical feeling of guilt. The illogical nature of the sensation does not reduce its intensity, and due regard must be paid to it; otherwise, the doctor may not be able to depend upon parental cooperation during treatment. The infant, apparently passive and incapable of understanding at this age, is peculiarly sensitive to the nonverbal signs of the parents' discomfort and is affected by the conflict between their protestations of love and their guilty behavior; at the same time, the physical effects of the treatment may be unpleasant.

It is not only with severe deformities that guilt may play a part. Many children brought to the doctor with a so-called foot problem have nothing wrong with them. The child's feet are normal, in the sense that he is not suffering from a disease but has merely one of the many variants of foot shape, size, or position of function that are common among the human body types. Surprisingly, when this is pointed out to parents, their response is often that they are aware that they have similar legs and feet, which have never caused *them* any trouble: "We did not think that anything was really wrong. We simply wanted to make sure that we could not be accused later of not having done the right thing."

If the doctor does nothing else, he can take the burden of responsibility on his own shoulders, with the knowledge that the child has had a competent examination.

Parental Insecurity. Where a child suffers from nothing more than one of the common variations in size and shape of the legs and feet, and where there is no sign of any disease, hereditary, congenital, or acquired, what brings parents to the doctor is usually a feeling of insecurity about the future development of the child. There may be a family history of deformity or disease. The chance remark of a neighbor or relative may be responsible. In the author's experience, there is one situation in which a surprising number of families seek help: in the case of an adopted child. This is understandable. However close the bond between parents and child, however secure the relationship, there is always, in such cases, a mystery in the minds of the new parents. The genetic inheritance of the child is unknown to them. There are few societies in the developed world in which the anonymity of the adopted child's real father and mother is not maintained. Any apparent deviation of growth on the part of the child from other children is cause for concern.

The medical practitioner has an important part to play in allaying fears in these and similar cases. It is crucial for him to state firmly, once he has examined and investigated the child, that there is no sign of any disease. If he then explains the difference between congenital malformations or disease, and the normal variations that occur in families, he can overcome the fears of the parents and put an end to their insecurity.

Parental "Games." There are times when the medical practitioner becomes involved in a complex situation with the family and his patient. He may find it distasteful, especially if his role is that of umpire between members of the family. He ought not to feel degraded: his first concern is the child. Behind the mother's or father's apparent flippancy lies a genuine sense of insecurity, or a significant conflict between the parents. In one case, he has it in his power to allay their concern by reassuring them, while in the other he can protect the child from a situation that manifests an apparent concern for the child but which might lead to a break-up of the family unit, or even to child battering. It is not suggested that the surgeon has the expert knowledge to deal with such psychological problems. If he becomes aware of them he can, however, initiate steps to bring in the necessary specialists.

CLUBFOOT (TALIPES EQUINOVARUS)

Talipes equinovarus is a complex, fixed deformity of the foot that is always present at birth.[4] It may be unilateral or bilateral, and is not necessarily inherited. The foot is characterized by an equinus (horse-foot) position, caused by a tight Achilles tendon; an inverted hindfoot, particularly the heel; and inversion of the forefoot (Fig. 8-1). The hallmarks of the condition which are always present to some degree, are listed below.[5]

Signs of Talipes Equinovarus

A **"pipe-stem" calf:** the term accurately describes the narrow, underdeveloped calf muscles, especially on the medial side. It also implies, correctly, that the abnormality is not confined to the foot alone but includes the distal part of the limb from the knee downward, on its medial aspect.

A **short Achilles' tendon,** giving rise to the fixed, equinus deformity.

A **prominent distal fibula**

A **small, varus heel,** with the fat pad displaced medially.

"The devil's thumbprint," excessive soft tissue on the lateral side of the foot, especially below the lateral malleolus and lower end of the fibula.

An **inverted forefoot,** the main component of the varus deformity.

A **short, wide foot**

A **short first metatarsal ray**

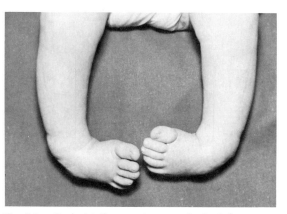

Fig. 8-1. Typical talipes equinovarus in the infant.

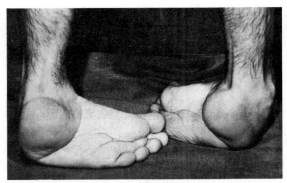

Fig. 8-2. Untreated clubfoot in an adult. All the hallmarks are present, including forefoot varus, heel varus, equinus deformity with a tight heel cord, and "pipe-stem" calves. The need for treatment in childhood is obvious.

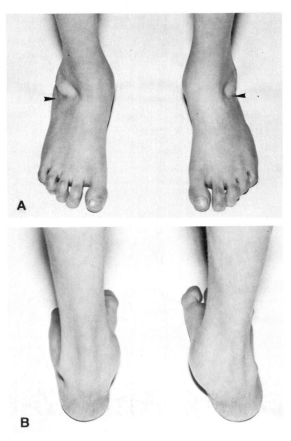

Fig. 8-3. Anterior (*A*) and posterior (*B*) views of a child who had undergone soft-tissue correction for clubfoot with tendon transplant. The result is a calcaneovalgus foot, but the signs of clubfoot are present, including "the devil's thumbprint" on each ankle (*arrows*). The feet are comfortable and function well, despite overcorrection.

Absence of these stigmata indicates not only that the deformity is of mild degree but also that the condition is benign and amenable to simple treatment. In a few cases it may even correct spontaneously within a year. When the stigmata are obvious, the clubfoot will be refractory; seldom responding to nonoperative treatment. In severe cases with the stigmata described above the condition will continue to recur until the child has finished growing (Fig. 8-2). Treatment, which should be started at birth, will usually include one or more operations, and follow-up must continue until the child stops growing.

Even in those patients in whom operation has been too assiduous, so that the child is left with the opposite deformity, a fixed, calcaneovalgus foot (a better outcome of treatment than having the foot varus and the heel elevated), the stigmata will be visible for the rest of the patient's life (Fig. 8-3).

It is possible that the mild cases, with a benign outcome within a few years of birth, represent uterine compression in the last trimester of pregnancy, while severe deformity is rather the effect of an hereditary or congenital disease that has been present since conception.

It is rare these days, in the developed countries of the world, to see people with the untreated deformity. Figure 8-4a-d shows one such person, and it serves to remind us that, even if the effect of all our treatment is merely to mask the deformity and to give the sufferer a "foot-shaped" foot, the efforts are well worthwhile. Untreated, the patient will be left with a severe deformity that makes walking difficult and may require a special boot. It leads to abnormal weight bearing, with resulting callosities on the outer side of the foot and, in the worst cases, severe crippling.

Treatment[6]

In Mild Cases. Treatment is begun soon after birth. The rationale is to stretch a foot that has been squeezed into an equinovarus position. This can sometimes be achieved by having the parents perform passive stretching exercises for the child.

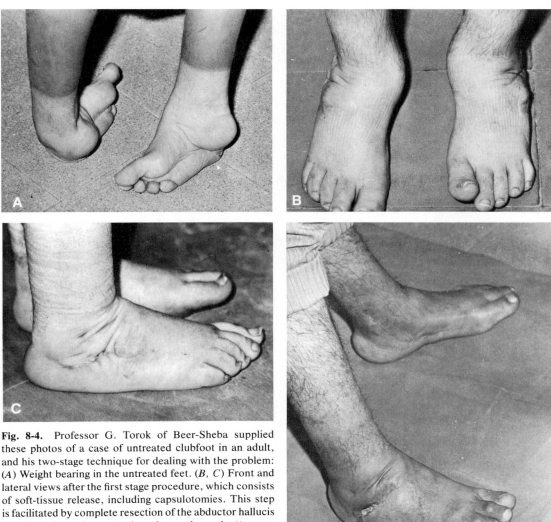

Fig. 8-4. Professor G. Torok of Beer-Sheba supplied these photos of a case of untreated clubfoot in an adult, and his two-stage technique for dealing with the problem: (*A*) Weight bearing in the untreated feet. (*B, C*) Front and lateral views after the first stage procedure, which consists of soft-tissue release, including capsulotomies. This step is facilitated by complete resection of the abductor hallucis muscle and opening up to the sole to release the "master knot" of Henry. Thereafter the plantar structures are safe. (*D*) The final result of late surgery.

STRETCHING EXERCISES. The mother is instructed in how to grasp the lower end of the affected leg with one hand while holding the foot with the other. She then moves the foot gently but firmly from its varus, toward a valgus position, thus stretching the contracted medial structures. Only when the exercises have succeeded in obtaining the limit of valgus in the range of motion should an attempt be made to stretch the equinus component. Any attempt to overcome the fixed equinus before the varus will result in twisting the foot inward and increasing the varus component.

Manipulation alone may be sufficient in the mildest cases. In most, however, the stretched position should be maintained by splinting. Of the many available forms of splint, the author favors the use of strapping with ½-inch zinc oxide plaster.

TECHNIQUE OF SPLINTING. The technique will be described in detail (Fig. 8-5), as it requires experience and meticulous attention to detail to be effective. If splints are applied

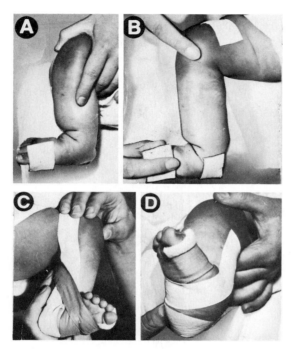

Fig. 8-5. Strapping for talipes equinovarus. (*A*) The application of the medial pad of felt. (*B*) The valgus strap for the heel has been applied. (*C*) The forefoot strap is in position. (*D*) The mid-foot U-strap has been applied, and the foot is well splinted in full calcaneovalgus position.

incorrectly or too tightly, ulceration of skin may easily occur; if applied too loosely, the splinting will not achieve its objective.

Two squares of adhesive-backed, elephant felt are required, together with six lengths of $\frac{1}{2}$-inch gauze bandage. The two squares of elephant felt are stuck to the foot; one anteriorly on the medial border, over the neck of the first metatarsal, and the other laterally, over the bone of the fifth metatarsal and extending onto the sole of the foot as far back as the heel. They are placed to protect the skin from the stretched edge of the strapping.

The first length of strapping is applied to pull the forefoot into valgus. It extends from the dorsum of the front of the foot, laterally, over the head of the first metatarsal (which is protected by the elephant felt). From there it crosses the transverse arch of the foot to the outer side of the leg. The plaster, which has no inherent elasticity, is stretched tightly to hold the forefoot at its limit of valgus, and

stuck to the outer aspect of the leg as far as the knee.

A second strip is applied to the medial aspect of the skin overlying the heel, extending under the heel (across the second felt square) and is similarly stuck to the outer side of the leg. The purpose of this strap is to hold the heel in the greatest possible valgus.

A U-shaped, third strip is then stretched under the longitudinal arch and up both sides of the leg for the maximal gain against the equinus and varus elements of the deformity.

No more is required, but to prevent the strapping from working loose too quickly, the foot and leg are then bandaged in a figure-of-eight manner with a 1-inch gauze bandage. Finally, a second series of three plaster strips, exactly like the first three, is applied over the bandage to buttress them.

If applied correctly, strapping will maintain the position of the foot for up to a week. Its main advantage is that the parents can perform manipulation three times a day with the strapping in place.

The purpose of manipulation is not to stretch tight structures: it is not possible to do so unless sufficient force is applied to tear fibrous tissue. Usually, with excessive force, the lower tibial epiphysis will be displaced first (equivalent to a fracture of the tibia) or the talar condylar epiphysis will be squashed. It is probable that manipulation works by the application of intermittent force to underdeveloped connective tissue, which stimulates growth in the tissue cells. In this way the tissue lengthens, and the fixed deformity is overcome.

The technique is not without its dangers. Stretching of the medial structures of the ankle and the foot, of necessity, affects all structures. The most vulnerable are the arteries. In severe deformity, especially soon after birth, any stretching may cause spasm of the arterial supply to the foot. The toes become white and totally avascular. If it is left, the condition may end catastrophically in distal gangrene. Fortunately, there is usually recovery within a few minutes, which can be aided by keeping the child warm, holding the limb in a dependent position, and even by gently rubbing, tapping, or flicking the affected toes with the tip of the surgeon's finger. Recovery is often sudden, and the toes become engorged with blood and bright red. When it occurs, strapping may be impossible, and the onset of treatment may have to be delayed for a few days. Gentle stretching by midwife or doctor may help overcome the spasm. Similarly, there may be arterial compression after the application of the strapping. It is even more dangerous than pure spasm, because the circumferential constriction of the strapping may be the cause. For this reason the foot must always be observed for 20 minutes after the application of strapping, to make sure it is not too tight, before the child is allowed home. The parents must be instructed to bring the child back if the toes turn white or blue or begin to swell. They should also be shown how to remove the strapping and bandage, should the need arise. If the toes do turn white, the leg should be treated in the way described for arterial spasm: the child is kept warm, the foot hung in a dependent position, and the skin rubbed, tapped, or flicked gently. In most cases the color soon returns. Blue toes signify venous, rather than arterial, constriction caused by strapping that is too tight. It should be removed and reapplied. Persistent avascularity should make the surgeon abandon the treatment.

The child should find the strapping comfortable. Persistent crying is never normal. Usually it means that the strapping is too tight or that there is a local constriction. After a few hours the pain stops, not because the pressure has eased, but because the area of skin has become anesthetic. Blisters will form; full-thickness loss of skin may occur, requiring grafting. The prevention of such a catastrophe depends upon careful application of the strapping and on parental vigilance. The task of explaining this to a mother, who is naturally apprehensive about her child, without alarming her is a formidable one for the doctor.

In mild cases of clubfoot, strapping is repeated, daily at first, then twice a week, then weekly, until the deformity has been fully overcome and the foot can be placed in the

extreme opposite of calcaneovalgus. Examination of a normal neonatal foot reveals that the forefoot can be everted until the dorsum touches the lateral side of the leg. This position should be the aim of manipulative treatment. Once attained, it is held by strapping until the child is 3 months of age, after which the foot can be left free. In the author's experience, persistent deformity after this age cannot be overcome by external splintage. Operation is required.

During the period of splintage, the most trying aspect is that the baby cannot be placed in a bath. With care, fecal and urinary soiling of the strapping can usually be avoided, but the bandages invariably become stained, and the skin thickened and unpleasant. A good bath, and a few hours of freedom, work wonders. If the child is attending a weekly clinic, it is the author's practice to advise the mother to remove the strapping and bandages the night before the visit. The baby can enjoy a bath and freedom for the night; the mother can see what degree of recovery has taken place during the week.

In Severe Cases. In most cases, severe clubfoot can be diagnosed at birth, not only by the severity of the deformity, but by the presence of the stigmata to a marked degree. The lack of calf development is particularly obvious and a significant internal tibial torsional element is added to the other deformities.

Few cases respond satisfactorily to conservative (manipulative) treatment.[7] In recent years, therefore, surgery has become the definitive treatment rather than a salvage procedure. In theory, the earlier the operation is performed, the better; however, few surgeons have performed adequate series of what is, after all, a major operation in the first 6 weeks of life. Today there is no bar to surgery at this age, as far as the anesthesia is concerned, but it is a far cry from advocating such a step for a life-threatening condition such as congenital obstruction to bowel, to doing so for a limb deformity that presents no such immediate hazard.

The authors consider it expedient to plan to

operate when the child is between 3 and 6 months of age. Once this has been decided upon, and discussed with the parents, a mode of treatment should be instituted within the first few days of life: otherwise the deformity will increase and make the surgeon's task more difficult. Manipulation and strapping is therefore begun immediately and continued in the way described before, until the child is admitted to hospital for operation. It is wise, however, to abandon the treatment at least a week before admission so as to allow the skin of the foot to return to normal and so obviate the greater chance of infection that exists when surgery is performed through flaking or peeling skin.

Occasionally the foot responds unexpectedly well to manipulation and strapping, and the parents are relieved that the child does not have to undergo major surgery. At this age, the bones of the foot are mainly in cartilaginous form, and in some cases soft-tissue correction is all that is required. If it is not sufficient, or if the child is treated later, bony correction may be necessary.

The Surgery for Persistent Talipes Equinovarus

Soft-Tissue Correction. The principle of soft-tissue correction is the cutting or lengthening of all connective tissues that, by their contracture, are causing the fixed deformity. This means treating tendons, ligaments, and abnormal fascial planes, as well as mobilizing the tarsometatarsal joints by capsulotomy.

A vertical incision is made on the medial side of the Achilles tendon, extending to the heel. The tendon is lengthened by Z-plasty. It will be found that equinus cannot be overcome until posterior capsulotomy of the ankle joint is performed. The tendon is sutured at its new length and the skin closed. A second incision is then made on the medial side of the foot, and capsulotomy is performed on the talonavicular, and any other, joints that are tight. The medial tendons, especially the tibialis posterior and flexor hallucis longus, are lengthened. The abnormal connective tissues on the medial side of the foot are then released, great care being taken to avoid damage to the medial

vessels and nerve. At the completion of the operation the foot should be floppy and completely correctable.

The foot is placed in a calcaneovalgus position in a well-padded above-knee plaster cast, with the knee flexed to 90 degrees. A below-knee cast is inadequate, since it tends to slip. The author has seen children who managed to rotate the leg completely within the plaster by constant wriggling. This may compound the deformity; it may even cause skin necrosis. By applying an above-knee cast slipping is prevented. The plaster is split along its length, to facilitate removal if abnormal swelling makes this course of action necessary.

The child is allowed to go home in the cast when the general effects of the operation have subsided, and he is readmitted 2 weeks after the operation for a change of plaster and removal of sutures. Another cast is applied. This is best performed under a general anesthesia, for the comfort of the child, provided such anesthesia can be administered by adequately trained anesthetists in the safety of a hospital. After 4 weeks the plaster is removed, and the child's feet are left free to recover mobility.

The deformity does not usually recur by the time the child begins to stand. With the development of the reflexes for walking, a major factor in the prevention of recurrent clubfoot deformity is the effect of the forces of gravity, which tend to keep the sole of the foot on the ground and so discourage the recurrence of varus or equinus deformity.

The inequality of growth persists and should be monitored over a period of time, until all growth of the foot has come to an end, at about the age of eighteen. Generally, even in severe cases of talipes equinovarus, no further treatment is required, but the stigmata of the condition remain. If the clubfoot is unilateral, there remains a persistent inequality between the feet, the affected one being shorter and wider. The difference may be as much as one shoe size, even in comparatively young children. The parents must be warned of this because, although the shortness of the foot means that there is unlikely to be pressure on the affected toe, the greater width may cause lateral constriction as the foot grows to fit the shoe (Fig. 8-6A).

Although operation gives a "foot-shaped" foot (Fig. 8-6B&C), there is usually persistent stiffness in the heel and forefoot, either from the original contracture or as a result of operative scarring. Studies of weight bearing in persons who have undergone such surgery reveal that the pattern is never normal. It depends upon the new balance of muscular and ligamentous support of the longitudinal and transverse arches of the foot. Provided the maximal weight-bearing points are supported by skin that can bear the weight, abnormal callosities will not develop, and the patient will have a comfortable stance and gait.

The author has seen a young man of 19 years who was capable of playing professional soccer with a surgically corrected clubfoot. Even the underdeveloped "pipe-stem" calf was not a hindrance, although he required specially-made boots, based on a proper last.

Calcaneal Osteotomy. In some feet, soft-tissue correction alone cannot give a satisfactory shape; in particular, when the heel is not only in varus position but curved inward and is much smaller than normal. No amount of soft-tissue release can overcome this. Bony correction is required. Dwyer's osteotomy is the operation of choice.[8] A medially based, opening wedge osteotomy is performed, and a bone graft (from the upper tibial shaft) is inserted to eliminate the varus deformity while at the same time increasing the height of the heel. The operation, based as it is on correct anatomical principles, is highly successful. Postoperative weight bearing applies compression to the graft and so aids bone union. The only difficulty is that, since the height of the medial side of the heel is raised, great care must be observed in planning the skin incision, so that closure of the wound is not made unnecessarily difficult.

The Dilwyn-Evans Operation. For cases in which severe forefoot adduction cannot be fully overcome by soft-tissue correction alone or when the deformity recurs, an operative

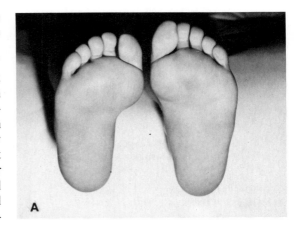

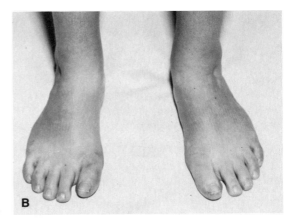

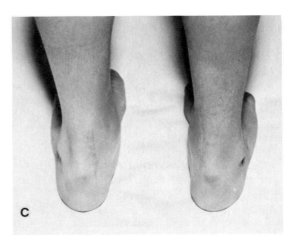

Fig. 8-6. (*A*) The affected right foot is shorter and wider than the left. (*B*, *C*) Two views of the feet of a boy who underwent soft-tissue correction for clubfoot years before. The result is good, although the stigmata of clubfoot, including thin calves and short first metatarsals, remain.

procedure has been designed to reduce further growth of the lateral side of the foot. It relies on arthrodesis of the lateral tarsal joints to prevent recurrence.

Wedge Tarsectomy. In late childhood, soft-tissue correction of the forefoot adduction may be impossible. A laterally based wedge tarsectomy allows the forefoot to be placed in an abducted position. The deformity is overcome, and a normal shoe can be worn, but the foot is certainly not normal, being smaller and permanently stiff.

Triple Arthrodesis. When growth is complete, residual deformity can be overcome by arthrodesis of the hindfoot. The operation includes arthrodesis of the posterior and anterior subtalar, and the talonavicular and calcaneocuneiform joints. Excision of bone results in a reasonably normal-shaped foot, in which weight bearing is concentrated upon those elements designed for that purpose. Abnormal callosities do not occur, and a normal shoe can be worn.

The Outcome of the Treated Clubfoot

As has been described, gentle, assiduous treatment allows the sufferer from clubfoot to have an almost normal childhood, even if the planned treatment includes operative interference. Furthermore, the adult who has undergone such treatment should have a comfortable foot of acceptable shape, even if it is never entirely normal. There are complications of the treatment that can hinder such an outcome.

Inadequate Correction. Persistent equinus deformity prevents the patient from bringing the heel to the ground. This is of little significance when high-heeled shoes are worn. Walking barefoot is another matter. If many sufferers find the current fashion in high-heeled shoes suitable for their feet, such heels have their drawbacks. The weight of the body is thrown forward onto the front of the foot; the abnormal weight bearing can lead to callosities beneath the metatarsal heads; which, in any case, are not normal, owing to their reduced mobility. The continual wearing of high heels can lead to further contracture of the calf muscles, enhancing the equinus deformity. The

patient may be consigned to wearing increasingly high heels.

In some cases, the tight heel cord of a partially corrected foot in a growing child or adolescent can apparently be overcome by ''bow-stringing'' of the tendon. If the heel is still in a varus position, the Achilles tendon slips medially to the longitudinal axis of the foot, whereas, if reduction of the heel is complete, it slips laterally. In this way, the heel can be brought to the ground without trouble, but at the cost of the position of the forefoot, which is held in persistent varus in the former case, or in an exaggerated valgus position in the latter. This bow-stringing may cause no symptoms for many years, until the abnormal weight bearing takes its toll on the skin under the affected areas; but the tendon may easily rub against the back of the shoe, causing pressure points or even adventitious bursae. Further growth often leads to an increase of the deformity of the front of the foot because of the tight tendon. If the deformity is varus, there are invariably symptoms, but, as has been stated, a fixed valgus deformity is compatible with a comfortable foot, even if it does not look attractive.

Scarring. Scars, especially those resulting from necrosis of skin due to injudicious strapping, can cause contractures in their own right. They occur in regions of the skin vulnerable to rubbing from the patient's shoes. At times the problems can be severe enough to warrant the use of full-thickness skin flaps. Surgical scars usually cause contractures of the skin only, and not of the subcutaneous tissues. This, itself, may constitute a problem, if such a scar is in a vulnerable site. It applies, usually, to the scar on the medial side of the foot. Occasionally, the use of Z-flaps may be required. Mostly, this can be prevented if the skin incisions employed are curved or S-shaped. All wounds are subject to contraction as the collagen of which they are composed becomes mature. In a straight incision, longitudinal contraction may be the outcome. If the incision is curved or S-shaped, the effect of collagen contraction is to convert the curve to a straight line. Contracture does not occur.

The most serious damage the surgeon can do is to cause trauma to the blood supply or the nerves of the foot. The former, while it rarely leads to gangrene, may easily result in Volkmann's contracture in the foot. In this condition, muscle necrosis occurs and the elastic muscle bellies are replaced by inelastic fibrous tissue. The patient develops a stiff clawfoot, which is easily subject to pressure from walking. Injury to sensory nerves creates areas of anesthesia on the foot. Loss of protective sensation is a disaster, leading to recurrent ulcers from unfelt pressure, and consequent amputation of the insensitive parts.

Rocker-Bottom Foot. This condition will be dealt with in greater detail in the section on the condition known as *vertical talus* (Chap. 6), but it is worth recording here that an unpleasant deformity results if the forefoot is reduced while the heel is allowed to retain its equinus position. The bones in the midtarsal region protrude into the sole, so that instead of an arch there is a bony prominence that develops callosities beneath it. The foot is difficult to fit into a normal shoe, and is seldom symptom-free.

Flat-top Talus. If a clubfoot is subjected to overzealous manipulation, the condition known as *flat-top talus* can develop.[9] Its name is derived from the characteristic radiographic appearance. The lateral view of the ankle shows a typical flattening of the curved, upper talar condyles that make up the distal articulation of the ankle. Whether this two-dimensional appearance is merely the result of flattening of the upper surface of the talar epiphysis, as a superficial examination of the radiographs suggests, or whether it is a more complicated lesion, is a matter of some debate. It has been pointed out, with good evidence to support the contention, that if further views of the ankle are taken, in different degrees of rotation, an aspect can be found in which the talus does not appear flattened. It is likely, therefore, that the radiographic appearance represents a more complex rotational injury. Two characteristics of the condition are, however, not in doubt: flat-top talus follows overforceful manipulation; damage to the talus

is of clinical significance, leading to loss of movement of the ankle joint owing to the distortion of joint surfaces, and, in the end, to degenerative osteoarthritis in adult life.

CALCANEOVALGUS DEFORMITY OF THE FOOT

Clinical Presentation

In contradistinction to clubfoot, the congenital deformity of calcanovalgus is nearly always benign in nature. It may be considered the opposite of equinovarus; the foot presenting with the heel (hence the name, calcaneus). Both the heel and the forefoot are in the extreme valgus position, so that the child is born with the foot squeezed against the lateral side of the shin. It is probable that the theory that the deformity is caused by pressure and "crowding" in the womb is a correct one. The posture of the foot, as well as the ease with which the condition can be treated, suggests that the deformity is not inherent in the growth of the limb before birth. The theory that the condition is due to late intrauterine pressure is more plausible. A first child in a tight intrauterine cavity may suffer disproportion, as may a large baby, or a degree of oligohydramnios may be responsible. The deformity may be unilateral or it may affect both feet. In the neonate with valgus and varus deformities, it is often possible to fold the whole child into a position resembling the shape of the uterus, when it will be seen that the legs and feet assume the valgus and varus positions.

Some children, especially those with long, thin feet, adopt a posture of calcaneovalgus naturally, but the condition is of no consequence unless the foot is stiff in this position. Examination shortly after birth differentiates between a posture and a deformity. The former can be left alone, since it is a variant of normal.

Treatment

If the foot cannot be placed into the alternative position of equinovarus, it ought to be treated. Manipulation is usually all that is required. It should be performed by the nurse or doctor, while the child is in a maternity unit. The task of stretching the foot should be taken over by the parents, once they have been taught the method and are confident of their ability to do it correctly. They are instructed to perform such stretching whenever the child's diaper is changed and to continue until there is no residual trace of the deformity; in most cases, this takes only a few weeks.

Sometimes the condition is so severe that stretching is not enough; it is then important to hold the position gained by each manipulation. Zinc oxide strapping is not very effective, because it is difficult to hold a foot in equinovarus. There is no area of skin on the leg to gain a purchase for this position. The foot is, therefore, best held in plaster-of-Paris.

After manipulation, the leg is held in as much equinovarus as can be obtained by stretching, with the knee at right angles. A well-padded cast is applied, with great care taken to prevent pressure points in the plaster. The incorporation of the flexed knee prevents the cast from slipping. The toes are left free, so their color can be observed. Spasm and avascularity are seldom a problem, presumably because, when the foot is held in the equinovarus position, the posterior tibial artery is relaxed, (unlike the situation that obtains in club foot).

The cast is changed twice a week for 2 weeks, then at weekly intervals; the child is bathed in the clinic at the time of each cast change. The use of the electric, power-driven plaster-cutter is contraindicated because of the distress to the infant. It is better to remove the plaster with hand tools, even if it takes a bit longer and more effort. The best tool is the long-handled plaster cutter, the guide of which can be slipped under one edge of the plaster, between the plaster shell and the cotton. In experienced hands, a 12-inch carpenter's tenon saw is an excellent tool, but the limb must be held quite still and the sawing motion must be gentle.

Treatment continues until the deformity can easily be overcome and full equinovarus is possible. Thereafter, the foot is left alone. Further treatment is seldom required (unlike

in the true club foot), but the child should be followed in the clinic for a few months.

Although it is rare indeed for operation to be required, Figure 8-7 shows a foot in such a case. An 11-month-old boy had persistent, fixed, severe calcaneovalgus deformity of one foot. It could not be overcome by manipulation or serial plasters. No other abnormality was present. In particular, nerve conduction studies and electromyography showed no neurological lesion. Operation was indicated.

METATARSUS ADDUCTUS

Clinical Presentation

Metatarsus adductus (or varus) is a congenital deformity confined to the forefoot.[10] It is always present at birth and may be uni- or bilateral. Since it is a mild condition, children who suffer from it may not have medical attention until they are some months old. The heel is normal.

The deformity (Fig. 8-8) is characterized by an inward curve of the forefoot, mainly of the shafts of the metatarsals. As a result, the front of the foot is rotated inward; but it is not the sole cause of the child's toeing-in. Many children of this age, and perhaps those with metatarsus adductus more than most, have the combination of internal tibial torsion and persistent fetal alignment (that is, internal rotation of the upper end of the femur), so that the whole leg is rotated inward as well.

A second feature of the deformity, present in severe cases, is an oblique groove on the medial side of the foot at the level of the tarsometatarsal joints (Fig. 8-9). The groove represents the area of underdeveloped soft tissue that is the main deforming force of the lesion. The size of the groove is directly related to the severity of the deformity. The mildest cases may have hardly any groove, in which case the only feature of the condition is hallux varus of a type that may be described as "muscular" (Fig. 8-10). At rest the foot may appear almost normal, but when the child stands or walks (and such children seldom appear in the orthopaedic clinic before they

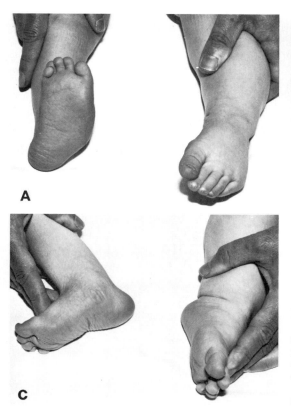

A

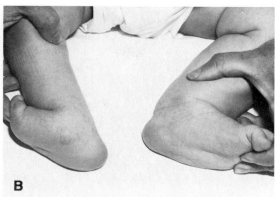

B

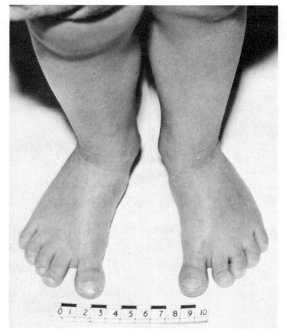

C

Fig. 8-7. Photographs of a severe case of talipes calcaneovalgus, in which there was unusual stiffness of the foot, show all the features of the condition: (*A*) Notice the natural posture adopted by the abnormal right foot, compared with the left which is normal. (*B*) The range of dorsiflexion of each foot is shown. The right foot packs very firmly against the calf. (*C*) Passive flexion of the right foot does not even reach the mid-position.

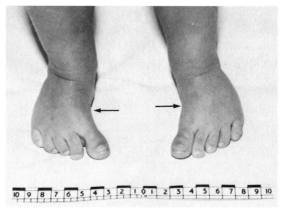

Fig. 8-8. (*Left*) Mild bilateral metatarsus adductus.

Fig. 8-9. (*Right*) Severe bilateral metatarsus adductus. The arrows show the oblique medial grooves.

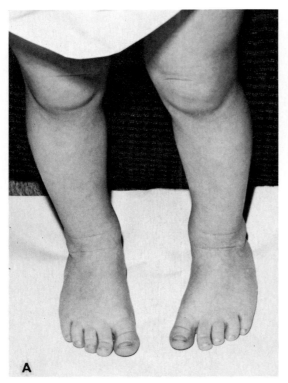 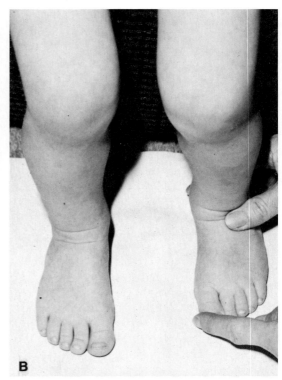

Fig. 8-10. (*A*) Muscular metatarsus adductus. (*B*) The deformity can be easily overcome by stretching the medial muscles of the big toe.

are old enough to walk) the big toe is held in a varus position by contraction of the abductor hallucis muscle. It is probable that underdevelopment of this muscle is the cause of the deformity in such feet.

Metatarsus adductus occurs approximately once in 1000 live births. It often occurs without cause, in which case it may be unilateral, but there is sometimes a family history. The problem of etiology is made more difficult by the comparatively late presentation for treatment. There is some evidence that the incidence of the condition is increasing, but it is not proven. It has been suggested that the modern practice of letting children sleep face-downward exacerbates the condition. If the infant is born with internal tibial torsion, or some degree of metatarsus varus, the weight of the feet on the bed when the child is sleeping prone may be enough to increase a congenital deformity, or even to initiate a mild case.

This may account for the different types of the condition. The severe form may be congenital, arising from intrauterine pressure, for example, while the mild, "muscular" variety may occur in susceptible children who often sleep in the prone position.

Treatment

Very few adults present with residual metatarsus adductus deformity, from which it has been inferred that no treatment is required for the condition. This is certainly not so. Figure 8-11 shows the feet of an African man who had never worn shoes. The residual metatarsus varus can be seen. One can draw the inference that the wearing of shoes plays a part in the resolution of the condition.

In general, this is all that is required for treatment. Once the child begins to walk and is given proper shoes, the metatarsus adductus tends to settle. Few mild cases are still visible after the age of five. The process can be hurried if valgus shoes are used or, indeed, if the shoes are worn on the opposite feet.

About one patient in ten has a severe form of the condition. Such children require treatment early in life. Splinting, either by valgus plaster casts or Denis-Browne splints, may overcome the deformity sufficiently for normal shoes to be fitted at the appropriate age. Operation is indicated if the deformity persists. It is best performed between the second and third year of life; not only so that the child has recovered well before nursery school, but because, at this age, soft-tissue correction is sufficient.

The procedure consists of lengthening of the medial muscles of the foot, transection of persistent fibrous bands, followed by mid-tarsal capsulotomy, to abduct the forefoot. For 6 weeks after operation, the foot is maintained in the fully corrected position, the casts being changed at 2 weeks for removal of sutures. Results of operation are good.

ARTHROGRYPOSIS

This profound, congenital disease of all four limbs is always present at birth (Fig. 8-12). The head and trunk are normal, and children suffering from the condition are mentally normal, tending, perhaps, to be above average in intelligence. There is generalized deformity and lack of development of all the limbs, from the shoulders and hips downward (Fig. 8-13). The lesion appears to be confined to the connective tissues of the limbs, which are quite abnormal. There are no subcutaneous creases around the joints, an indication of lack of fibrous tissue differentiation. Similarly, the separate muscle bellies are not clearly developed and may be represented in part by undifferentiated sheets of muscles. The bones and joints are also inadequately formed, so that movements of all the joints are reduced, both by abnormality in the shape and contractures by poorly developed capsular tissue. Michele has suggested that the basic defect is in growth of the limb bud, which fails to undergo the repeated foldings that result in the

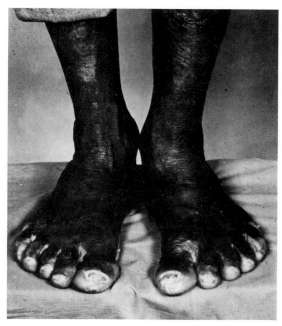

Fig. 8-11. Residual metatarsus varus in a man who has never worn shoes.

normal shape of the structures of the limb at birth.

In the lower limb the deformities are progressively more severe, from proximal to distal, so that the feet are profoundly abnormal. Severe, intractable talipes equinovarus is present. The knees are in valgus position and stiff, and the hips are so markedly anteverted that dislocation may occur.

Such children have great difficulty in walking. Treatment must be prolonged and assiduously conducted, since deformities may recur until growth stops. It consists of operations for straightening and stabilizing the proximal joints, followed by soft-tissue or bony correction of the clubfoot.

Carefully chosen surgery gives a leg of acceptable shape which can be suitably splinted by proper orthotic apparatus to allow the child to walk. The limbs will, of course, never function normally, and the patient will need a protected environment for life. Children with arthrogryposis, adequately treated, respond in a most gratifying manner because of their mental abilities.

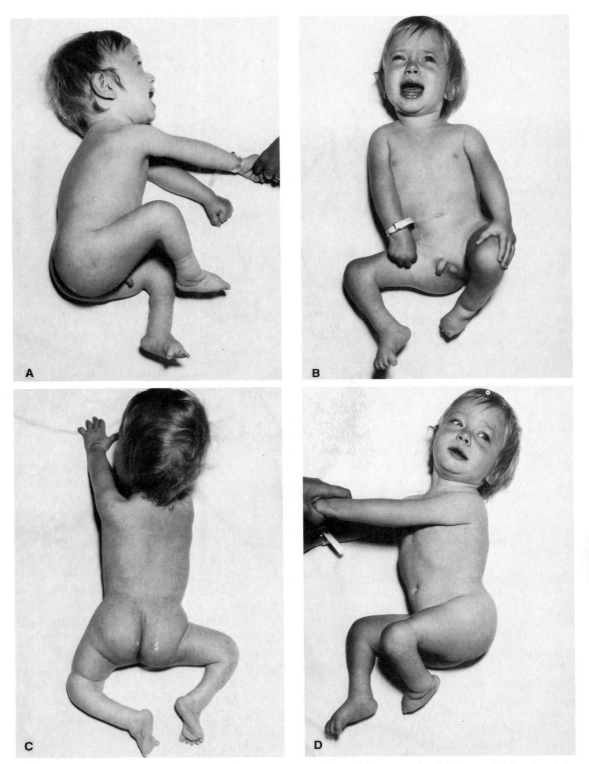

Fig. 8-12. This young boy shows all the features of arthrogryposis multiplex congenita. Stiffness and deformity of the joints of the limbs is accompanied by abnormal connective tissue development. Skin creases are notably absent. The trunk is normal and the child appears intelligent. Clubfoot is present.

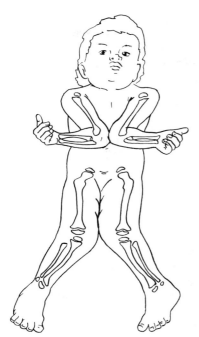

Fig. 8-13. Drawing of the pattern of limb deformities seen in arthrogryposis.

SOME OTHER DEVELOPMENTAL ABNORMALITIES OF THE FOOT AND LEG

Any combination of abnormalities may occur in the lower limb, from the most minor deviations to severe deformities; even complete absence of the limb. The most severe may yet be ameliorated by a wise combination of surgery, orthotic splinting, or prosthetic replacement. Only a few, with special features, will be described.

Hypoplasia of the Lower Limb

Nobody has legs exactly equal in size and shape, but in some people the inequality amounts to a deformity. Abnormal increase in the size of a limb occurs in two conditions, both rare: congenital arteriovenous fistula and a few cases of neurofibromatosis.

Hypoplasia is much more common. Usually, one leg only is involved, and the deformity is present at birth. The affected limb is smaller than the one on the other side, although each of its parts is in proportion. The difference in size is small, but as the child grows, the

inequality in the legs increases until such time as growth is complete.

There are two clinical problems: a short-leg limp and difficulty in obtaining shoes. The first can be alleviated by adjusting the heel of the child's shoe, while the latter, at the worst, entails buying two pairs of shoes of different sizes. Fortunately, some shoe stores will sell single shoes of different sizes.

In rare cases, the difference in length is sufficient to warrant leg equalization, either by planned epiphyseal stapling of the normal leg during growth, or shortening in the adult. Leg lengthening is seldom justified, unless the adult patient is so short of stature that he will not contemplate further shortening of the normal leg, since the procedure is difficult and occasionally associated with disastrous complications. Surgery is never advised for the foot, since the function is normal.

Duplication of the Hallux

A fairly common congenital abnormality, duplication of the hallux, is not uncommon. It is usually partial; varying from a longitudinal ridge in the nail, with a widened distal phalanx, to complete duplication of the tip. Some cases require surgery, either for its cosmetic effect or to fit into shoes, but the production of a good-looking toe is not always easy and should be performed by an experienced plastic surgeon.

Sixth Toe

Many babies are born with a sixth toe. It may vary from a tiny appendage on the lateral side of the foot, sometimes near the base of the fifth metatarsal, to a properly functioning, extra toe. Surgery is indicated in most cases, not only for ease of fitting shoes: the presence of an extra toe is usually a cause of great concern to the parents, since it is easily visible, and most laymen have a horror of congenital abnormality.

Absence of Metatarsal Rays

Congenital absence of metatarsal rays is uncommon. That usually seen is complete absence of the fifth, including the toe. There is surprisingly little visible abnormality; merely a long, narrow foot. Few lay observers notice that there is no fifth toe unless it is pointed out to them. No treatment is required, apart from the correct fitting of shoes (for which a lateral inset may be required) since the function of the foot is normal.

The Lobster-Claw Foot

In contrast to the shape produced by absent rays, the splitting of the foot longitudinally at the metatarsal level, often with duplication of metatarsal rays, results in a horrifying deformity: the so-called lobster-claw foot, which might, more expressively, be termed "chameleon foot." The function may not be se-

verely disturbed, but the appearance is most unpleasant, and the fitting of reasonable footwear almost impossible without complex reconstructive surgery. Such feet never function completely normally.

Fibular Agenesis

Sometimes the distal part of the fibula fails to develop or is represented only by a fibrous band.[11,12] The child is born with a severe valgus deformity of the ankle, owing to lateral tethering, and further growth of the limb causes progressive deformity, since the lateral side of the ankle fails to keep pace with the medial.

Treatment is surgical.[13] A series of opera-

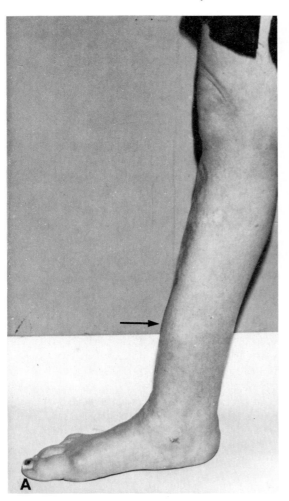 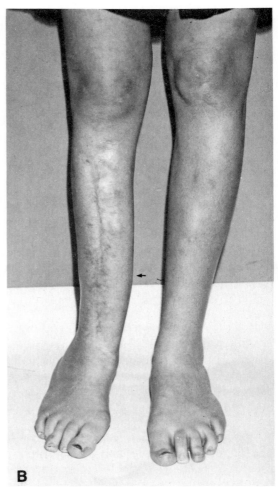

Fig. 8-14. This 18-year-old girl had congenital pseudarthrosis of the right tibia; it has united following bypass grafting. There is a valgus and flexion angulation deformity in the tibia (*arrows*) and, consequently, a deformity of the foot.

tions may be required to excise the fibrous bands and so allow the tibia to grow normally. The surgery may be extensive and seldom results in a normal leg, but the leg does grow reasonably straight and can be supported by adequate orthotic splinting.

Pseudarthrosis of the Tibia

This rare, congenital abnormality (Fig. 8-14)[14] is seldom visible at birth. Sometime during childhood the patient develops a pathological fracture of the lower third of the tibia. It may unite or break down again, or it may progress to nonunion. The affected part of the tibia is abnormal, showing radiographic changes such as sclerosis, abnormalities of shape, and irregular ossification in that region of the diaphysis. The underlying disease is thought to be localized neurofibromatosis.

Clinically, the pseudarthrosis is associated with localized forward bowing of the tibia; the deformity is often very severe. Over the years, treatment has proved difficult. Surgery offers the only means—not always successful—of obtaining bone union.[15] Excision of the lesion and bypass grafting has proved effective, although there is usually a modicum of residual anterior bowing and some permanent deformity.[16] Repeated operations are worth attempting if the patient is not to be condemned to wear a leg-iron for the rest of his life.

REFERENCES

1. Klaus, M. H., and Kennel, J. H.: Parent-to-infant attachment. *In* Recent Advances in Paediatrics. Edinburgh, Churchill Livingstone, 1976.
2. Solnit, A. J., and Stark, M. H.: Mourning and the birth of the defective child. Psychoanal. Study Child, *16:*523, 1961.
3. Hare, E. H, Lawrence, K. M., Paynes, H., and Rawnsley, K.: Spina bifida cystica and family stress. Br. Med. J., *2:*7, 1966.
4. Kite, J. H.: The Club Foot. New York, Grune and Stratton, 1964.
5. Fripp, A. T., and Shaw, N. E.: Club Foot. Edinburgh, Churchill Livingstone, 1967.
6. Blockey, N. J., and Smith, M. G. H.: The treatment of congenital club foot. J. Bone Joint Surg., *48B:*660, 1966.
7. Ono, K., and Hyashi, H.: Residual deformity of treated congenital club foot. J. Bone Joint Surg., *56A:*1577, 1974.
8. Dwyer, F. C.: Osteotomy of the calcanum for pes cavus. J. Bone Joint Surg., *41B:*80, 1959.
9. Dunn, H. K., and Samuelson, K. M.: Flat-top talus. A long-term report on twenty club feet. J Bone Joint Surg., *56A:*57, 1974.
10. Kite, G. P.: Congenital metatarsus varus. J. Bone Joint Surg., *49A:*388, 1967.
11. Coventry, M. B. and Johnson, W.: Congenital absence of the fibula. J Bone Joint Surg., *34A:* 941, 1952.
12. Thompson, T. C., Straub, L. R., and Arnold, W. D.: Congenital absence of the fibula. J. Bone Joint Surg., *39A:*1299, 1957.
13. Serafin, J.: A new operation for congenital absence of the fibula. J. Bone Joint Surg., *49B:* 59, 1967.
14. Eyre-Brook, A. L., Baily, R. A. J., and Price, C. H. G.: Infantile pseudarthrosis of the tibia. J. Bone Joint Surg., *51B:*604, 1969.
15. Boyd, H. B.: Congenital pseudartharosis treatment by dual bone grafts. J. Bone Joint Surg., *23:*497, 1941.
16. Boyd, H. B., and Sage, F. P.: Congenital pseudarthrosis of the tibia. J. Bone Joint Surg., *40A:*1245, 1958.

9 Research into the Cause of Clubfoot

J. E. HANDELSMAN

Clinicians have disagreed about the cause of clubfoot since the time of Hippocrates. True clubfoot is always a rigid deformity, even at birth. The heel equinus, forefoot adduction, and whole-foot varus cannot be passively corrected (Fig. 9-1). However much a deformity looks like true talipes equinovarus, if it can be overcorrected without effort it should be regarded as a different entity, probably a consequence of the intrauterine position of the fetus. A rigid deformity is always associated with the stigmata described in Chapter 8. The most notable of these is the lack of the posterior calf musculature.

ETIOLOGICAL FACTORS

Not only does the cause of true clubfoot remain controversial; even the underlying pathology is obscure. A racial tendency has been recorded in the condition, and a broad hereditary factor has also been described.[1] Aberrations of the attachment of tendons have been evoked by several authors:[2,3] medial insertion of the Achilles tendon, tethering of the peroneus longus tendon in the sole of the foot, and variations of the insertion of an abnormally short, thick tibialis posterior tendon have been described. All these abnormalities, in particular those of the peroneus longus tendon, have been seen in otherwise normal feet in cadaveric dissections.

Nichols (1897) first noticed anomalies of the tarsal bones present at birth.[4] These have since been described by other authors, but there is no convincing evidence that they are the fundamental factors in clubfoot.[5]

Diminution of the bulk of the calf muscle (Fig. 9-2), on the other hand, is a constant finding.[6] The affected extrinsic muscles on the posterior and medial side of the foot are fibrosed, with loss of stretch of the muscle bellies. Small differences in the power of muscles acting on joints regularly produce a disproportionately severe degree of deformity.

It seems logical to postulate that clubfoot is the result of a form of muscle malfunction and imbalance. The presence of the deformity at birth would then be secondary to the existence of such a muscle anomaly from an early intrauterine stage.

Furthermore some conditions in which muscle imbalance is present, such as poliomyelitis and myelomeningocele (Fig. 9-3), often cause a deformity of the foot that is very much like talipes equinovarus. This view is supported by the fact that the calf muscles in severe clubfoot clinically resemble those in arthrogryposis multiplex congenita, a condition commonly associated with an unresilient equinovarus deformity (Fig. 9-4).[7–9] The possibility that arthrogryposis may have a neurologic basis is supported by similar clinical findings in the feet of patients suffering from lumbosacral

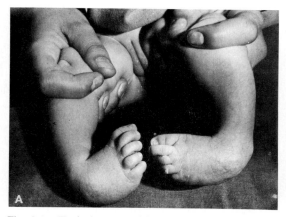 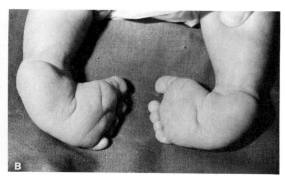

Fig. 9-1. Typical severe rigid clubfoot soon after birth. (*A*) Anterior view, showing equinovarus deformities. (*B*) Posterior view, showing varus of the heels and thin calves.

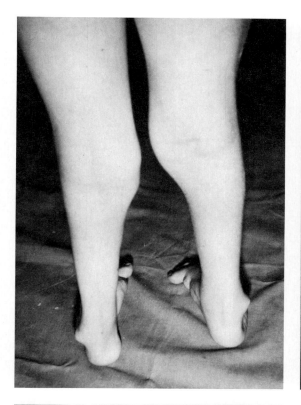 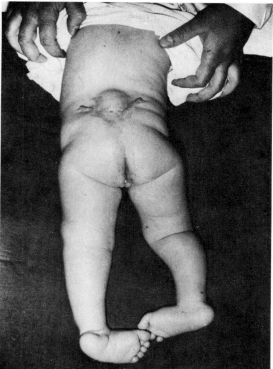

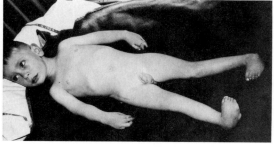

Fig. 9-2. (*Top left*) Thin calves in clubfoot.

Fig. 9-3. (*Top right*) Equinovarus feet in myelomeningocele.

Fig. 9-4. (*Left*) Arthrogryposis with severe talipes equinovarus.

agenesis (Fig. 9-5), in whom the motor nerve supply to the limb is known to be deficient or anomalous. Eighteen such patients have been examined, and their feet were found to be clinically indistinguishable from those of patients with the fibrous type of arthrogryposis. The majority presented with a rigid bilateral equinovarus deformity.

Based upon these considerations, a project of research was undertaken to examine the hypothesis that the affected muscles in children with clubfoot deformities would show characteristic features of neuromuscular disease.[10] Bechtol and Mossman studied such muscles in two fetal specimens with bilateral clubfoot deformities. They found muscle degeneration resembling arthrogryposis. their work supported our hypothesis that the thin calf asso-

ciated with clubfoot is a localized form of arthrogryposis and that the etiological factors and basic pathology of the two conditions are similar.

Histologic examination of muscle fibers, using conventional stains such as hematoxylin and eosin, cannot show pathological changes due to neuromuscular damage. On the other hand, histochemical stains that are specific for oxidative and glycolytic enzyme systems have been able to differentiate between two types of fibers in mammalian muscle tissue.

The slow-twitch, Type I muscle fibers utilize oxygen and are rich in the oxidative enzymes commonly found in mitochondria. The Type II, fast-twitch fibers derive their energy from stored glycogen. In many mammals the two types of fibers tend to occur in separate muscle

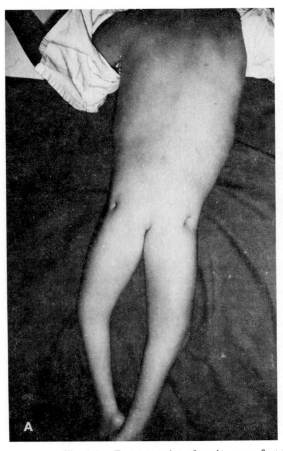
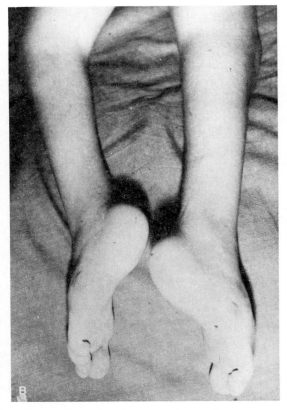

Fig. 9-5. Two examples of equinovarus feet in patients suffering from lumbosacral agenesis.

bellies (Table 9-1). By contrast, all human skeletal muscles contain both Type I and Type II fibers in a regular ratio of 1:2.

HISTOCHEMICAL STAINS

Type II fibers stain dark, whereas Type I fibers stain lighter. Normal human muscle presents a typical "checkerboard" effect because of this (Fig. 9-6).

Histochemical Stains

Type I, slow-twitch fibers were demonstrated by:
  NAD (NADH diaphorase)
  Mitochondrial ATPase reaction incubated at *p*H 4.5

Type II, fast-twitch fibers were revealed by:
  PAS for glycogen
  Phosphorylase for glycolytic enzymes
  ATP (myofibrillar ATPase) incubated at *p*H 9.5

Significance of the Histochemical Differences

The metabolic differences that distinguish the two muscle fibers types are not inborn but depend entirely upon the characteristics of their nerve supply. This was established by Buller, Eccles, and Eccles and confirmed by Dubowitz, who performed nerve cross-over experiments in the domestic cat.[11–13] By severing and cross-anastomosing the adjoining nerve supplies to the slow-twitch soleus muscle and the fast-twitch flexor hallucis longus muscle, he showed that a reversal of both enzyme content and fiber characteristic resulted.

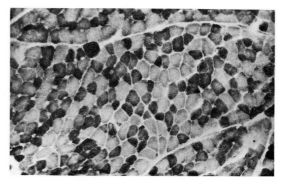

Fig. 9-6. Typical mosaic pattern of human muscle stained histochemically. Type I fibers stain light and Type II, darker.

These experiments suggest that the action of a nerve on a muscle is twofold. Its obvious function is the transmission of excitatory stimuli, causing muscle contraction; but every nerve has several important secondary trophic effects on the muscle fiber it supplies: first, a trophic type factor which determines the enzyme content and therefore the staining characteristics of the fiber and, second, a trophic size factor which regulates the size of muscle fibers. The latter may be the cause of the unusually large fibers found in myopathies such as myotonia congenita. A third trophic factor controlling fiber direction and alignment may also exist.

The reversal of recognized enzyme patterns, variations in the size of muscle fibers and disruption of the alignment of fibers are evidence of disturbance in the motor nerve supply.

A feature of partly denervated muscle is its ability to stimulate the axones of adjacent healthy motor units to divide, penetrate, and reinnervate its nonfunctioning fibers. Since the enzyme function of a muscle fiber is determined by its nerve supply, the reinnervated fiber always takes on the characteristic of the invading axon. Thus, previously denervated muscle that subsequently recovers function always contains fiber of a single type. In man the typical "checkerboard" effect is lost as all the fibers stain uniformly (Fig. 9-7). The resulting appearance is termed *grouping,* and is evidence of denervation and subsequent reinnervation of an area of muscle (Fig. 9-8).

Table 9-1.   Muscle Fiber Types

Characteristics	Type I	Type II
Contraction	Slow-twitch	Fast-twitch
Macroscopic type of muscle	"Red meat" fibers	"White meat" fibers
Metabolism	Uses oxygen	Uses stored energy (glycogen)
Contained enzymes	Oxidative enzymes	Glycolytic enzymes, phosphorylase and ATPase

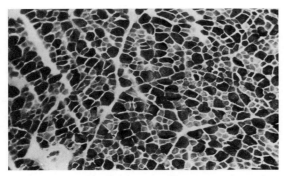

Fig. 9-7. Atrophy of Type II fibers, which stain pale, with resulting loss of the normal "checkerboard" effect. Variations in size of the residual Type I fibers can be seen.

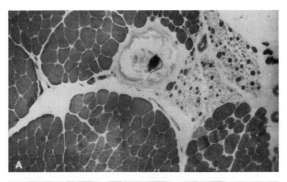

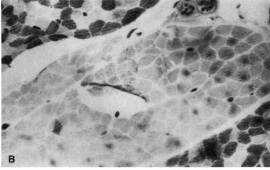

Fig. 9-8. Examples of grouping: (*A*) Type II grouping. (*B*) Type I grouping.

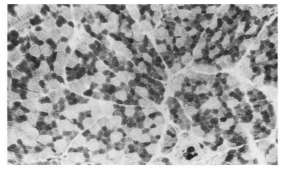

Fig. 9-9. Smallness and angularity of fibers.

Histochemical stains are able to demonstrate other anomalies of the fibers, such as smallness and angularity, which are also trophic-dependent (Fig. 9-9). Furthermore, they show alterations in the total fiber population. Degenerate or nonfunctioning fibrils in the center of a muscle fiber do not stain at all, so producing a bullseye targetlike appearance.

Material

Muscle specimens were taken from 46 patients undergoing corrective surgery for clubfoot. The operations were, therefore, not performed for experimental purposes. The majority of patients were under the age of 5 years at the time of surgery. Sex distribution was equal. Eighty-seven specimens were obtained for histochemical examination. Of these, 49 were taken from the posteromedial group of muscles, that is from those muscles that are clinically affected in clubfoot. Table 9-2 shows the number of specimens taken from individual muscles. Thirty-five specimens were similarly taken from the opposing muscle group, that is, from the peroneal muscles. Since these muscles are not subject to contracture in talipes equinovarus, these biopsies were used as controls. The muscle bellies were approached through a small incision in the interosseous membrane.

Method

Biopsy Technique. Excision of the muscle specimens was facilitated by placing a suture in each end of the tissue to be excised. The use of a sharp blade reduced the tissue trauma. Muscle for histochemical analysis was maintained at its resting length by using the sutures to tie the specimen longitudinally on to a wooden spatula with notches cut at each end. The specimen was kept moist by covering it with a damp saline gauze swab. Processing was undertaken within 30 minutes. Specimens

Table 9-2. Muscles from Which Specimens Were Taken

Muscle	Number
Tibialis posterior	24
Gastrocnemius	11
Flexor hallucis longus	6
Flexor digitorum longus	7
Abductor longus	1

were orientated, secured in gum tragacanth on cork discs, and rapidly frozen to −160°C. Sections were cut to a thickness of 10μ; histochemical staining was undertaken, and the fibers were identified according to the classification of Dubowitz and Pearce.

Results Of the 87 biopsies examined histochemically, no apparent abnormality could be detected in 17 specimens. However, measurement of both Type I and Type II fibers in this group revealed that these were smaller in size than in average muscle (Fig. 9-10).

Obvious abnormalities were present in the remaining seventy biopsy specimens. In many instances, more than one anomaly was evident in the same section (Fig. 9-11). The main deviations are summarized in Table 9-3. All are evidence of major neurogenic disease. Table 9-4 shows the presence of lesser abnormalities. All suggest faulty innnervation. In eight cases there was an increase in the number of central nuclei; evidence of intrinsic muscle disease which may be neurologically determined.

Fibrosis was not a feature of the muscle biopsies studied. Blood vessels in the muscle and surrounding tissues were completely normal. Muscle spindles were encountered in many sections, and all presented a normal appearance.

The general pattern of abnormalities seen in the peroneal muscles was similar to that of the posteromedial group. Nine of the 17 specimens in which no apparent abnormality was found, came from peroneal musculature. In order to compare the two groups more directly, 18 specimens each of tibialis posterior muscle and peroneus muscle sampled were examined in detail. It was found that the actual fiber size in nine tibialis posterior biopsies were smaller

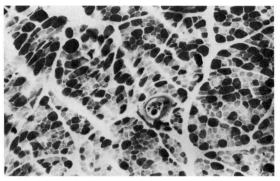

Fig. 9-10. Smallness in size of both Type I and II fibers.

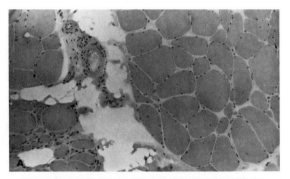

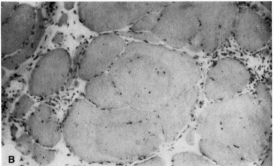

Fig. 9-11. Two examples of extreme variation in fiber size.

than those in the peroneal group.[14] The remainder were similar in other respects, except that the total muscle bulk, as determined by the number of muscle fibers in a comparable section, was greater in all the peroneal muscle specimens.

Conclusion

Biopsy revealed specific abnormalities in 70 specimens. Although superficially normal, the fiber size in the remaining 17 biopsies was smaller than would be expected in normal muscle, so that these, too, are mildly affected.

Table 9-3. Main Abnormalities

Type	Number
Grouping of individual fiber types	19
Type I fiber atrophy	20
Type II fiber atrophy	3
Profound loss of fiber direction	25
Associated smallness and angularity of fibers	7
Presence of target cells	4

Table 9-4.   Lesser Abnormalities

Type	Number
An absolute increase in Type I fiber population	10
An absolute increase in Type II fiber population	1
Scattered degeneration of individual fiber types	6
Areas of fiber regeneration	4
An increase in the number of central nuclei	8

In many of these 70 specimens, more than one anomaly was seen. Major evidence of neurogenic disease was seen in 78 instances, and changes strongly suggestive of faulty innervation were evident in 21 other preparations. Possible evidence of intrinsic muscle disease was seen on eight occasions, but this may in fact be neurologically determined.

The findings in the 35 peroneal muscle biopsies followed the same pattern as those in the 49 specimens taken from the posteromedial muscle group, but individual fibers were larger and the total muscle bulk greater in the peroneal biopsies. This finding suggests that the peroneal muscles, although obviously abnormal, are less affected than those in the posteromedial group. Muscle imbalance may therefore play a role in the production of clubfoot deformity.

The study supported the contention that the extrinsic musculature in talipes equinovarus is abnormal. It was concluded that an underlying neurogenic pathology, producing changes in calf musculature, is a dominant factor in the etiology of common clubfoot.

ELECTRON MICROSCOPIC STUDIES

To confirm the histochemical abnormalities, 53 more specimens were obtained for electron microscopic studies.[15] An approximately equal number of specimens were taken from the clinically affected tibialis posterior, soleus, and long toe flexor muscles, and from the peroneal muscle group.

Method

The muscle biopsy was peformed with a fresh scalpel, and the specimen was held at its resting length in a cooled double-arm clamp fixed in 5-per-cent glutaraldehyde at 4°C. The muscle was subsequently washed in phosphate buffer and post-fixed in 1-per-cent osmic acid. The preparation was embedded in Araldite-Epon and sections were cut on a Reichert ultramicrotome and then stained with uranyl acetate and lead citrate. Sections were viewed on a Siemen's Elmiskop ultramicroscope.

Results

The ultramicroscopic appearance of normal muscle is of myofilaments which lie in parallel rows, forming myofibrils. These exhibit recurring light and dark bands, the I- and A-bands respectively. The I-band is divided by a dense, broad Z-line, and down the center of the A-band is a lighter zone, the H-zone, which itself is bisected by a dark M-line. The length of the A-band is fairly constant at 1.5μ, but the I-band shortens with muscle contraction. The myofibrils are separated by mitochondria, glycogen granules, some triads and occasional lipid bodies. Type I and Type II muscle fibers are not easily distinguishable with the electron microscope. However, Type I fibers tend to have more mitochondria and thicker Z-lines.

Every specimen examined showed significant anomalies. Disorganization of myofibrils was found in the majority. Myofilaments could not be seen, and Z-material was scattered in a haphazard fashion. Excessive folding of the basement membrane occurred frequently, often blurred in outline with unformed Z-material and sometimes a total loss of myofibril structure. Loss of fiber direction was particularly common (Fig. 9-12). Myofibrils were present both longitudinally and end-on in the same section. Streaming of Z-material or more complete disorganization of this structure associated with irregular fiber formation was seen. Marked distension of mitochondria was also observed.

In some areas, satellite muscle cells, an attempt at regeneration, could be seen developing in disintegrated areas (Fig. 9-13). Tubule formation where fibers had disintegrated, leaving empty spaces, and T-tubule formation caused by an extension of sarcolemma penetrating into degenerate muscle, were both in evidence. Elongated degenerate nuclei with no muscle fiber formation occurred, and hyper-reactive nuclei with muscle formation were also seen. Excessive lipid formation often accompanied disorganization. The relative absence of fibrous tissue at the ultramiscroscopic level was a feature of this study.

Correlation between source of the biopsy and of the anomalies seen electron microscopically established that there was no significant difference between peroneal and posteromedial musculature.

Discussion

The histochemical analysis of the same muscles examined in this study showed major and also lesser abnormalities, the latter in some instances being no more than an alteration of fiber size. The ultramicroscopic examination, however, has revealed that every fiber is abnormal and that the changes are significant. Major disorganization of myofibrils and total loss of fiber direction, both common, would appear to be incompatible with normal function.

The histochemical studies suggested that peroneal musculature was less affected than the posteromedial group, but no such distinction could be made electronmicroscopically. The histochemical evidence that the changes in muscles have a neurogenic basis is supported to some extent by the study at the ultramicroscopic level. Although most of the anomalies are consistent with both myopathic and neuropathic lesions, the nuclear changes

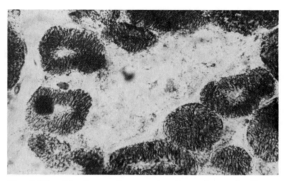

Fig. 9-13. Electron microscopic view of muscle fibers, showing abnormal attempts at regeneration, with "target cell" formation.

and Z-line disturbances in particular, favor an anomaly of motor nerve supply.

It has been suggested that these histochemical and electron microscopic changes may be the result of the period of immobilization, stretching of the tight posteromedial and relaxation of the peroneal muscles that preceded the surgical correction at which the biopsies were obtained. To reproduce the conditons that pertain during cast correction in clubfoot patients, baboons, whose musculature closely resembles humans', were chosen for experiemnt.

Material and Method

Four young baboons, aged between 6 and 36 weeks, were used. One foot in each animal was immobilized in a below-knee cast in an attitude of calcaneovalgus, in order to stretch the posteromedial extrinsic muscle group and relax the peroneal muscles. The opposite foot was left free as a control. Glass fiber Litecast, which is durable and impervious to water, was used in place of plaster-of-Paris. No anesthetic was given, but careful padding with foam and nylon stockinette was used under the Litecast.

The first baboon, aged 6 weeks, died from unrelated causes soon after the cast was applied. For this reason, the second animal, also 6 weeks old, was immobilized for two periods; for 8 weeks and then for another 7 weeks, after a rest period of a fortnight. The older animals were both 36 weeks old when the casts were applied, and were immobilized for 17 and 25 weeks, respectively.

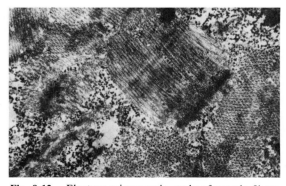

Fig. 9-12. Electron microscopic study of muscle fibers. The view shows marked alteration in fiber direction, even at this magnitude.

Thereafter, the animal was anesthetized with ketamine and the cast was removed. Biopsies were obtained from the flexor digitorum longus and an unselected peroneal muscle from both the immobilized and the control limb. Two biopsies were taken concurrently from each muscle, one for histochemical and the other for electron microscopic examination, so that a total of eight biopsies were obtained from each animal. The technique followed was exactly the same as that used for biopsy of the patients with clubfoot.

None of the baboon muscles studied histologically, in either the immobilized muscles or control muscles, showed any anomaly when stained histochemically. There were no abnormalities in the electron microscopic studies of baboon muscle taken from either the immobilized or control hind limb.

There was thus no significant change in either muscle group of the immobilized or control leg in any of the three animals up to 25 weeks of immobilization.

This complete normality of every baboon specimen of muscle subjected to varying periods of immobilization and either stretching or relaxation, is in sharp contrast to the appearance of some of the biopsies taken from the same muscles in children with clubfoot.

This series suggests that the quite specific anomalies in clubfoot musculature are characteristic of that condition and that the basic abnormality is probably due to an underlying neurogenic defect, as indicated by the appearance of the anomalies. The conclusion from this work is that the immobilization and correction of a clubfoot by serial plaster casts plays no part in the production of muscle changes observed in the condition.

REFERENCES

 1. Wynn-Davies, R.: Family studies on the cause of congenital club foot. J. Bone Joint Surg., *46B:*445, 1964.
 2. Flinchum, D.: Pathological anatomy of talipes equinovarus. J. Bone Joint Surg., *35A:*111, 1953.
 3. Singer, M.: Tibialis posterior transfer in congenital club foot. J. Bone Joint Surg., *43B:*717, 1961.
 4. Nichols, E. H.: Anatomy of congenital equinovarus. Boston Med. Surg. J., *136:*150, 1897.
 5. Elmslie, R. C.: The principles of treatment of congenital talipes equinovarus. J. Orthop. Surg., *2:*669, 1920.
 6. Irani, N. N., and Sherman, M. S.: The pathological anatomy of club foot. J. Bone Joint Surg., *45A:*45, 1963.
 7. Otto, A. G. [Cited by James, T., (1951)]: Multiple congenital articular rigidities. Edin. Med. J., N.S., *58:*565, 1841.
 8. Pena, C. E., Miller, F., Budzilovich, G. N., and Feigin, I.: Arthrogryposis multiplex congenita. Neurology (Minneapolis), *18:*926, 1968.
 9. Lebenthal, E., et al.: Arthrogryposis multiplex congenita: Twenty-three cases in an Arab kindred. Pediatrics, *46:*891, 1970.
10. Isaacs, H., Handelsman, J. E., Badenhorst, M., and Pickering, A.: The muscles in club foot—a histological, histochemical and electron microscopic study. J. Bone Joint Surg., *59B:*465, 1977.
11. Buller, A. J., Eccles, J. C., and Eccles, R. M.: Differentiation of fast and slow muscles in the cat hind limb. J. Physiol, *150:*399, 1960.
12. Dubowitz, V., and Pearse, A. G. E.: Reciprocal relationship of phosphorylase and oxidative enzymes in skeletal muscle. Nature (London), *185:*701, 1960.
13. Dubowitz, V.: Cross innervated mammalian skeletal muscle: histochemical, physiological and biochemical observations. J. Physiol., *193:*481, 1967.
14. Brooke, M. H., and Engel, W. K.: The histographic analysis of human muscle biopsies with regard to fibre types. Neurology (Minneapolis), *19:*591, 1969.
15. Afifi, A. K., Smith, J. W., and Zellweger, H.: Congenital nonprogressive myopathy. Neurology (Minneapolis), *15:*371, 1965.

10 Developmental Conditions of the Feet

PES CAVUS

A fixed, high, longitudinal arch deformity of the foot is known as pes cavus. It is always significant, and the foot can never be regarded as normal, not only because it usually gives rise to symptoms at some time during the patient's life, but because the causes of the condition are potentially serious.

Pes cavus usually manifests itself in childhood, often by the age of four. Very rarely, it may be present from birth. The condition is nearly always bilateral, and the deformities of the two feet symmetrical, but occasionally one foot is more severely affected than the other (Fig. 10-1).

Pes cavus may vary from a very mild, to a very severe, disease. It may be familial. The elements of the deformity are as follows: a high, longitudinal arch to the foot, especially the medial, longitudinal arch; poor development of the intrinsic muscles of the foot, amounting in some cases to a fibrous thickening that can be felt beneath the plantar fascia as a tight band (Fig. 10-2) prominence of the metatarsal heads in the sole of the foot; a greater or lesser degree of varus deformity of the heel; and dorsally curled toes. In the most severe cases there may be contracture of the calf muscle, so that there is an element of equinus deformity as well; however, in many patients the contracture is confined to the front of the foot, a deformity more correctly described as plantaris.

As the child grows, the condition usually worsens, until, at the age of seventeen or eighteen, a final stage is reached. Thereafter the shape of the foot changes only if there is further atrophy of muscles with increasing stiffness (Fig. 10-3), or the onset of degenerative changes within the tarsal and metatarsal joints in middle age (Fig. 10-4).

Pes cavus may be caused by several diseases, which are either neurologic or muscular in origin; all are important. Peroneal muscle atrophy (Fig. 10-5), a familial disease with muscle wasting and contractures, is probably the most common, but rare conditions, such as Frederick's ataxia and muscular dystrophy, also cause pes cavus. Other neurologic conditions, such as missed poliomyelitis, may very rarely present as a cavus foot, and high arches certainly exist in myelomeningocele and cerebral palsy; but the underlying disease is usually evident on examination. One condition may easily be missed. Diastematomyelia, in which an abnormal, midline, bony projection in the spine results in traction injury of the cauda equina as the spine grows. Although it is rare, the condition should always be borne in mind, since it is amenable to surgical cure.

Brewerton has shown that in at least one third of cases of pes cavus no underlying disease can be found.[1] Such cases are usually familial, and the condition may represent the result of inadequate development of the lower segments of the spinal cord, so that an imbal-

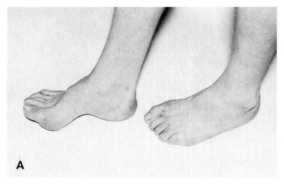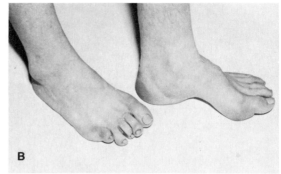

Fig. 10-1. Two views of the feet of a young man with moderately severe bilateral pes cavus. The right foot is more severely affected than the left. The high arch, tight heel cord, and clawtoes can be seen.

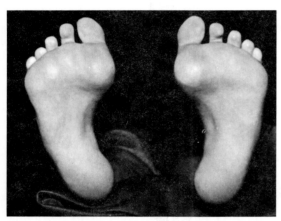

Fig. 10-2. Severe pes cavus. The prominent metatarsal heads of the transverse arch can be seen, as well as the tight fibrous band of the plantar fascia, which is not covered by the usual intrinsic muscle layers.

ance between the extrinsic and intrinsic muscles of the feet exists.

The child may have difficulty with walking and running and may be poor at games because of inadequate muscle control secondary to the underlying disease. The fitting of shoes may be a problem, and the child may develop metatarsalgia at an early age; in adults, it is almost universal in pes cavus. Callosities and adventitious bursas may be severe beneath the metatarsal heads.

Careful neurologic examination should be performed, and in many cases specialist investigation is required, both for prognostic purposes and for the rare cases in which exploration of the spinal cord is indicated.

Management

Patients with pes cavus require foot care throughout their life. Attention to the fitting of shoes must begin at an early stage and can never be relaxed. Many adults need custom-made shoes with appropriate insoles. For adults, chiropody is essential to cope with callosities.

Soft-Tissue Operations

Sometimes surgery is indicated, mainly to improve the shape of the foot and so enable footwear to be fitted. In children, soft-tissue correction is sufficient in most cases. This includes Steindler's operation, in which the proximal attachment of the plantar fascia to the under-surface of the heel is transected, so that the plantar contracture can be released. If there is an element of equinus deformity, lengthening of the heel cord is required. Finally, deformity of the toes may be overcome by flexor-extensor tendon transplants.

Flexor-Extensor Tendon Transposition.[2] The clawtoe deformity may be very severe in young people, without secondary degenerative changes in the joints leading to stiffness that can only be rectified by arthrodesis. The deformity is due to imbalance between the flexor and extensor muscle groups. It can be overcome, at least as far as the second to fifth toes are concerned, by detaching the extensor tendons from their origin, detaching the flexor tendons from their insertions, and suturing the proximal ends of the flexor tendons to the distal ends of the extensor tendons. When the patient wakes and tone returns to the muscles, the flexor muscles pull the extensor tendons, and thus, instead of tending to flex the toes into a claw deformity, they become extensors; that is, they straighten the toes. The operation is technically difficult.

Bone Operations

Bone operations include Dwyer's calcaneal osteotomy,[3] if there is severe varus deformity of the heel; and ultimately, in some severe instances, triple arthrodesis of the hindfoot may be essential, during the course of which the cavus deformity can be overcome by appropriate excision of tarsal bones to reshape the foot.

BONY LUMPS

Congenital variations in the shape of bones of the hindfoot may give rise to lumps that lead to pressure from footwear.

Navicular Lumps

Elongation of the medial tubercles of the navicular bones, related to the attachment of the tibialis anterior and posterior tendons, commonly causes pressure from the shoes, leading to adventitious bursa formation. In some cases there may be separate accessory navicular ossicles. Pain from bursitis can be cured by excision of the bony lumps. Care must be taken to prevent detachment of the tibialis tendon insertions at operation.

Dorsal Tarsometatarsal Exostoses

In some patients a dorsal bony lump develops at the base of the first metatarsal, immediately related to the first tarsometatarsal joint. The swelling is very liable to pressure from the upper of the shoe. Not only is a bursa liable to form in this position, but the terminal branch of the cutaneous nerve may easily be injured with the formation of a traumatic neuroma. Surgical excision cures the condition, provided sufficient bone is excised from the opposing surfaces of the joint.

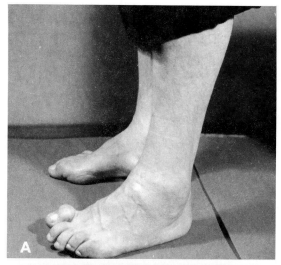

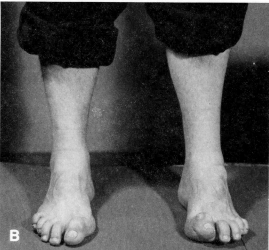

Fig. 10-3. In the adult, further muscle atrophy and pressure causes deterioration of the condition. Note the bursa over the dorsum of the left hallux.

Anterolateral Ankle Callosities

Occasionally, children or adolescents are seen with a thick callosity, lateral and anterior to the ankle joint. The cause may be difficult to understand, until it is seen that such patients habitually adopt a position of acute inversion of the foot when sitting. As a result the rim of the lateral talar condyle is pressed against the skin in this region, leading to the callosity.

The condition requires no treatment; the callosity soon subsides once the patient is

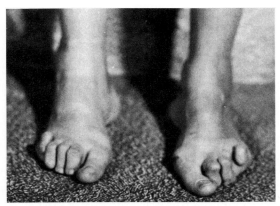

Fig. 10-4. Mild clawtoes have led, in middle age, to severe deformity. The left fourth toe has been amputated.

persuaded to stop the habit of leaning on the dorsum of the foot. Removal of the bony ridge is contraindicated, because it entails opening the ankle joint, and the lateral talar condylar ridge is essential for normal ankle function.

The "Winter-Heel" Syndrome

A relatively common developmental variation in the shape of the back of the heel bone is the presence of a lateral calcaneal ridge. Clinical observation suggests that this bony ridge occurs more commonly in girls than in boys. It must be emphasized that the ridge is a normal variation in the shape of the calcaneus. In itself it does not necessarily give rise to symptoms, even though the Achilles tendon runs over the superior dome of the calcaneus before attaching to the bone inferiorly. The cause of pain in patients with a calcaneal ridge is pressure from shoes; hence the name, *Winter-heel syndrome.*

Such patients have no trouble in summer when they choose to wear sandals, probably without backs because they know that they get pain when they wear shoes. The advent of cold and wet weather heralds the onset of symptoms. Pressure from a shoe on the bony ridge gives rise to swollen adventitious bursa in the overlying subcutaneous tissue. The overlying skin thickens and hardens by repeated rubbing, until a proper callosity is formed. The picture of the winter-heel syndrome is present. Since normal shoes do not accommodate the shape of such heels, the

patient is forced to seek surgical attention. The calcaneal ridges continue to grow until late in adolescence, and it is usually at this age that the patient presents for treatment.

Once symptoms are established, operation is the only solution and, if carefully performed, is curative. It consists of the removal of the bony ridge. The patient is positioned prone, when the feet turn naturally outward on the table. A vertical incision is made over the calcaneus, lateral to the Achilles tendon. The sural nerve is seen and protected before the periosteum covering the dome-shaped, superior eminence of the calcaneus, deep to the Achilles tendon, is incised vertically and stripped from the bone on its superficial and deep aspects, to expose the calcaneal ridge. It is covered with a layer of articular cartilage—an unexpected anatomical finding, because it is not part of any articulation. The offending bony lump is then excised by means of an oblique osteotomy, with care being taken to leave that part of the calcaneus to which the Achilles tendon is attached. The osteotome penetrates the full width of the bone, but extreme caution must be exercised not to strike the osteotome too hard with the hammer lest the sharp end of the instrument penetrate the other cortex unexpectedly or the medially placed, posterior tibial vessels may inadvertently be damaged. The osteotome is withdrawn and the skin edges opposed, so that the surgeon can palpate the lump of bone through the callosity, to ensure that no ridge is left. Usually this is felt transversely at the level of the uppermost part of the Achilles tendon attachment. Where necessary, any remnants are trimmed with a bone nibbler. The wound is closed in layers and care is taken to reconstitute the deep fascia with catgut sutures, to prevent the skin from adhering to the bone. Excision of the bursa is not required, since it will subside once the pressure point has been removed.

Postoperative care includes rest in an elevated bed and early exercise. Since the tendon has not been detached, and the weight-bearing part of the calcaneus has not been touched, prolonged avoidance of weight bearing is un-

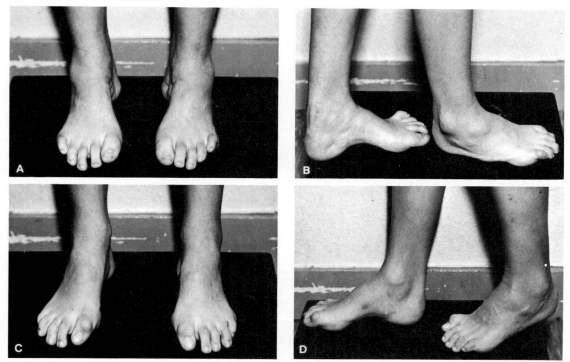

Fig. 10-5. (*A, B*) Front and side views of a young woman with severe pes cavus. She was found to be suffering from peroneal muscular atrophy. She had previously undergone bilateral Achilles tendon lengthening and Steindler's plantar fascial release. (*C, D*) Similar views of her teenage sister, who suffered from the same disease.

necessary. The patient can begin walking as soon as comfort allows.

In rare cases, the bony lump is so large that a more radical operation is required: an oblique, closing wedge osteotomy of the upper part of the calcaneus allows the bony ridge to be depressed away from the surface. The operation cures the condition, but since the Achilles tendon is attached to the proximal portion of the bone, either internal fixation or prolonged bed rest, until the fracture has united, is required to prevent displacement of the fragment by the pull of the calf muscles.

OSTEOCHONDRITIS

There is a group of conditions that occurs in growing bones, collected under the term, osteochondritis. The word implies, "an inflammation of bone and joint," which is something of a misnomer. What characterizes the lesions is that they show typical radiographic changes.

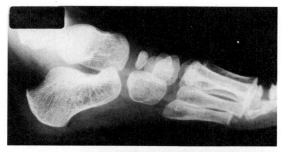
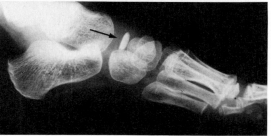

Fig. 10-6. Radiographs of the feet of a child with Köhler's disease. The one navicular ossification center is normal in size and density. In the other foot, the ossifying nucleus is smaller and denser (*arrow*).

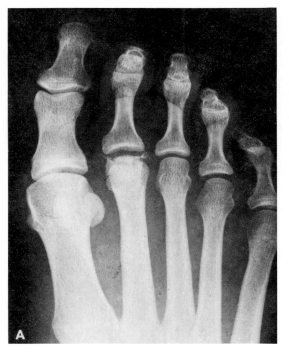

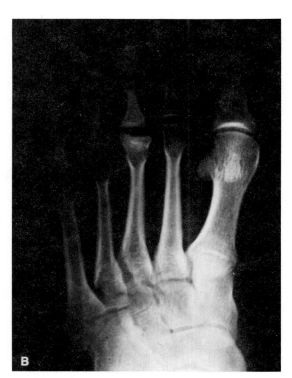

Fig. 10-7. (*A*) An example of Freiberg's disease of the second metatarsal head. (*B*) The third can also be affected.

(All were described within a short time of the advent of diagnostic radiography, just before World War I.) Changes visible on films are confined to the ossification centers within the epiphyses of growing bones and occur in a cycle: cessation of growth of the ossific nucleus, sclerosis, fragmentation, and finally, reossification. The primary lesion is probably avascular necrosis of part or all of the growing cartilage plate, of which the ossific nucleus is the visible radiographic component. Apley has classified the condition very practically into three groups, according to the nature of the injury to the epiphyseal cartilage, that is, into *crushing* osteochondritis, *splitting* (so-called osteochondritis dissecans), and *pulling* osteochondritis or traction apophysitis that occurs in those parts of an epiphysis into which a tendon is inserted.[4]

In the foot, examples of each type of osteochondritis can be found.

Crushing Osteochondritis

Köhler's disease (Fig. 10-6) is avascular necrosis of the epiphysis of the navicular bone.[5] It occurs in children between the ages of 3 and 5 years, and causes pain in the foot on weight bearing. It should always be included in the differential diagnosis of children of this age who are constantly whimpering and fractious, especially on excursions that involve much walking. Complete resolution takes place eventually, and distortion of the navicular bone is uncommon in adult life.

Freiberg's disease (Fig. 10-7) is a form of crushing osteochondritis of the head of the second metatarsal bone. (See Metarsalgia, Chap. 5.)

Splitting Osteochondritis

Two examples of osteochondritis dissecans occur in the foot:

Talar Osteochondritis Dissecans. Fragmentation of the lateral side of the lateral talar condyle occurs in mid-adolescence. Usually, one large, loose body is found. It may be completely asymptomatic, or the patient may have episodes of recurrent locking of the ankle

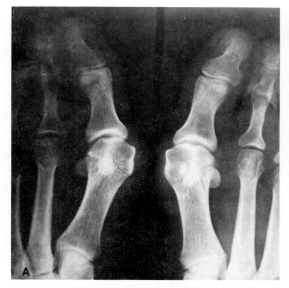

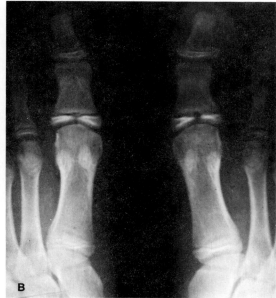

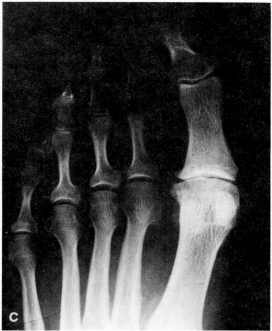

Fig. 10-8. Hallux rigidus. (*A*) The usual lesion in the metatarsal head. (*B*) Occasionally the defect seems primarily to affect the basal phalangeal epiphysis. (*C*) The result is osteoarthritis.

joint as the loose body shifts within its bed. In that case it requires surgical incision.

Hallux Rigidus. The primary lesion in hallux rigidus (Fig. 10-8) is a splitting osteochondritis of the growing cartilage on the dorsal aspect of the head of the first metatarsal. It usually happens in mid-adolescence. (See Acquired Conditions, Chap. 11.)

Traction Apophysitis.

Sever's disease (Fig. 10-9) is a form of pulling osteochondritis of the calcaneal apophysis to which the Achilles' tendon is inserted.[6] Diagnosis does not depend upon radiographic changes, because similar sclerosis and fragmentation is commonly seen on films of the other heel. It depends on tenderness in the

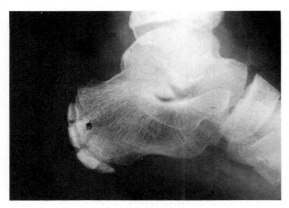

Fig. 10-9. Sever's disease. The calcaneal apophysis is seen to be sclerosed, flattened, and fragmented.

heel, with pain on excessive walking. It occurs most commonly in children of about 8 to 12 years of age, and the apophysis recovers spon- taneously in a year or two. Symptoms can be reduced if the child is allowed to wear a slightly raised heel to prevent recurrent traction injury to the epiphysis.

REFERENCES

1. Brewerton, D. A., Sandifer, P. H., and Sweet- nam, D. R.: The aetiology of pes cavus. Brit. Med. J., *2:*659, 1963.
2. Taylor R. G.: The treatment of claw toes by multiple transfers of flexor into extensor tendons. J. Bone Joint Surg., *35B:*539, 1951.
3. Dwyer, F. C.: Osteotomy of the calcaneum for pes cavus. J. Bone Joint Surg., *41B:*80, 1959.
4. Apley, A. G.: A System of Orthopaedics and Fractures. ed. 5. London, Butterworths, 1977.
5. Cox, M. J.: Kohler's disease. Postgrad. Med. J., *34:*588, 1958.
6. Lewin, P.: Apophysitis of the os calcis. Surg., Gynecol. Obstet., *41:*579, 1925.

11 Acquired Deformities of the Toes

HALLUX VALGUS

Hallux valgus is the commonest affliction of the normal adult foot.[1] It is significant only when it gives rise to symptoms, but in the end most patients suffer at least some discomfort and seek expert attention. The condition has a complex etiology, as far, at least, as the symptomatic syndrome is concerned.

ETIOLOGY

Hereditary Factors

Hallux valgus is seen more commonly in women than in men. There is often a familial history in such patients; many women recall similar trouble in the feet of their female relatives.

The condition may be present in childhood; often in combination with a short, big toe that adopts a valgus position from the early years (Fig. 11-1). Such toes usually have a valgus shape to the distal phalanx as well.

Flatfoot

More commonly, slight congenital hallux valgus is aggravated by an associated plano-valgus foot (Fig. 11-2). In this condition, discussed elsewhere, an outward-tilting (valgus) heel causes the weight to be borne on the inward-rolled foot, especially along its medial border. This pronated foot, within its shoe, causes the patient to throw the weight of the body onto the medial border of the big toes when standing and in the push-off phase of walking. Since the first metatarsophalangeal joint has lax collateral ligaments, the counter pressure of the medial border of the shoe or the ground itself, if the individual is walking barefoot, forces the big toe to adopt an habitual valgus position when bearing weight. At the same time the hallux is rolled laterally by the pronation of the forefoot so that, during the push-off phase of normal walking, the toe is not so much extended passively, as it should be, as strained into further valgus.

Metatarsus Primus Varus

Congenital hallux valgus is, in most cases, associated with congenital splaying of the five metatarsal rays of the foot (Fig. 11-3). Such feet are usually of the large-boned variety. As a result of the splaying of the rays there is a wide transverse metatarsal arch. (Fig. 11-4). Part of this shape is an exaggerated metatarsal primus varus, in which the first metatarsal is splayed medially. It is not only the wide spread of the metatarsal bones that causes this varus: it is the shape of the first metatarsal bone itself.

Metatarsal primus varus means that the metatarsophalangeal angle is large to begin with, so that any factor that adds to the valgus distortion of the big toe will aggravate the condition.

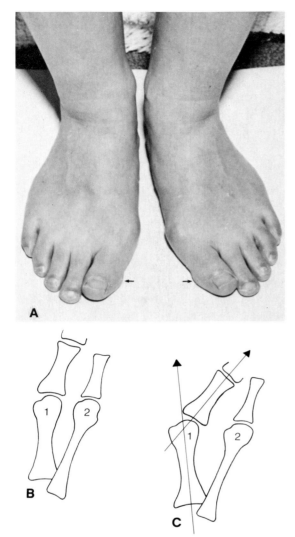

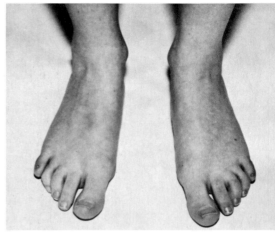

Fig. 11-2.   Long, thin, planovalgus feet, with early hallux valgus.

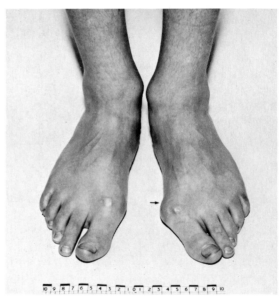

Fig. 11-1.   (*A*) Familial hallux valgus, associated with a short first toe; the second toe is the longest. Some degree of pronation of the foot is present, as well as valgus position of the distal phalanx (*arrows*). (*B*) Diagram of normal bony relationships. (*C*) Hallux valgus.

Fig. 11-3.   Hallux valgus with congenital matatarsus primus varus in the left foot (*arrow*).

The Vagaries of Fashion

A shoe that pinches the toes will add to the valgus strain on the big toe and increase the deformity. There has rarely been a fashion in women's shoes (or, for that matter, in men's) for many years that has been designed to protect the toes. The term *fashion* has become synonymous with *discomfort*. The ubiquitous high heel throws the weight of the body onto the front of the foot. Whatever the reason for the fashion (in men, presumably to add to their height and in women, to make the calves appear more "attractive") the result is the same: further crowding of the toes (Fig. 11-5). Since, even in the highest heels, little attempt is made to design a horizontal platform for the back of the foot to give the heel an adequate purchase for weight bearing, excessive weight

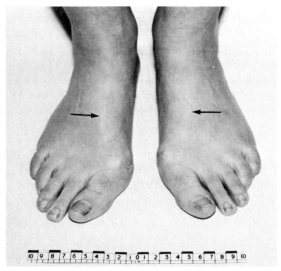

Fig. 11-6. Tendon bow-stringing can be seen (*arrows*). Early callosities are visible overlying the bunions.

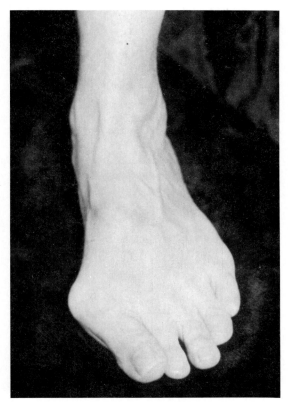

Fig. 11-4. The wide transverse metatarsal arch associated with hallux valgus. It can be seen that the deformity of the big toe is rotational as well as angular.

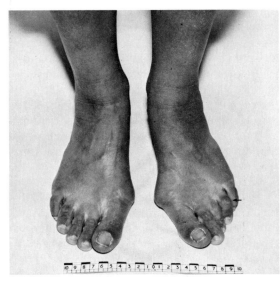

Fig. 11-5. Hallux valgus with crowding of the toes and dorsal callosities, especially of the left fourth toe (*arrow*).

is borne beneath the metatarsal heads. The recent return of the pointed toe in shoes, reminiscent of the excesses of the so-called "winkle-picker" shoes of a few years ago, bodes ill for the toes of the public. Even without such pointed toe caps, the fashion for shoes with high, platform heels and hard uppers of the toecaps is bringing increasing numbers of young people with painful hallux valgus, pressure points, adventitious bursas, and even premature onychogryphosis and separation of the nail of the big toe, to orthopaedic clinics and podiatrists. The shoe, itself, may not be the only deforming force. Tight stockings or elastic tights may be the extrinsic cause of continuous pressure on the big toe, increasing the valgus force applied to the hallux.

Tendon Bow-stringing

Once the hallux has been forced into a valgus position, the tone of the long extensor muscle causes gradual loosening of the soft connective tissue that binds its tendon to the dorsum of the first metatarsophalangeal joint. Since there is no true tendon sheath in this region, the tendon gradually moves laterally until it begins to have a bow-string effect upon the big toe (Fig. 11-6). It becomes another deforming force on the hallux, adding to the valgus imbalance. Without a retaining anatomical structure to limit the bow-stringing effect, the extensor tendon continues to act as a deforming force for the rest of the patient's life. In old age the degree of hallux valgus can reach extreme proportions of 90 degrees or more. The axis of the adductor hallucis muscle is perfectly placed to add to the valgus deformity.

PATHOGENESIS

Medial Collateral Ligament Strain

Increasing valgus strain of the toe gives rise to stretching of the medial collateral ligament of the first metatarsophalangeal joint. As a result, what began as a valgus, strained position of the base of the proximal phalanx ends as lateral subluxation.

The collateral ligament attachment to the medial side of the first metatarsal head gradually becomes thickened by repeated rupture of collagen fibers and is replaced by a thickened mass of fibrous tissue.

Formation of a Medial Osteophyte

This lump of fibrous tissue soon becomes tender, owing to repeated inflammatory reaction at the site of the ligament insertion. Eventually, a periosteal reaction occurs, leading to new bone formation on the medial side of the first metatarsal head. The bony lump enlarges.

Development of a Bursa

As in other parts of the body, when constant pressure is applied to the skin, a subcutaneous bursa develops, probably because the pressure of the shoe against the medial side of the toe causes shearing strains in the subcutaneous connective tissue. There is a consequent separation of collagen fibers into two planes, with fluid between. In time, the tissues develop an adventitious bursa. At first the bursa is protective in function, allowing compressed skin to slide easily over the underlying bone; but in the end, continued pressure results in repeated inflammatory reactions in the bursa, which itself becomes painful. Instead of pro-

tecting the toe, the bursa becomes a cause of symptoms. With increasing fibrosis of the bursa, the symptoms change from intermittent to continuous pain.

In extreme cases, continuous pressure may even lead to necrosis of an area of skin overlying the bursa. Pressure ulcers usually heal if the pressure is relieved, unless synovial fluid from an underlying bursitis prevents this. Once a fistula has been created, the synovial fluid tends to prevent healing of the ulcer, probably not only because of the physical presence of the fluid, but because its chemical nature includes anticlotting, heparinlike substances which prevent clotting, so that fibroblasts are unable to fill the defect and allow epithelialization.

A draining sinus is one way of dealing with the situation, provided the fluid secreted by the bursa continues to drain. Changes in pressure may cause a reverse flow of fluid, in which case infection is a constant threat, since it may spread. In old people with a diminished vascular bed or diabetes wet gangrene may ensue at any time.

Osteoarthritis

Further distortion of the joint results in osteoarthritis (Fig. 11-7). In the early cases this usually begins on the medial side of the joint. Examination of the cartilage of the metatarsal head shows a vertical pattern of erosion in this area, which, in the normal toe, is opposed by the cartilage-covered base of the proximal phalanx. In the valgus-strained toe, however, it is exactly this region of the metatarsal head that is uncovered by the phalanx. Instead, cartilage is constantly exposed to the medial synovium, which probably starts the erosion of articular cartilage. Later, the erosions spread and become generalized. The secondary capsular reaction that occurs in this condition increases the fibrosis around the joint and fixes the deformity. Eventually, osteophytes form on the lateral side of the metatarsal head and, in particular, circumferentially around the base of the phalanx. Impingement of the osteophytes may lock the

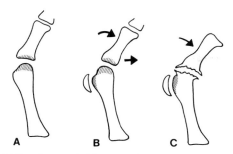

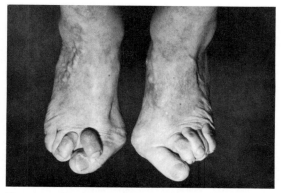

Fig. 11-7. Osteoarthritis secondary to hallux valgus. (*A*) The normal first metatarsophalangeal joint. (*B*) In hallux valgus, lateral angulation (*curved arrow*) is followed by lateral subluxation (*straight arrow*). A bursa forms over the prominent medial "osteophyte." (*C*) Secondary degenerative changes occur in the joint, with loss of articular catrtilage and osteophytosis.

Fig. 11-8. Crowding of the toes. On the right, the second toe is dislocated dorsally over the hallux, with severe pressure upon its proximal interphalangeal joint. On the left, severe crowding has caused dorsal corns on all the toes.

subluxed joint, leading to further stiffness and constant pain.

Crowding of the Toes

The big toe is the strongest digit, and as it goes over into valgus deformity it pushes the other toes outward (Fig. 11-8). The pattern of deformity that develops in the toes depends on the width of the transverse metatarsal arch, the shape and length of the individual toes, and the design of the footwear.

Often the second toe is pushed dorsally until it comes to lie above the first when the patient is walking. In rare cases it may come to lie beneath the big toe (Fig. 11-9). The third, fourth, and fifth toes are usually forced to adopt a valgus position. Increasing crowding leads to callosities wherever the shoe presses, usually on the outer side of the fifth toe but occasionally on the tips of the third and fourth.

Hammer Deformity of the Second Toe

In some respects, the deformity that the second toe adopts is in a special case, since it occurs so commonly.

To understand the development of fixed deformity in the second toe, the transverse metatarsal arch must be considered not as a row of metatarsal heads bearing weight in one plane, but as a true arch. While there has been argument as to whether an arch exists during the push-off phase of weight bearing or whether

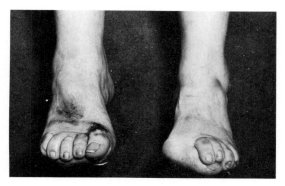

Fig. 11-9. Poor foot care and hygiene have led to a different pattern of crowding in each foot. The left hallux is completely displaced beneath the second and third toes.

all the metatarsal heads are pressed in one plane onto the ground, what is not in doubt is that, when the foot is fully relaxed and bearing no weight, an arch does exist. Observation of the second toe with the foot in this position shows that it is straight. During walking, the toes are flexed by action of the long flexor tendons, especially the sublimis, when they grip the ground. With the arch pressed flat and the toes flexed, the second metatarsophalangeal joint is forced into hyperextension; also, if, as commonly happens, the second toe is the longest of the five, active flexion forces the metatarsophalangeal joint into greater hyperextension.

In time, especially if the second toe is crowded between the first and third by hallux valgus, the position of hyperextension of the metatarsophalangeal, flexion of the proximal interphalangeal, and hyperextension of the distal interphalangeal joints is habitual. Capsular stretching in this exaggerated position leads to gradual subluxation followed by dorsal dislocation of the base of the proximal phalanx, fixed flexion due to adhesions in the proximal interphalangeal joint, and subluxation and fixed hyperextension of the distal phalangeal joint.

The typical, established picture of fixed hammer deformity of the second toe is now present. Finally, the dislocated head of the second metatarsal causes increasing pressure to be concentrated beneath it, with the gradual development of a thick callosity in the skin and an underlying subcutaneous adventitious bursa. The latter causes symptoms by developing repeated inflammatory bursitis, while the hardened pearl of skin in the center of the callosity is a potent source of pain leading, in some cases, to extravasation of blood intradermally, due to rupture of capillaries by pressure.

Similarly, the fixed deformity of the proximal interphalangeal joint leads to a dorsal callosity caused by the pressure of the shoe, while a callosity may form on the tip of the toe if dislocation of the metatarsophalangeal joint does not weaken the digit. A result of such a distal callosity is gradual elevation and deformity of the nail of the second toe.

Hammer Deformities of Other Toes. Deformity is not necessarily confined to the second toe following hallux valgus. Sometimes the third, fourth, and even the fifth toes may become hammered and may have the same problems as the second.

MANAGEMENT OF HALLUX VALGUS AND RELATED DEFORMITIES

As in all other painful, or potentially painful, conditions of the feet, the management ranges from prevention to amelioration by conservative means, including protection of pressure points, strengthening of muscles to improve

weight bearing, care of the feet, and the choice of proper shoes. Only when such measures fail should operation be contemplated.

Congenital Hallux Valgus

In the rare case of congenital hallux valgus there is usually abnormality of the distal phalanx as well. Such feet are by no means always painful, provided care is taken to choose shoes that are neither too short (in which case pressure on the toes causes premature callosities) nor too long and wide (when sliding movements within the shoe usually cause blisters on the skin).

If it is not possible to obtain properly fitting shoes, osteotomy of the neck of the first metatarsal may be required to improve the shape and direction of the hallux. It is often necessary to perform a medially based wedge osteotomy of the base of the distal phalanx as well, to overcome the deformity of the distal part of the toe. Occasionally the latter alone is required.

Hallux Valgus in Childhood

Some degree of hallux valgus exists in all human feet and there is a spectrum of variation in the general population. Those children who were born with a moderate degree of hallux valgus, usually accompanied by some degree of metatarsus primus varus, may have the condition aggravated if they suffer from pes planus as well. They tend to roll the forefoot into pronation because of the absence of the longitudinal arch, and consequently press the toe into an increasing valgus deformity. Any support of the longitudinal arch will prevent the latter complication.

The authors favor the use of the Helfet heel seat for this condition, for reasons which are explained in the section on flatfoot. The use of this heel support controls the hallux valgus satisfactorily and allows the toe to continue growing straight.

In Adolescents[2]

It is difficult to be sure if this condition is more common in young women than in men, but it is certain that more females request treatment. It may follow pes planus in childhood, but most cases in mid-adolescence are of the variety accompanied by marked metatarsus primus varus.

Poorly designed footwear may lead to symptoms of pain in the first metatarsophalangeal joint, even at this age. There may be a bunion. The prime task of the medical adviser is to persuade the patient to wear proper shoes. These should be of the correct length, and in particular, the width of the shoe must be adequate.

Physiotherapy, in the form of foot strengthening and toe mobilizing exercises, may help overcome the patient's symptoms, while the use of intraarticular steroid injections may sometimes be required to overcome traumatic synovitis in the first metatarsophalangeal joint.

Operation may be necessary for two reasons: to relieve painful symptoms, or for cosmetic purposes. The patient may be unable to obtain adequate shoes, despite every effort. It might be argued that the operation is required, not because of the abnormality of the foot, but because of the inability of a society to supply correct footwear for one of its members; in any event, economic considerations are a factor. The patient may request operation, even if there are no symptoms from the condition, because the shoes that can be worn are so unsightly as to constitute a real cause of distress. A woman, in particular, may be so sensitive about the shape of her feet that nothing can persuade her to show them in public. The cosmetic problems are by no means insignificant to the patient; the surgeon has to decide whether they justify surgery.

The authors feel that a young adult has the right to decide to undergo the discomfort and transient disability of a foot operation to improve the shape, provided all has been fully and carefully explained, with particular reference to the length of time required before full recovery takes place. A major problem for the surgeon is the possibility of some complication arising. If he does not mention this to the patient, he is being less than fair; if he overemphasizes the chances of infection, delayed wound healing, nonunion of the osteo-tomy, deep vein thrombosis, or the uncommon, but serious, problems resulting from anesthesia, he makes it difficult for the patient to make an objective decision.

The dilemma is capable of resolution only if the surgeon satisfies himself that the subject is not undergoing surgery for inadequate or neurotic motives. Some degree of narcissism is part of normal ego development in adolescence, but it may be converted to an abnormal hatred of a particular feature. The self-absorption common at this age sometimes shows itself in an unjustified sensitivity about hair color, or the shape of ear, nose, or, in this case, feet. The transient and illogical nature of such feelings makes them invalid reasons for operating. They may change arbitrarily and lead to an equally irrational disappointment with the results of operation.

The patient's youth is an advantage, for as a rule neither ligament stretching, subluxation, nor secondary degenerative changes are present within the metatarsophalangeal joint. The problem is one of the position of the toe in relation to the foot. Surgery can therefore be directed to "putting the toe on straight." This can be accomplished by performing osteotomy of the neck of the first metatarsal, just proximal to the joint, but not opening it.

Metatarsal neck osteotomy was described by Mitchell and Wilson.[3,4] Many variations have been reported,[5,6] but all are based on the same principle of straightening the toe and reducing the medial bony lump without opening the metatarsophalangeal joint. The Crawford-Adams procedure will be described.[7] One of the authors has performed over 100 such osteotomies. There has been no case of infection or nonunion; the only complication occurred in two patients, both adolescent and therefore still growing, who developed recurrent valgus deformity, despite union of the osteotomy.

The Crawford-Adams Osteotomy In this procedure (Fig. 11-10), a *wedge osteotomy* of the neck of the first metatarsal is performed: a medially based wedge of bone is excised, with its apex at the lateral cortex, just proximal to the capsular attachment of the joint. The angle

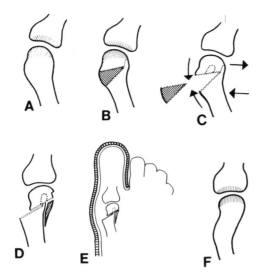

Fig. 11-10. Technique of the Crawford-Adams osteotomy. (*A*) The first metatarsophalangeal joint before operation. (*B*) A medially based wedge is cut in the neck of the metatarsal and a lateral spike is left in the proximal phalanx. (*C*) The wedge is removed and the distal fragment tilted to overcome the valgus deformity of the toe (*curved arrows*) and displaced laterally to correct metatarsus primus varus. (*D*) The excised bone is broken up and packed laterally around the osteotomy site. (*E*) The shape and position of the plaster-of-Paris splint. (*F*) The result, after union of the osteotomy.

of the apex is carefully measured to be exactly that required to straighten the toe. A spike of bone is fashioned from the lateral point of the proximal fragment of the metatarsal shaft. A hole is drilled into the medial part of the metatarsal head. The osteotomy is completed, and the wedge is closed; at the same time, the head is displaced laterally and the spike fitted into the drill hole in the metatarsal head.

In this way, the toe is straightened the medial bony projection sunk into the foot by lateral displacement of the head, and the osteotomy fixed by the spike; so that no screw, wire, or complicated form of immobilization is required. The only splinting needed is a U-shaped plaster-of-Paris slab, molded into varus to maintain the position of the toe. (Fig. 11-10E).

The patient bears no weight on the foot for 10 to 12 days, after which the splint is changed and the sutures removed. He is allowed to walk in soft shoes until the osteotomy has united, 6 weeks after operation. Thereafter,

rehabilitation follows a course similar to that in other operations on the hallux.

In Adults

Once secondary changes have begun within the joint, osteotomy to straighten the toe is no longer adequate to overcome the pain.

The "Spoke-Shave" Operation. In young women, particularly; before the valgus is too severe, and while the main problem is the presence of a bunion; excision of the medial bony lump alone may put an end, for a time, to the inflammatory bursitis. It is a simple operation, satisfactory in carefully selected cases, but the surgeon must make it plain that the valgus distortion of the toe has not been changed, and the process of subluxation, tendon bow-stringing, and osteoarthritis will continue, so that a second operation may be required later in life.

Combined Operations. Many combinations of soft-tissue and bone procedures have been advocated. All are capable of giving good results if carefully planned and competently performed. None is invariably successful. Apart from nonunion of osteotomies and infection of the wound, there is one complication that is worthy of mention:

A common feature of the combined procedure in the adult hallux valgus is basal osteotomy of the first metatarsal to overcome the common, underlying metatarsus primus varus.[8] Normal function of the transverse metatarsal arch depends largely upon weight bearing by the first metatarsal head. After osteotomy of the base of the first metatarsal, the shaft of the bone can be displaced upward, so that the head no longer reaches the ground. Within a few months, severe metatarsalgia sets in beneath the heads of the second, third, fourth, and fifth metatarsal heads, progressively; a most unfortunate outcome of the surgery. Kilikian regards this complication as so serious that he advocated that basal osteotomy of the first metatarsal should never be performed.

Figure 11-11 shows, in diagrammatic fashion, the combined operation of basal osteotomy and excision of the medial exostosis.

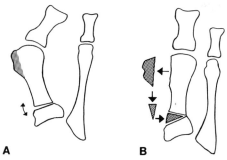

Fig. 11-11. Excision of the exostosis and basal osteotomy of the first metatarsal. (*A*) An opening osteotomy of the base. (*B*) Excision of the exostosis; the bone is trimmed and inserted into the osteotomy as a bone graft.

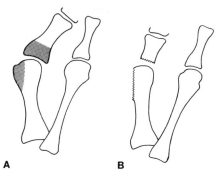

Fig. 11-12. Keller's arthroplasty. (*A*) The amount of bone to be removed from the metatarsal head and the base of the phalanx is shown. (*B*) The postoperative position of the bones.

Osteotomy can similarly be combined with tendon transplant or with excision arthroplasty. None of these operations should be attempted by the occasional surgeon.

Keller's Arthroplasty. The wide choice of operations available to the surgeon is an unhappy reminder that no operation is generally applicable or universally successful. A basic requirement of surgery remains: if a shoe cannot fit the foot, the foot must be shaped to fit a shoe.

Correction of the valgus deformity is common to all procedures. Excision arthroplasty has a further effect: when the toe is shortened the bow-stringing effect of the tendons is overcome, and the deformity does not recur. Provided the operation succeeds, the toe will remain comfortable for the rest of the patient's life. The authors find that Keller's operation is the simplest to perform, and in their hands they find it successful in most cases. It must be emphasized that orthopaedic surgical opinion is not unanimous on this point.

Keller described the operation in 1904.[9] In essence, it consists of excision of the base of the proximal phalanx to create an excision arthroplasty; that is, a loose, fibrous joint in which the gap between the bones is sufficient to prevent bone meeting bone. It soon fills with hematoma, which is converted to fibrous tissue. The medial third of the head of the first metatarsal is then removed, including the so-called exostosis that develops in this region in hallux valgus (Fig. 11-12).

Preoperatively, the procedure is explained to the patient, with particular emphasis on his or her role in the postoperative recovery of muscle power and movement by conscientious exercise. A reasonable plan consists of 2 weeks' rest with elevated foot, the patient being allowed up for toilet and gentle indoor walking with the weight borne on the heel of the affected foot; 2 weeks with firm bandaging in soft shoes, but with the patient able to leave the house; and 2 weeks to get back into conventional shoes.

TECHNIQUE. The operator stands at the foot of the table, and a dorsal, curved incision is made, medial to the long extensor tendon, down to bone. It extends from the shaft of the first metatarsal, through the metatarsophalangeal joint, and well into the shaft of the proximal phalanx. The soft tissues are reflected medially, to expose the exostosis on the metatarsal head. Spikes are passed around the base of the proximal phalanx, and the capsule is detached from it, the toe being progressively flexed until it is circumferentially exposed. The base is excised by transverse cross-section of bone, approximately 1 cm. distal to the joint. Care is taken to prevent injury to the flexor hallucis longus tendon on its plantar aspect.

The toe is held in flexion, and the medial third of the head of the metatarsal is excised with an osteotome; inadvertent fracture of the metatarsal shaft and damage to the circumferential artery that runs around the neck from its inferior surface are carefully avoided. The extensor tendon is then lengthened and the wound sutured in layers while the assistant holds the toe straight.

After operation, the toe, which should maintain its position without support, is carefully bandaged, to hold it in that position. On rare occasions this is achieved by inserting a Kirschner wire across the joint, but it has the side-effect of preventing early mobilization and should be removed after 21 days to allow rehabilitation to take place. A 4-inch crepe (Ace) bandage is used, beginning around the forefoot, and thence around the hallux to fix it in a straight position, in slight plantar flexion. The bandage is then brought around the ankle to prevent slipping. Several layers can be applied, but there is no reason to make it too tight. It merely causes pain and may damage the skin flap.

The patient is advised to keep the foot elevated and begin early calf exercises to prevent venous thrombosis. He may sit in a chair next day, and can begin bearing weight on the heel, assisted by crutches, when the foot is comfortable. After bilateral operation, this is seldom achieved before the 8th day. Weight bearing should be restricted until the wound has healed, but from the day after operation, the patient should be instructed to practice active plantar flexion. This is a difficult movement to regain with any strength. In climbing, walking, or other sports where powerful propulsion is required, there is strong plantar flexion of the first toe.

Dorsiflexion is basically a passive movement during walking, and recovery of this movement is best accomplished by passive stretching when the wound has healed.

The plantar flexion exercises should have an isometric element; that is, the patient should feel that the toe is being shortened against the resistance of the bandage as it is flexed. The object of the exercises is a firm, fibrous union of exactly the right length, and this is achieved by adaptive shortening of the long flexor and extensor tendons, which is evident when stable, powerful movement is possible.

COMPLICATIONS OF KELLER'S OPERATION. Not all patients are satisfied with the procedure.

Too Much Shortening. If too much bone is removed from the base of the phalanx, the patient is left with a floppy toe and persistent weakness (Fig. 11-13). Although the pain is relieved and a normal shoe can be worn, this is not a good outcome of the operation.

Relative Lenghtening of the Second Toe. If the second toe was the longest before operation, the patient may be left with a toe that is so long that it soon undergoes hammer deformity, requiring a second operation. For this reason, it is sometimes necessary to shorten the second toe and perform arthrodesis at the time of the Keller's operation, even if there is no deformity of the toe.

The Dorsally-Displaced Hallux. Excision arthroplasty always causes readjustment of the tone of the associated tendons. If the extensor tendon is not lengthened, the patient is left with an unpleasant-looking, dorsally displaced phalanx. This responds to subcutaneous extensor tenotomy.

Rotational Deformity. In some cases, the intrinsic muscles of the foot can rotate the toe so that the nail is pressed against the ground. Bandaging can overcome this deformity, but the occasional case requires lateral intrinsic tenotomy at the time of operation.

Sudeck's Atrophy is moderately common in the foot following any operation, and leads to persistent redness, pain, swelling, and stiffness (see Swollen Feet, Chap. 19).

HALLUX RIGIDUS

The second common disorder of the metarsophalangeal joint of the big toe is hallux rigidus. The term denotes a clinical syndrome that usually begins in early adult life and runs a course of increasing signs and symptoms, leading to considerable disability. The pathology is one of osteoarthritis, manifesting in a characteristic way.

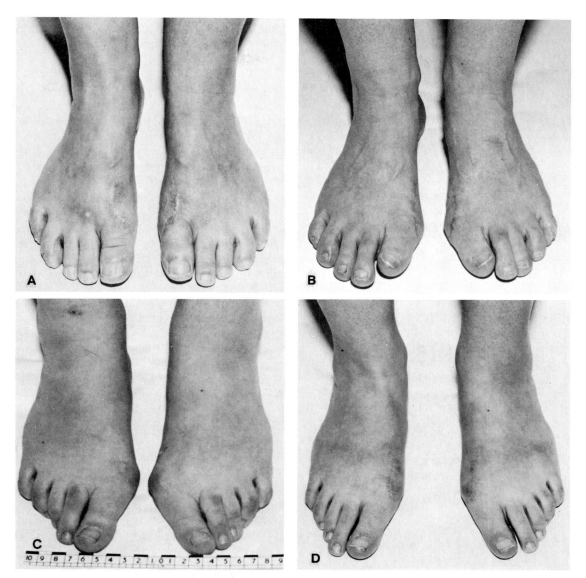

Fig. 11-13. (*A*) The result of Keller's arthroplasty—the toes are straight and comfortable. (*B*) The result of a Keller's operation that left both big toes, especially the left, short and medially rotated. The second toes are now the longest. (*C*) Another case of bilateral hallux valgus before operation. (*D*) The same case after operation.

ETIOLOGY[10]

In the authors' experience, the syndrome is equally common in men and women, suggesting, perhaps, that the cause of the joint degenration is different from that in hallux valgus. Since florid cases are seen as early as the end of the third decade, it is probable that in many cases, if not most, it begins in adolescence.

From the way the condition develops, it is likely that the primary lesion generally occurs in the head of the metatarsal (Fig. 11-14). What evidence is available suggests that the damage to the articular cartilage of the head is traumatic in origin. Occasionally, the patient gives a history of a specific injury, but it is more common for the doctor to hear a story of

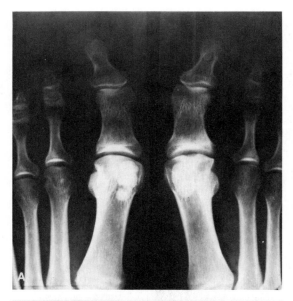

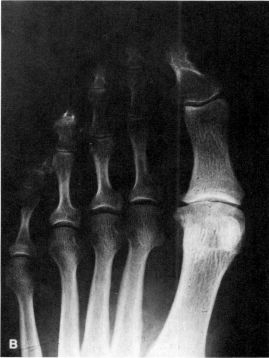

Fig. 11-14. Hallux rigidus. (*A*) Radiograph of a foot in which the epiphyses have recently fused shows a typical osteochondral defect of the head of the first metatarsal, as described by McMaster. (*B*) A similar case, years later, with developing osteophytes, especially laterally, but dorsally as well.

multiple minor injuries. Teenagers playing constant football, or running habitually in soft shoes, are at risk, as are ballet dancers.

PATHOGENESIS

The adolescent may complain of pain and intermittent swelling of the first metatarsophalangeal joint. Often this recurs with each episode of hard physical activity and settles with rest. There is seldom any radiographic change in the first metatarsal head to begin with. Later, changes are clearly visible. McMaster, in an excellent article, describes a characteristic lesion on the apex of the dome of the metatarsal head, extending onto its dorsal margin.[2] It consists of a flap of articular cartilage. The process is one of posttraumatic osteochondritis dissecans. In some cases the toe remains clinically normal, but in others the base of the proximal phalanx becomes distorted because of wear. Years later, the resulting incongruity of the joint surfaces leads to a pattern of erosion of the articular cartilage of both surfaces of the joint. The process of osteoarthritis, once begun, runs its inevitable course: further loss of articular cartilage, development of osteophytes and recurrent inflammation, leading to fibrosis of the capsule. The result is increasing pain and stiffness in the joint.

The development of the deformity has a typical pattern. The edge of the base of the phalanx develops a circumferential rim of osteophytes, and the characteristic lesion is the formation of a dorsal crown of osteophytes on the metatarsal head. In time, such osteophytes pile up until a transverse ridge of bone can be felt through the overlying skin. Pressure on this ridge by the patient's shoe leads to the development of a dorsal bursa, itself a cause of pain. The pattern of deformity in the osteoarthritic process of hallux rigidus is different from that occurring in hallux valgus. In the latter condition, the state of the joint is one of increasing instability, while in hallux rigidus, the joint becomes increasingly rigid. The rigidity follows a characteristic pattern, probably dependent on the original crushing lesion of the metatarsal head. The normal metatarsophalangeal joint has an arc of flexion-extension of about 90 degrees; flexion being, in most cases, about 10 degrees and extension, 80 degrees (Fig. 11-15).

Passive extension (or dorsiflexion, as it is commonly called) is the most important movement of the joint, since it is on this that the normal take-off depends during walking. Unfortunately, dorsiflexion is gradually lost in hallux rigidus. As a consequence, the patient develops pain on walking at an early stage. At first the loss of dorsiflexion is just a few degrees, and the pain is present only at the extreme of passive dorsiflexion, but gradual dorsal fibrosis and osteophyte formation progressively decreases the dorsal arc of movement. Episodes of pain are more frequent.

The full-blown clinical picture is one of complete loss of dorsiflexion of the first metatarsophalangeal joint, leading, in many cases, to a fixed plantar flexion (Fig. 11-16). This is associated with a large, dorsal, transverse ridge of osteophytes with an overlying traumatic bursitis. Any attempt at normal gait is impossible, and the patient has a constant limp. Ultimately, abnormal strain is placed on the inferior capsule of the interphalangeal joint of the big toe. The capsule becomes stretched by constant passive dorsiflexion during walking. The toe adopts a characteristic posture of abnormal dorsiflexion at rest, indicative of the degree of unstable passive hyperextension during walking.

Such a florid deformity of the big toe, occurring as it does in healthy young adults, usually requires treatment.

SURGICAL TREATMENT

Pain from hallux valgus is due to passive dorsiflexion while walking. The patient can proceed comfortably only by hobbling on the heel. A transverse metatarsal bar on the sole of the shoe (Fig. 11-17) will result in a calcaneal gait, but it is functionally not comfortable for long, and few patients can put up with such a bar permanently. Operation is the only alter-

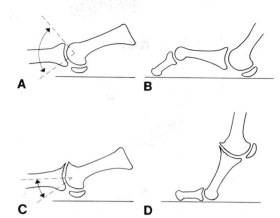

Fig. 11-15. Hallux rigidus. (*A*) The curved arrows show the normal range of extension and flexion of the metatarsophalangeal joint seen from the side. (*B*) The position of the joint when the patient is standing on tiptoe, bearing weight on the metatarsal head and the tip of the toe. (*C*) The range of motion in hallux rigidus is limited; dorsiflexion is lost. (*D*) The patient can stand on tiptoe only by hyperextending the interphalangeal joint.

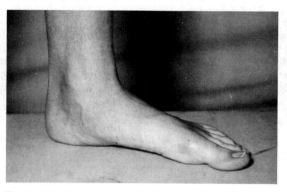

Fig. 11-16. An example of early loss of dorsiflexion of the big toe.

native. Three procedures are available; each has its advocates.

Kessel Osteotomy[11]

Kessel described a dorsally based wedge osteotomy of the base of the proximal phalanx (Fig. 11-18).[12] By closing the wedge the proximal phalanx is angulated dorsally. By this means the reduced arc of movement is transferred to a more useful range for passive dorsiflexion. Provided secondary osteoarthritic changes are not severe, osteotomy has

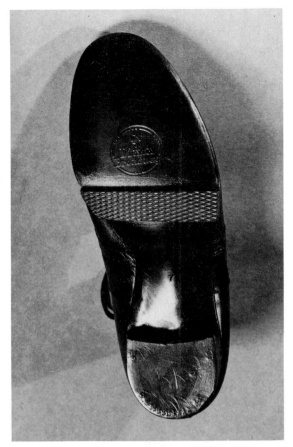

Fig. 11-17. A transverse metatarsal bar has been added to the sole of this shoe.

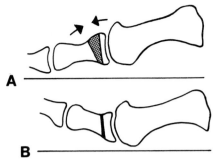

Fig. 11-18. Kessel osteotomy of the proximal phalanx. (*A*) A lateral view of the hallux shows the site of a dorsally based osteotomy. (*B*) After removal of the wedge, the osteotomy is closed to hyperextend the toe.

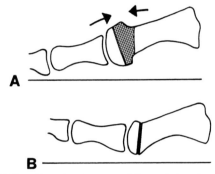

Fig. 11-19. Dorsal osteotomy of the metatarsal neck. (*A*) The dorsally based wedge. (*B*) After closure of the osteotomy.

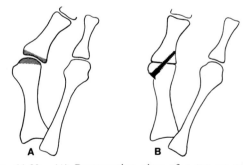

Fig. 11-20. (*A*) Preoperative view of a toe on which arthrodesis was performed. Excision of the articular cartilage of the joint was followed by screw fixation (*B*).

a useful place in the treatment of hallux rigidus. A second operation may be required later.

Dorsal osteotomy of the metatarsal neck may also be performed (Fig. 11-19) but it is technically more difficult and may affect the weight-bearing ability of the transverse arch leading to metatarsalgia.

Arthodesis

Many orthopaedic surgeons have held the opinion that arthrodesis (Fig. 11-20) is the only operation that works in hallux rigidus.[13] It is certainly true that arthrodesis offers certain advantages. Bony fusion of the joint overcomes the pain completely; the toe is stable and strong. Professional soccer players, for example, require arhtrodesis to enable them to kick a football. The procedure has its problems. It does not always succeed, and there is no foot more painful than that with a failed bone fusion. Repeated grafts may be necessary to overcome this complication.

For arthrodesis to be comfortable, the joint must be fixed in some degree of dorsiflexion: otherwise, the take-off phase of walking can only take place by abnormal hyperextension of the interphalangeal joint. There is no difficulty in fixing the toe at the correct angle of dorsiflexion, but this entails its being dorsally angulated for life. Shoes must at least have soft uppers and, especially, soft toe caps. Sometimes custom-made shoes are required.

Keller's Operation

If the authors' experience, Keller's arthroplasty is a perfectly satisfactory operation to overcome hallux rigidus, provided care is taken to trim all dorsal (and, in some cases, laterally circumferential) osteophytes from the metatarsal head. At times, arthroplasty appears to be more successful in hallux rigidus than in hallux valgus, provided the operation is performed meticulously, and careful physiotherapy and rehabilitation are used to bring about a reasonable degree of passive dorsiflexion.

VARUS DEFORMITY OF THE FIFTH TOE

Congenital varus deformity of the fifth toe is more common in males than in females (Fig. 11-21). It is usually associated with large feet with wide transverse arches and spread metatarsals. Just as the metatarsus primus varus results in hallux valgus, the fifth toe is often packed into marked varus. This foot shape is a normal variant, but the wearing of shoes may easily cause pressure on the lateral side of the fifth metatarsal head, with consequent bursa formation; hence the name *bunionette* for the condition.

Suitable shoes may be very difficult to find, and operation may be necessary. Excision of the fifth metatarsal head removes the lump, but it leaves a floppy fifth toe, with pressure points, and the authors regard such an operation as deforming and do not recommend it.

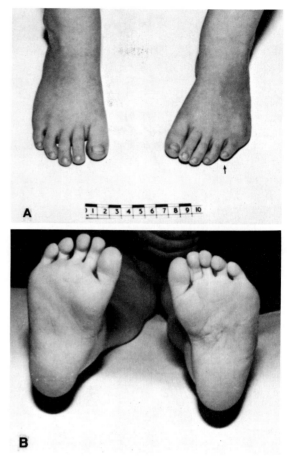

Fig. 11-21. Congenital varus deformity of the fifth toe. (*A*) Dorsal view of both feet. The left little toe is affected (*arrow*). (*B*) Plantar view of the "bunionette."

Osteotomy of the neck of the fifth metatarsal, on the other hand, gives a highly satisfactory result.[14] Performed through a small dorsal incision, an oblique osteotomy (similar to Wilson's osteotomy of the first metatarsal neck) allows the toe to be straightened immediately. The position can be retained merely by postoperative bandaging with the toe straight. The patient requires bandaging for 4 weeks for union to take place, but is allowed to bear weight, wearing a soft slipper, after 4 or 5 days.

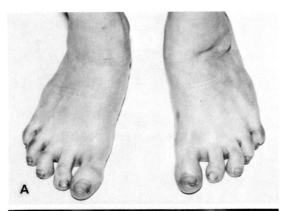

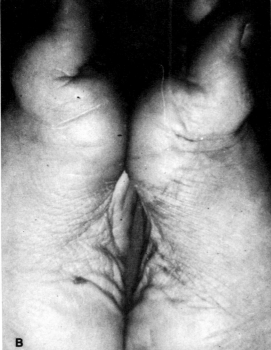

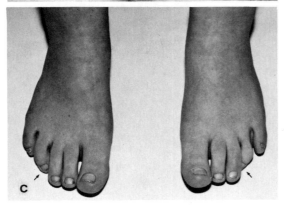

Fig. 11-22.   Variations in the shape of toes. (*A*) Congenital curly toes. (*B*) Congenitally clawed big toes. (*C*) Congenitally long, varus fourth toes, worse on the left (*arrow*) than on the right.

OTHER TOE ABNORMALITIES

Variation in the shape, mobility, and function of the toes is very common, occurring more often and with greater severity from the medial to the lateral side of the foot (Fig. 11-22). The causes are manifold, ranging from a familial tendency alone to severe secondary deformities, depending on extrinsic factors in the rest of the foot (such as neurologic imbalance) or external pressure on the foot itself. Variations or deformities may be described as mobile or fixed. They may have been present at birth or acquired later.

CONGENITAL DEFORMITIES OF THE TOES

Partial or Complete Absence

Any variation of aplasia or hypoplasia of the toes may occur, either individually or as part of a general digital abnormality of the hands and feet. Figure 11-23 shows a child born with abnormalities of the fingers and toes. There were severe cutaneous fibrous constriction rings around the ankles. These were treated by plastic surgery, in which the scar was excised and the constriction overcome by Z-plasty.

Such variations of the toes are usually of little practical importance, except cosmetically, unless one or more toes projects far ahead of the others, giving rise to pressure effects in normal shoes. Surgical trimming may be required for ease in fitting footwear. Cosmetic improvement can be obtained at the same time.

Syndactyly

Partial or complete fusion of toes occurs commonly, usually between the second and third. It does not usually extend as far as the distal phalanges, and is of no significance to the patient, unless accompanied by abnormal shape of the toes.

Polydactyly

Duplication of the Hallux. This condition, present from birth, is immediately obvious to the parents, who usually press the surgeon to do something active. There may be duplication of the terminal part only of the distal phalanx or of both phalanges of the toe. The mildest cases may be of duplication of the nail with its underlying bed, or even merely of a wide, flattened, unpleasant-looking distal phalanx and a longitudinal ridge or groove on the nail. Most cases need surgical treatment of some sort, either to prevent pressure on an abnormally shaped toe, or for cosmetic reasons.

In complete duplication of the hallux, surgical excision may be simple, but the broad, flattened, duplicated toenail may require a carefully planned plastic surgical procedure by an experienced specialist. There are no symptoms from the abnormality itself, provided care is taken with the fitting of shoes.

The Sixth Toe. Many children are born with a sixth toe on one or both feet. The extra digit may vary in size, from a small fragment of tissue, without bony structure but surmounted by a spike of nail, to a completely normal extra toe. The latter may fit neatly with the other toes into a normal shoe, but in many cases, the sixth toe projects from the rest of the foot, either at the level of the metatarsal head which is duplicated or even, occasionally, from the base of the fifth metatarsal.

A vestigial sixth toe may simply be brushed off the feet at birth by a wise midwife or obstetrician, in which case the parents may never be aware of the condition. An anatomically complete, projecting toe may require planned amputation under general anesthesia and bloodless field. This is probably best performed when the child is 3 months old, but certainly before the age when shoes are fitted. This minor abnormality carries an extraordinary stigma in the eyes of many people, and the parents are only too eager, as a rule, to have the operation performed.

Abnormalities of the Packing of the Toes

Minor abnormalities in the shape and size of the individual toes do not affect the function

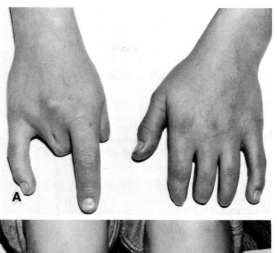
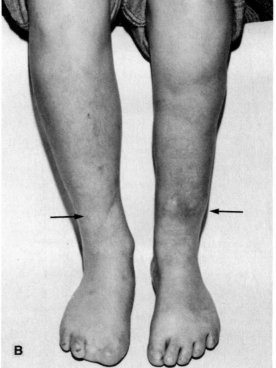

Fig. 11-23. (*A*) Congenital abnormalities of the fingers. (*B*) The legs in the same case. The arrows indicate the circumferential scars following plastic surgery for congenital constriction rings in the calves.

of walking. In the end, however, such abnormalities do give rise to symptoms owing to pressure from shoes. What is required of the five toes is that they fit together "like a good bunch of bananas" within the toe cap of the shoe. Of the many congenital variations in the shape of the packed toes that give rise to pressure, three are most common.

Mallet Deformity of the Distal Phalanx (Fig. 11-24) Congenital flexion contracture of the distal phalanx of the second or third toe is usually associated with a long toe. The second toe is normally longer than the rest, but the fixed flexion deformity is not due to pressure and may be seen soon after birth. What may be called the mallet deformity of the toe may give rise to pressure symptoms in childhood, or they may be delayed until adult life.

In the end, the patient develops a terminal callosity on the tip of the toe and distortion of the shape of the nail, which is either lifted up or pressed flat, depending on where the weight is borne. Treatment is by operation. Either the tip of the toe is amputated or, if the patient wants to retain the nail, and the nail bed has not been too severely distorted, arthrodesis of the terminal phalangeal joint (after wedge excision of the joint) is carried out to overcome the mallet deformity. Arthrodesis in this way has the advantage of shortening the toe as well as straightening it.

The Varus Underriding Toe. The fourth toe, or in some cases the third, may come to lie habitually beneath the next toe on walking (Fig. 11-25). Pressure on one or another of the adjacent toes is inevitable because of the wearing of shoes.

The basic abnormality is not only the flexion and varus deformity of the underriding toe, but also that the medial, adjacent toe does not pack neatly against it. It is as though there are two independent "bunches of bananas," the one consisting of the first, second and third toes, and the other of the fourth and fifth. The two "bunches" are mutually incompatible within the shoe.

In the authors' view, attempts at splinting the toe to overcome the deformity do not work, and operative correction of the underriding toe is required.[15] This should be undertaken whenever the symptoms of pressure warrant it. Usually this is in childhood or adolescence in severe cases, but minor degrees

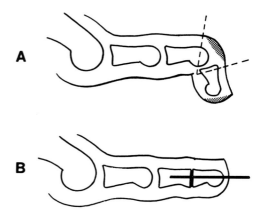

Fig. 11-24. (A) Diagram of a mallet deformity of the distal phalanx. (The strippled line indicates the wedge to be excised for distal interphalangeal arthrodesis.) (B) The postoperative position with the Kirschner wire in situ.

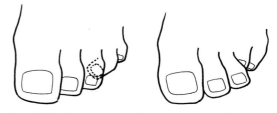

Fig. 11-25. Two varieties of underlying varus fourth toes.

of the condition may not require surgery until later.

The Congenitally Overriding Fifth Toe (Fig. 11-26). Congenital dislocation of the fifth toe is usually bilateral, although one side may be much more severe than the other. Often there is a family history of the condition. An interesting feature is that, despite the uselessness of the little toe and its severe displacement, many patients are in no hurry to have it operated upon, unless they develop pressure from shoes. In the end, most come to surgery.[17]

The operation is by no means straightforward, unless the toe is merely amputated. Since removal of the toe leaves a poor cosmetic result because of prominence of the fourth toe, it should not be performed unless other procedures have failed.

At operation, all elements of the toe that contribute to the deformity require correction.

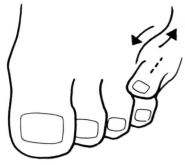

Fig. 11-26. The congenitally overriding fifth toe. The arrows indicate how the skin flaps should be slid to avoid postoperative contracture.

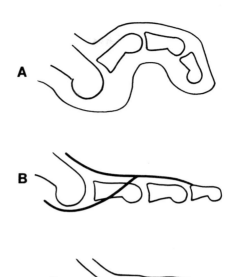

Fig. 11-27. (*A*) Clawtoe deformity. (*B*) The effect of flexor-extensor tendon transplant. (*C*) Arthrodesis of the interphalangeal joint and excision of the metatarsal head.

The extensor tendon is lengthened, and total circumferential capsulotomy of the fifth metatarsophalangeal joint is performed. The toe can then usually be brought to lie next to the fourth, but the base of the proximal phalanx may have become so splayed by the habitually dislocated position that, in its new situation, it forms a bony lump. Occasionally, excision of the base of the proximal phalanx is necessary, but it leaves a loose, floppy toe that is easily displaced.

Attention must be given to the skin on the dorsum of the fifth metatarsophalangeal joint, through which the incision has been made. This skin may easily become a deforming force since it, too, is contracted. Care must be taken in the placing of the incision, and it must be sutured without contracture, either by means of a V–Y-flap[16] or a sliding Z-flap.

For the outcome to be successful, at the end of the operation the fifth toe must lie easily next to the fourth, without any tendency to dislocate dorsally.

ACQUIRED DEFORMITIES OF THE TOES

The Clawtoe

The two common patterns of fixed deformity in the toes differ in their etiology. Clawing of the toes (Fig. 11-27) results from neuromuscular imbalance between the extrinsic and intrinsic muscles of the feet. Many causes of upper motor neuron paralysis of the legs result in clawtoes, as one of the variants of muscle disease. In pes cavus, a high longitudinal arch and dropped metatarsal transverse arch is accompanied by typical clawing of the toes. In children and young adults, the toes may be mobile or at least capable of passive stretching. Later the deformities become fixed, with resulting pressure points at the areas of vulnerability within the shoe; that is, there is usually a thick callosity beneath the metatarsal head and a corn on the tip of the toe. Tight shoes may cause a third callosity on the dorsum.

Conservative management is by meticulous chiropody and carefully fitted shoes which, in severe cases of clawing, often must be custom made. Figure 11-27 shows that, as well as fixed flexion deformities of the interphalangeal joints, the condition includes hyperextension of the metatarsophalangeal joint. Surgical correction must deal with the proximal joint of the toe as well.

The Haig Forefoot Suspension. The Forefoot Suspension devised by Dr. Armen Haig* is of

*Haig Suspension supplied by Yorke Dynamold Shoes, Inc., 118-07 Queens Boulevard, Forrest Hills, N.Y. 11375.

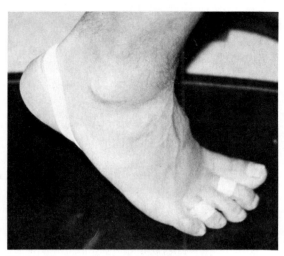

Fig. 11-28. The Haig forefoot suspension.

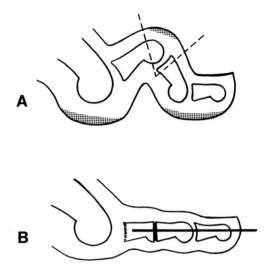

Fig. 11-29. Hammer toe. (*A*) A diagram to show the deformity indicates the pressure areas. The stippled lines show the amount to be excised for proximal interphalangeal arthrodesis. (*B*) Excision of the base of the proximal phalanx and arthrodesis of the proximal interphalangeal joint, held with a Kirschner wire.

considerable value in the treatment of metatarsalgia due to clawtoes. It is, in principle, a dynamic replacement of the action of the interossei muscles (see Dysfunction, Chap. 5).

An oblong piece of soft material under the ball and arch of the foot anchors non elastic toe-retaining loops for the second and fourth toes. An elastic loop from the base of the pad encircles the heel under medium tension.

In walking, tension is transmitted to the toe loops as the heel rises, so extending the proximal interphalangeal joints (Fig. 11-28). The device, therefore, reinforces the plantar aponeurosis and the extensors of the interphalangeal joints. Weight is distributed, as it should be, to the ball of the foot and the straightened toes.

In mobile toes, operation is directed to restoring the balance of the muscle tone. (See Pes Cavus, Chap. 10). When the deformity is fixed, the interphalangeal joints are straightened and arthrodesis is performed, the toe being fixed by the insertion of an intramedullary Kirschner wire. The metatarsophalangeal joint requires mobilization, not stiffening. In some cases, extensor tenotomy and capsulotomy is sufficient, but excision arthroplasty may be necessary, either by removal of the base of the proximal phalanx or even, occasionally, by excision of the metatarsal head.

The Hammer Toe. Figure 11-29 shows the deformity usually described as hammer toe. It is caused by external compression; in particular, of a long second toe (see Hallux Valgus, Chap. 11). The collapsed metatarsal head causes hyperextension of the metatarsophalangeal joint. The pattern of deformity is thus, typically, fixed hyperextension, leading to dislocation of the metatarsophalangeal joint and hyperflexion of the proximal and hyperextension of the distal interphalangeal joint.

Surgical treatment is, again, by arthrodesis and straightening of the proximal (and, if necessary, of the distal) interphalangeal joint, while the metatarsophalangeal joint must be mobilized, either by soft-tissue correction or by excision arthroplasty.

REFERENCES

1. Kelikian, H.: Hallux Valgus and Allied Deformities of the Forefoot. Philadelphia, W. B. Saunders, 1965.
2. Cholmeley, J. A.: Hallux Valgus in Adolescents. Proc. Roy. Soc. Med., *51:*903, 1958.
3. Mitchell, C. L., Fleming, J. L. Allen, R., Glenny, C., and Sandford, G. A.: Osteotomy bunionectomy for hallux valgus. J. Bone Joint Surg., *40A:*4, 1958.

4. Wilson, J. N.: Oblique displacement osteotomy for hallux valgus. J. Bone Joint Surg., *45B:*552, 1963.

5. Gibson, J., and Piggott, H.: Osteotomy of the neck of the first metatarsal in the treatment of hallux valgus. J. Bone Joint Surg., *44B:*349, 1962.

6. Carr, C. R., and Boyd, B. M.: Corrective osteotomy for metatarsus primus. J. Bone Joint Surg. *50A:*1353, 1968.

7. Adams, J. C.: Osteotomy of first metatarsal neck for hallux valgus (discussion). J. Bone Joint Surg., *49B:*197, 1971.

8. Bonney, G., and MacNab, I.: Hallux valgus and hallux rigidus. J. Bone Joint Surg., *34B:* 366, 1952.

9. Keller, W. L.: Surgical treatment of bunions and hallux valgus. New York Med. J.: *80:*741, 1904.

10. Goodfellow, J.: Aetiology of hallux rigidus. Proc. Roy. Soc. Med., *59:*821, 1966.

11. Kessel, L., and Bonney, G.: Hallux rigidus in the adolescent. J. Bone Joint Surg., *40B:*668, 1958.

12. Heaney, S. H.: Phalangeal osteotomy for hallux rigidus. J. Bone Joint Surg., *52B:*799, 1970.

13. Harrison, M. H. H., and Harvey, F. J.: Arthrodesis of the first metatarsophalangeal joint for hallux valgus and hallux rigidus. J. Bone Joint Surg., *45A:*471, 1963.

14. Leach, R. E., and Igou, R.: Metatarsal osteotomy for bunionette deformity. Clin. Orthop., *100:*171, 1974.

15. Sweetnam, D. R.: Congenital curly toes. An investigation into the value of treatment. Lancet, *II:*398, 1958.

16. Wilson, N. N.: V-Y correction of varus deformity of the fifth toe. Brit. J. Surg., *41:*133, 1953.

17. Cockin, J.: Butler's operation for an overriding fifth toe. J. Bone Joint Surg., *60B:*78, 1968.

12 Other Painful Conditions of the Feet

The foot is a complex structure, and any of its anatomical constituents—skin or bone, tendons, tendon sheaths, bursas, or joints—may give rise to pain. The diagnosis of the cause, whether traumatic, inflammatory, degenerative, or neoplastic disease, depends upon the taking of a detailed history and on precise examination of the foot.

TRAUMATIC LESIONS

The Achilles Tendon

There is no synovial sheath around the Achilles tendon; merely a fine, fibrous structure, the paratenon, loosely attached to it. This paratenon is capable of inflammatory reaction similar to, but less florid than, true tenosynovitis. It may result from direct or indirect injury. The patient feels pain when the calf muscle is contracted on walking, especially on slopes and stairs. On examination, local tenderness is elicited at the site of injury. The sheath of the tendon may be swollen.

Sub-Achilles Bursitis. This condition, always due to an indirect injury such as repeated irritation following unusual amounts of walking, may be misdiagnosed as paratendinitis.

Treatment is similar to that of other inflammations of fibrous tendon sheaths: rest, aided by a firm elastic bandage and a raised heel on the shoe or steroid injection around, but not into, the tendon. Physical therapy, such as ultrasound, may be beneficial because the tendon is near the surface.

Injury to the Musculotendinous Junction. Avulsion of fibers at the musculotendinous junction of the Achilles tendon is the usual manner of disruption of the calf muscles. The medial head of the gastrocnemius is more frequently involved than the lateral. Avulsion may occur during normal activity, but more often during an unusually strenuous physical effort, such as lifting an unexpectedly heavy object, playing a difficult shot at tennis, or suddenly stretching the muscle by a slip on the floor or a stair. The patient feels as if he has been struck on the calf, turns around, and is astonished to see no one there. Injuries to the muscle occur mostly in the younger age groups; tendon rupture, (described below) more often in people over the age of 35.

Muscle avulsions are never complete and are usually limited to one side of the calf, most often the medial, so the lopsided calf simplifies the diagnosis. Swelling is almost immediate, and ecchymosis tracks down the calf, becoming visible under the skin a few days later.

The patient finds it too painful to put the heel to the ground, and can hardly walk. With rest, the tear will heal, although the calf will never return to its former shape completely. Strapping the leg, raising the heel, and injecting local anesthetic to overcome the pain, followed by physical therapy, will accelerate recovery.

138

Rupture of the Achilles Tendon. Disruption of the tendon usually takes place approximately 2.5 to 5 cm. above its insertion into the calcaneus. When the swelling subsides, the gap, by then only slightly tender, is palpable. The deep flexor muscles can provide only limited power for plantar flexion, and this is reflected in the push-off phase of walking and in a rather shuffling gait. The heel hardly leaves the ground.

Complete rupture of the tendon may result from direct trauma, but it also happens occasionally in healthy athletes at a time of extreme fatigue. Patients on corticosteroid medication are also subject to sudden disruptions due to fibrous tissue softening. Most cases, however, result from indirect trauma during sporting activity.

As is only to be expected from the largest tendon in the body, and the one that bears the full weight on active exercise, the Achilles tendon does not rupture without signalling the event by immediate pain to the unfortunate sufferer. The story is such a common one that most medical practitioners have encountered cases. A healthy man or woman, often in the late thirties or early forties, is exercising vigorously. Often the patient has taken up some sport after years of inactivity. Suddenly, a sensation likened to a blow on the back of the ankle, (or even, occasionally, described as a feeling of being shot in the leg) is experienced. The patient is stopped in his or her tracks and can walk only with great difficulty, and with a limp. The older the patient, the less the force required to rupture the Achilles tendon.

Total rupture causes less pain, local tenderness, or immediate disability than partial tears or avulsions of muscle fibers. Whereas a sufferer from a partial tear seeks medical attention within a short time, a complete tear may not be diagnosed until the swelling and bruising have subsided, days or weeks later. There is often a delay before a doctor is seen, and—even more surprising—the lesion is not always diagnosed at the first visit. This happens if the calf is not adequately examined at the time.

To diagnose rupture of the Achilles tendon,

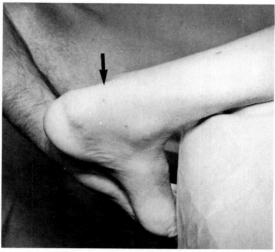

Fig. 12-1. Photograph of the left leg of a patient with a ruptured Achilles tendon. The arrow indicates the defect in the tendon. A circumferential hematoma is present around the heel. The tone of the calf muscle is lost.

the patient should be examined in the prone position. Unless the leg is examined immediately after the injury, local edema is present. The hematoma extends gradually down to the foot around the heel because of the effect of gravity (Fig. 12-1). It subsides in a week or two. The swelling persists for many weeks, but in the end it, too, disappears.

In late cases, the gap in the Achilles tendon is often obvious at a glance. It is possible to palpate this gap immediately after the rupture and, whatever the extent of the edema, the defect remains palpable.

The diagnosis is confirmed by the muscle squeeze test described by Thompson and Doherty and by Simmonds.[1] The latter author described the test (Fig. 12-2) with the patient lying prone on the examination table, while the first two advised that the patient kneel on a chair. In either test, the foot and ankle project over the edge. When the calf is squeezed on the normal side, the ankle undergoes plantar flexion, whereas on the injured side the ankle remains inert.

TREATMENT. Without treatment the tendon heals inadequately, and with sufficient lengthening to cause permanent loss of power of the calf and permanent lameness. Immobilization

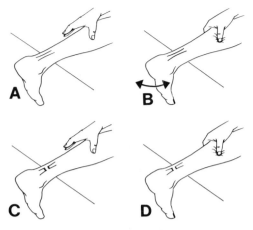

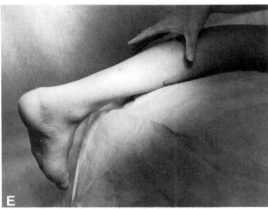

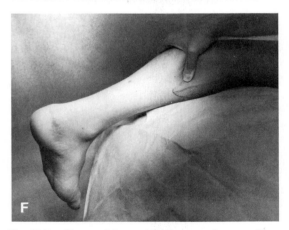

Fig. 12-2. Simmonds' test. (*A*) Diagram of a normal leg, with the patient lying prone. The examiner's hand can be seen over the calf muscle. (*B*) When the calf is squeezed, the foot tilts downward (*arrow*). (*C*) A leg with a ruptured Achilles tendon. (*D*) However hard the calf is squeezed, the foot remains still. (*E*) Photograph of the patient shown in Figure 12-1. (*F*) Simmonds' test is positive.

of the foot in equinus fosters healing without much lengthening, but the fibrous scar between the two ends of the tendon is often inadequate and may have an hourglass shape. There is therefore a greater chance of recurrence of the tendon rupture after conservative treatment.[3] Even the most favorable outcome is likely to leave the patient with a mechanical disadvantage, so that the calf does not recover full power, however assiduous the exercise program. The authors therefore recommend meticulous suture within a reasonable time of the injury.

Immediate suture is not obligatory in this condition, and most cases can safely be left to the next routine operating list. Some surgeons even consider that the suture is facilitated if a short delay is allowed before operation; this provides for some scarring of the tendon ends, which prevents the sutures from cutting out. If the delay is too long, however, muscle wasting and adhesion of the tendon can make operation difficult.

TENDON SUTURE. The tendon is exposed through a lateral incision parallel to its fibers (Fig. 12-3) and the paratenon is dissected after vertical incision, to allow separate closure and so prevent adhesion of the skin to the tendon. Thick, chromic catgut (size 0 or 1) is used for the suture, since braided silk may cause inflammatory swelling, while monofilament stainless steel or nylon may be palpable and tender.

Zig-zag Bunnell sutures[4] are inserted (Fig. 12-4) to obtain a firm grip on the axial fibers of the tendon, and the knots are buried. Paratenon and skin are sutured separately. A "non-weight-bearing," split plaster cast is applied, with the ankle in full equinus. This is changed on the 10th to 12th day, to allow removal of skin sutures. It is replaced by a weight-bearing cast with the foot in full equinus, with incorporated heel. An equal raise is fitted to the heel of the opposite shoe and the patient is allowed to walk. After 8 weeks, when the cast has been removed, provided the tendon feels intact, the patient continues to wear equal raises on both heels for another 3 or 4 weeks. Gentle, active, non-weight-bearing exercises are performed to overcome the equinus. Thereafter, the height of the raises on the heels is halved, and 2 weeks later they are removed entirely.

If operation has been delayed for any reason, the ends of the tendon must be dissected sufficiently to allow full apposition before they are sutured. This dissection may have to be extensive, but always within the sheath of the paratenon. At a later stage, where there is a palpable, non-tender gap, it may not be possible to approximate the tendon ends. In that case the scar tissue should be excised, the ends freshened, and the gap bridged, using the plantaris tendon and strips of aponeurosis if required.

Injury to Other Tendons in the Foot and Ankle

Indirect injury can occur to tendons other than the Achilles, but it is much less common. Severe, twisting movements, especially of inversion, may rupture the tibialis anterior or posterior tendon. On rare occasions, a direct stubbing injury to the hallux will cause snapping of the long flexor or extensor tendon, which should be sutured. Avulsion of the peroneal insertion into the base of the fifth metatarsal is discussed later.

Instability of the Ankle and Subtalar Joints

Repeated, sudden "giving way" of the foot and ankle into inversion is a common complaint. The condition occurs at any age, but is

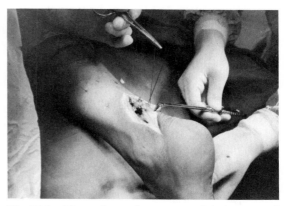

Fig. 12-4. The tendon ends are opposed during Bunnell suture. The tone of the calf is present, as shown by the position of the foot.

common in adolescence, and again at the age of about 40 years. It is more common in women than in men. In such cases there may be a history of a preliminary injury, but not necessarily so. While walking, or at least taking the weight on a leg, the foot and ankle suddenly collapse into inversion and the patient drops to the ground, experiencing a feeling of severe insecurity, with pain lasting a few minutes or longer, if there is associated bruising and swelling.

Three distinct anatomical problems cause inversion instability. Since the treatment is not the same in each, accurate diagnosis is essential.

Peroneal Tendon Dislocation. Inversion injury of the ankle may result in rupture of the fascia covering the peroneal tendon sheath. Recurrent dislocation of peroneal tendons follows. (See section on The Running Foot).

The Tilting Talus. Severe inversion injuries of the ankle can cause complete rupture of the lateral ligament of the ankle joint. This injury is probably best treated by surgical suture, but the ligament can be made to heal without lengthening by careful application of a plaster cast in eversion compression. If the ligament is allowed to heal with laxity, abnormal talar tilting may occur precipitously when the foot is inverted a few degrees (Fig. 12-5). Ankle subluxation occurs suddenly and the patient falls.

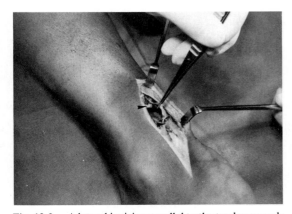

Fig. 12-3. A lateral incision parallel to the tendon reveals the wide gap in the Achilles tendon (*arrows*).

Precise diagnosis is essential, and can be made by taking anteroposterior radiographs of both ankles stressed into full inversion. On the affected side the talus is seen to be tilted into severe subluxation, whereas on the normal side the joint is merely opened up into inversion.

Surgery consists of re-forming the lateral ligaments of the ankle to prevent the extreme degrees of inversion. Watson-Jones described a technique in which the tendon of the peroneus brevis muscle is detached proximally as far as possible toward the muscle belly;[5] that is, 3 cm above the tip of the malleolus. A tunnel is then drilled through the fibula from front to back. The detached tendon is inserted through this tunnel, from back to front, and is then threaded through a vertical drill hole in the outer margin of the neck of the talus, laterally, and back into the tip of the malleolus, where it is sutured. The tendon therefore reconstitutes the lateral ligament of the ankle.

Harding has suggested that the first half of this operation is sufficient to prevent recurrent dislocation. After the procedure, the patient must spend 8 weeks in a below-knee walking cast, molded into eversion. The operation is technically difficult, but if successful, it prevents dislocation completely.

Peroneal Muscle Inhibition. In many patients, adolescents and older persons, recurrent "giving way" of the ankle into inversion, is caused neither by dislocation of the peroneal tendons nor by recurrent talar dislocation within the mortise of the ankle joint. The cause of the mechanical collapse is not immediately obvious.

Unless careful inversion stress radiographs are perfomed, it is easy to diagnose such cases as tilting talus. In this event the patient may be subjected to unnecessary surgery which may not prevent recurrence of the condition. A careful history will often reveal previous minor sprains of the lateral ligament of the ankle joint (see Chronic Sprains). It is probable that the course of events leading to such inversion collapse is as follows: a partial tear of the anterior fibers of the lateral ligaments

has healed, with slight stretching. The patient, especially when wearing high heels, is slightly less stable than if she were walking in a flat heel. The foot tilts into slight inversion and, instead of the normal increase in peroneal muscle tone to support the ankle, sudden total peroneal muscle inhibition takes place and the foot collapses into full inversion. It will be noted that the collapse takes place at the subtalar joint, unless the passive stretching is so severe that a further tear of the lateral ligament occurs.

Peroneal muscle inhibition is similar to the quadriceps inhibition that takes place in a knee subjected to sudden weight bearing when the quadriceps muscle is wasted or weakened, causing the knee to give way and the patient to fall to the ground. It should be treated in the same way; that is, by strengthening of the peroneal muscles through physical therapy. This can be performed most easily by active balancing exercises on a tilting board. Watson-Jones' operation may prevent the subtalar collapse by fixing the peroneus brevis to the lateral malleolus; however, it is using a hammer to crack a nut. In the most severely recurrent cases, a lateral flare on the heel of a flat shoe may prevent the subtalar joint from tilting into equinus.

Ankle Sprain

As described before, inversion injuries of the ankle usually result in partial tear of the lateral ligament. Anatomically the lateral ligament consists of vertical, anterior, and posterior oblique components; the whole constituting a fan-shaped ligament radiating from the tip of the lateral malleolus (see Chap. 3).

The term *sprain* is used to imply a partial tear of the ligament, without abnormal laxity. Most sprains heal within a few weeks; some leave sufficient laxity to allow peroneal reflex inhibition, while a few give rise to talar instability as described.

The ankle is particularly prone to strain and is perhaps the commonest site in the whole body. When trauma is mild the symptoms are, too. When, as commonly happens, it occurs as the result of a severe twist, usually into inversion, in the course of a warm game, the ankle feels as if it is "giving way," with an acute stab of pain. After a while the pain may subside, especially if the ankle is strapped. The player may be able to continue the game. It is only hours later as the joint cools or when the victim attempts to put the foot to the ground the next morning, that the now swollen ankle feels stiff and very painful.

Bruising and ecchymosis appear below and in front of the lateral malleolus. Tenderness may be elicited at the attachment of the ligaments to the lateral malleolus, to the lateral side of the calcaneus, or to the borders of the subtalar joint.

Distinction should be made between strains and ruptures of ligaments. Usually the sprained tissues are acutely tender and painful on any movement causing tension. Complete rupture of the ligaments results in gross local swelling, for the joint effusion leaks into the extraarticular tissues, but with little or no pain on passive movements, which may be in excess of the normal. As the ligaments may be ruptured in part, with adjacent areas of sprain, the signs may be mixed.

When there is doubt, the area of maximum tenderness or the joints themselves should be injected with local anesthetic, to permit stress radiography of the ankle and subtalar joints. The ankle is stressed into inversion while the foot is forcibly adducted, or everted and abducted. When the ligaments are ruptured, the talus tilts away from the malleolus, and the subtalar joint is seen to open on one side or the other.

After forcible eversion and abduction, the deltoid ligament on the medial side of the joint may be avulsed; the consequence is continuing disability until repair can be effected.

Forced dorsiflexion, especially when combined with rotation, may sprain a ligament at the apex of the longitudinal arch. A heel seat or arch support may be required after the acute symptoms have subsided.

For success, treatment of sprains should start early—if possible, immediately. Swelling is reduced by cold compresses and aided by support strapping, which, by limiting move-

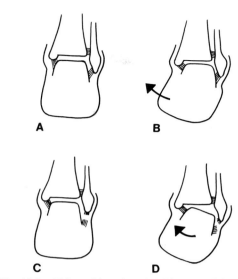

Fig. 12-5. Talar subluxation. (*A*) Diagram of the normal ankle showing intact medial, lateral, and inferior tibiofibular ligaments. (*B*) Despite forced inversion of the ankle, the talus remains stable within the mortise. (*C*) After disruption of the lateral ligament. (*D*) Forcible inversion causes abnormal talar tilt.

ment, also reduces pain and, after a minor injury, would allow walking. When the injury is more severe, crutches or a plaster cast may be necessary.

The treatment of sprains by immediate injection of procaine or similar local anesthetic was advocated by Le Riche over 30 years ago. He contended that the traumatic exudate contains metabolites that irritate the local sensory nerve endings. A reflex which causes further exudate and prolongs the process of pain and disability is established. The procaine anesthetizes the nerve endings, interrupts the reflex, and permits the swelling to resolve.

Immediate movement of the ankle joint is encouraged. If the injury is mild, an elastic or compression bandage is applied, and the patient is permitted full weight bearing; if the sprain is severe he should use crutches temporarily.

When the swelling is down, a corrective plastic heel seat curbs excessive or uncontrolled inversion.

Rupture of the Lateral Ligaments of the Ankle

When these ruptures go undiagnosed initially, they cause recurrent instability later, often severe enough to require surgery.

For ruptures of the ligaments of the ankle, reconstruction by the Watson-Jones tenodesis or the Osmond-Clarke realignment brings satisfactory stability and function. When the subtalar joint is involved, the Grice arthrodesis is usually the operation of choice.

Buckling or "Giving Way" of the Ankle

"Giving way" is a symptom of instability and may be due to any of the following causes:

1. Disruption of the capsular ligaments of the ankle or subtalar joints
2. Slipping peroneal tendons after rupture of the embracing retinaculum
3. Loose bodies from osteochondral fractures or osteochondritis dissecans
4. Paralysis of the peripheral muscles of the leg from nerve injury or following poliomyelitis
5. Severe fatigue may lead to loss of control of the ankle by the peroneal muscles.

Illusory "Giving Way." Severe sprains may leave a legacy of adhesions which manifest themselves by twinges or stabs of pain on certain movements. The sudden pain causes a momentary weakness which the patient may mistake for "giving way."

Chronic Sprain. In many cases, despite a stable joint, the patient is left with chronic sprain and swelling and local tenderness in the anterolateral fibers of the lateral ligament. There is usually local thickening of the synovium immediately beneath the injured part of the ligament. The condition responds to gentle exercises, local friction, or ultrasound therapy, but local injection of intraarticular corticosteroids and a local anesthetic agent usually brings the inflammatory reaction to a rapid end.

Stress Fractures in the Foot

Michael Devas, in his excellent monograph on stress fractures, commented that such "fractures occur in normal bones of healthy people doing every-day activities and with no injury."[6] By "normal" he meant that most patients who developed stress fractures were not suffering from any disease at the time. By definition, if there has been a history of injury, the condition is not one of stress fracture.

Failure of mechanical strength of a bone depends on two factors: the force applied and the strength of the bone itself. In stress fractures, repeated force on the structure, none in itself capable of damaging the bone, finally results in mechanical failure. What is an everyday amount of activity in one person may represent an unusual degree in another, and lead to a stress fracture.

With increasing age there is a decrease in bone strength; apart from that, there may be osteoporosis and osteomalacia. Stress fractures throughout the skeleton become more common. In the foot, however, stress fractures are common in healthy young people who subject their feet to unaccustomed exercise.

The fractures may result from repeated lateral strains on the bone, or by repeated and rhythmic muscle pull. Compression stress fractures are particularly common in many bones in older patients and in the calcaneus in young children. Distraction stress fractures, whether transverse or oblique, occur in long bones such as the metatarsals and the fibula, in both adults and children. The crack appears to start in the cortex away from that area to which the stress was applied.

At onset the symptoms may be vague, and only those aware of its possible existence will diagnose the condition. An ache or pain follows unusual or increased activity. Activity is always a precedent. Rest relieves the symptoms, but they recur when activity is repeated. An athlete will develop the symptoms regularly with each training session and so establish the diagnosis. For the ordinary person, whose activities vary from day to day, diagnosis may be elusive. Occasionally the onset is so abrupt that the patient cannot continue to run or play.

On examination there is local bony tenderness, and in superficial bones, redness and swelling may be visible. Applying stress to the bone causes tenderness localized to the site of the fracture. In time, radiography usually confirms the diagnosis, although at first the signs may be hazy and the fracture line ill-defined, especially in the case of the calcaneus. Callus, sometimes heavy, does usually, slowly encompass the shafts of long bones such as the metatarsals. The diagnosis in some cases depends upon the comparison of two radiographs taken a few weeks apart. If the first shows fluffy, ill-defined, subperiosteal new bone, while the latter shows well-consolidated cortical thickening, the diagnosis of stress fracture is certain.

In the early stages the condition may have to be differentiated from early nonarticular arthritis or gout. Both present with local signs and symptoms. Vascular conditions, such as varicose veins or even intermittent claudication, may cause symptoms related to activity, as may tenosynovitis.

Rest of the injured part, with or without splinting, and having the patient walk on crutches to keep active, but avoid bearing weight, is the treatment of choice. Healing is stimulated by isometrics and a program of contrast bathing, and "non-weight-bearing" exercises. An elastic bandage bound round foot and ankle is all that is required, but for fractures of the metatarsals, when displacement is threatened, or for the obstinate athlete, a plaster cast gives added security. Stress phenomena and fractures may be prevented, at the beginning of the season, by a training program of steadily increasing activity which avoids excessive muscular effort in the early stages. Stress fractures may occur in the calcaneus, the navicular, and in any of the metatarsals.

The Calcaneus. Of all stress fractures sustained by women recruits during training for the United States Marine Corps, 25 per cent occurred in the calcaneus.[2] The fractures can happen at any age and, as Devas pointed out, they often account for the painful heel that eludes diagnosis because of the vagueness of the symptoms and the lack of radiographic changes in the early stages. The calcaneus has, perhaps, the longest latent period in developing radiographic confirmation of a stress fracture. Three months is not too long to wait. We believe, with Michael Devas, that some

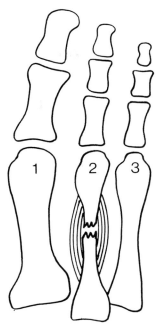

Fig. 12-6. When a healthy person develops pain and swelling in the foot after unusual exercise, march fracture should be considered.

cases of so-called traction apophysitis of the calcaneal tuberosity are actually stress fractures in the apophysis.

TREATMENT. A soft rubber pad in the heel of the shoe spreads the load and reduces weight-bearing pain. When necessary, the foot and ankle are strapped. These methods should be continued until all tenderness has disappeared. Raising the heel of the shoe reduces the compressive force of the calf muscles and plantar fascia, and is also beneficial.

March Fractures. Stress fractures of the metatarsals, usually involving the shafts of the second and third, are known as march fractures (Fig. 12-6).[7,8] They are normally readily diagnosed, especially in adults; but a young person who has engaged in unusual exercise—a fresh recruit in the army or an athlete on a new training program—may complain of aching and pain in the forefoot. The metatarsal shafts are tender and sometimes swollen. Symptoms are relieved by rest and by the support of an elastic bandage. Radiographs confirm the diagnosis, usually within 2 weeks. Healing is uncomplicated in most cases. Some few patients in the early stages may suffer severe pain on standing and walking and may compensate for the fracture by walking on the heel or outer border of the foot.

Inversion of the foot commonly results in the so-called Jones injury; that is, avulsion of the peroneus brevis insertion into the base of the fifth metatarsal. More often, there is an avulsion fracture of the base of the metatarsal. Occasionally these occur without one specific injury. In such cases, repeated minor traumatic episodes have resulted in a stress fracture.

The condition must also be distinguished from gout, rheumatoid arthritis, and traumatic osteoarthritis of any of the small joints of the foot.

The Navicular Bone. A compression stress fracture of the tarsal navicular bone resembles Köhler's disease of this bone in children. The navicular forms the apex of the longitudinal arch, and as such is subject to considerable stress on weight bearing. When the muscles which sustain the longitudinal arch become fatigued, compression in the arch is increased, and so is the ache and pain of the fracture. At such times, stress fracture may be difficult to distinguish from foot strain.

At first an elastic bandage, and then a plastic heel seat which takes the strain off the arch without pressure on it, is helpful.

INFLAMMATORY CONDITIONS

Bursitis

Habitual pressure on a bony protuberance leads to a cycle of pathological changes in the overlying soft tissues. Such bony prominences are vulnerable only when they are near the surface.

The first changes are in the skin. Thickening of the epidermis results in toughening of the horny layer until a callosity is present. At first it is protective, until central cornification forms pearls of dead tissue which cause pressure in their own right. In the underlying, subcutaneous tissue, repeated rubbing leads to a plane of cleavage in the collagen layers. Fluid is formed, or collects, in this space, and an adventitious bursa is created. In itself it may

have some protective function, but repeated trauma causes the lining of the bursa to thicken until a pseudosynovial membrane develops.

In the end, continued pressure causes an inflammatory reaction and traumatic bursitis is present. The inflamed bursa causes constant throbbing pain, and walking is difficult. In some cases bacteremia gives rise to septic bursitis. The abscess may burst, leaving a chronic sinus, or a surgical incision may accomplish this. In other cases, constant pressure on the skin overlying the bursa leads directly to necrosis and so to a noninfected sinus.

Such sinuses are difficult to close, since constant drainage of fluid keeps the stoma open. Bacteria may invade the bursa at any time and precipitate infection. To treat the bursitis one must treat the cause, which is abnormal pressure on the bony prominence. The hard skin should be removed by meticulous chiropody. Pads of felt, microcellular rubber, or padded leather protect the pressure point. Attention to the fitting of shoes is essential.

Often such conservative treatment is ineffectual and surgery is required. Excision of the bursa is seldom sufficient, and operation should include removal of the causal bony prominence. Any of the bony lumps in the foot, whether congenital or acquired, may give rise to bursitis. In the sections on hallux valgus, hallux rigidus, navicular lumps, and winter heel syndrome, typical examples of bursitis and their treatment have been discussed.

There are two bursas related to the heel that can cause pain. The subcutaneous bursa over the back of the calcaneus, whether due to a congenital calcaneal ridge or to abnormal pressure by shoes, has been discussed (see Winter Heel Syndrome, Chap. 10).

Retrocalcaneal Bursitis. The deep surface of the Achilles tendon is not attached to the upper end of the calcaneus, but gains a purchase fairly low down on its posterior surface. The retrocalcaneal bursa separates the bony prominence of the dome of the calcaneus from the deep aspect of the tendon. Like other bursas, it is liable to develop inflammation from abnormal friction; usually after excessive marching, mountaineering, or similar unusual activity.

A congenitally protuberant dome of the calcaneus is particularly suspect. During World War II, when a mountain division of the British Army was formed in Scotland, a surprising number of men developed retrocalcaneal bursitis. Unwonted dorsiflexion while climbing caused abnormal pressure and friction on the heel from hard army boots. Almost invariably a protuberant posterosuperior surface of the calcaneus was responsible. Excision of the protuberance prevented recurrence of the condition.

The operation is performed through an incision along the medial border of the Achilles tendon. A wedge of bone must be removed, including the protuberance, right down to the tendon insertion. Convalescence is relatively painless, and usually the patient can resume training some 10 to 14 days later. Fowler and Philip advocated splitting of the Achilles tendon, but we have not found it necessary.[4]

Tenosynovitis in the Foot and Ankle

Tendons, when injured by a direct blow, by exceptional acceleration in running, by prolonged exertion, or unwonted activity, may suffer strain. This may occur at the junction of the tendon and bone, at the attachments of the muscle fibers to the tendon, or in the tendon itself. Most often involved are the Achilles tendon, the tibialis anterior or -posterior, the peronei, and the tendon of hallucis longus.

Figure 12-7 demonstrates the anatomical fact that these tendons are enclosed within synovial sheaths as they run over the bony grooves in the ankle and foot, or are constricted beneath fascial retinacula. Injury to the tendon causes swelling of the surrounding sheath, with pain on movement of the tendon. There is marked local tenderness at the point of injury and less severe tenderness along the length of the swollen tendon sheath.

Synovial sheaths of the extensor digitorum longus tendons on the dorsum of the foot and of the flexor tendons behind the ankle and extending into the foot, being less vulnerable to injury are less often affected. So-called degenerative changes in the collagen fibers of tendons are common in people over the age of thirty-five. The change is probably responsible for painful tendinitis and similar conditions in many parts of the body. Supraspinatus tendinitis, bicipital tenosynovitis, tennis elbow, De Quervain's syndrome in the wrist, trigger finger, even ruptured Achilles tendon—all are examples of snapping of collagen fibers in tendons caused by this pathological process. Anatomical variations in the parts of the body account for the difference in clinical manifestation of the various conditions.

Tenosynovitis may also be a sign of a synovial inflammatory disease such as rheumatoid arthritis or gout. The resulting boggy thickening and synovial effusion cause pain localized to the sheath itself.

Variants, major or minor, of the rheumatoid process, may present as tenosynovitis. Diagnosis of the cause may be obvious, or it may require careful consideration. Lord Cohen, when Professor of Medicine at the University of Liverpool, demonstrated a relationship between oxaluria and seasonal multiple tenosynovitis. Oxalates crystallize in an acid urine when strawberries and tomatoes, among other vegetables, are in season. The tenosynovitis subsides rapidly after the urine is alkalized.

At the other end of the spectrum, patients with florid rheumatoid disease of the foot and ankle, including erosive disease of the joints, muscle contractures, generalized porosis, and even vasculitis with skin changes, may also suffer from generalized tenosynovitis. Unless this is appreciated, the surgeon may spend much effort in trying to make a stable, painless foot yet still have a patient complaining of localized pain and swelling. Early treatment to reduce inflammation and swelling is important, since adhesions from chronic fibrosis are difficult to treat conservatively.

Tenosynovitis and Stenosing Tenovaginitis of the Tibialis Posterior.
Tenosynovitis of the tibialis posterior is a cause of pain on the medial side of the foot. It may start after an

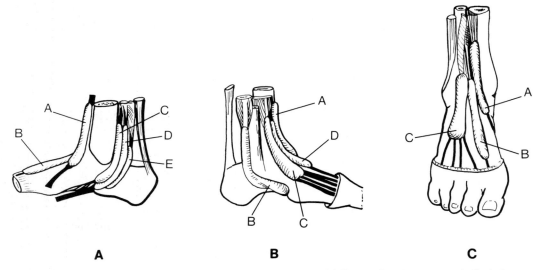

Fig. 12-7. Tendon sheaths of the foot and ankle. *Medial View:* A, tibialis anterior; B, extensor hallucis longus; C, tibialis posterior; D, flexor digitorum longus; E, flexor hallucis longus. *Lateral View:* A, tibialis anterior; B, peroneal tendon sheath; C, extensor digitorum longus; D, extensor hallucis longus. *Anterior View:* A, sheath of tibialis anterior; B, sheath of extensor hallucis longus; C, extensor digitorum longus.

eversion strain or a fatiguing run or march. Pain is felt behind and below the medial malleolus, extending into the arch of the foot.

The signs and symptoms resemble those of the tarsal tunnel syndrome, and the two may be associated. Walking is uncomfortable, or even painful, as are all active movements, such as inversion and eversion, which cause the muscle to contract and move the tendon through the inflamed sheath.

Patients in their forties or fifties develop tenosynovitis of the tibialis posterior muscle following relatively trivial injury, usually a valgus wrench, when descending stairs without care, or stumbling over a pebble in the dark. In this age group, symptoms tend to persist.

Rest is an effective treatment; this may be accomplished by immobilizing the foot and ankle in an elastic bandage and having the patient use crutches for walking. A heel seat or insole which prevents eversion of the heel may be helpful, as are antiinflammatory medications. The injection into the tendon sheath of a local anesthetic agent combined with an intraarticular corticosteroid may cure the condition, or at least alleviate it, but the substance

of the tendon itself must be avoided, as the steroid may soften the injured collagen fibers and cause them to snap.

Sometimes relief is achieved only by a plaster cast, worn for 2 or 3 weeks to prevent movement of the tendon within the sheath. If the inflammation does not settle, the tendon sheath may require surgical decompression, with excision of the affected synovium and repair of the tendon.

The Tibialis Anterior. The tendon of the tibialis anterior is more vulnerable than that of the tibialis posterior, and is more easily injured by a direct blow or a wrench of the foot into plantar flexion. It may be traumatized by repeated irritation of a shoe, or receive a direct injury from a boot.

Treatment, as for the posterior tendon, includes rest and protection.

Extensor Hallucis Longus. The tendon of extensor hallucis longus may be irritated by the osteophyte which forms on the dorsum of the medial midtarsal joint when the middle-aged foot sags. An inflamed bursa forms around the tendon and is irritated by the repeated pressure of the edge of the shoe. Felt pads may protect against pressure, but simple removal of the bony protrusion solves the problem.

Tenosynovitis of the Peroneal Tendons. Acute inversion injuries of the foot may cause traumatic tenosynovitis of the trouser-shaped tendon sheath surrounding the peronei, with or without damage to the tendons themselves.

Tenosynovitis in this region is less common than avulsion fracture of the base of the fifth metatarsal (Fig. 12-8). The latter, after such an inversion injury, presents as a painful swelling of the protuberance of the base of the metatarsal. Walking is painful; spreading echymosis is characteristic. Firm bandaging relieves the symptoms, but the pain may last for as long as 6 or 8 weeks. Even when the tenderness has subsided, the enlarged lump at the base of the fifth metatarsal may persist, with pressure from a shoe that previously fitted comfortably.

Any of the other tendon sheaths may be affected in people who engage in unusual occupations or sporting activities. A careful history of the onset of symptoms, or a description of the position of the foot at the time of injury, will help in diagnosis. Local palpation reveals tenderness of the tendon sheath, which confirms the diagnosis.

Three case histories illustrate the features of posttraumatic tenosynovitis:

CASE 1: A 15-year-old girl attending a school that specializes in training for the stage and ballet complained of recurrent pain behind the ankle, extending into the sole of the foot. Each episode followed a period of dancing practice, especially after exercising on point; that is, dancing on her toes while wearing a blocked ballet shoe. Examination showed slight swelling and tenderness localized to the sheath of the flexor hallucis longus tendon, extending from the groove on the posteromedial surface of the lower end of the tibia into the sole of the foot, toward the big toe.

Passive extension of the hallux reproduced the pain, which localized the synovial sheath involved. Infiltration of 3 ml. of 1-per-cent lidocaine (Lignocaine) abolished the symptom immediately, and injection of 60 mg. of an intraarticular steroid (methylprednisolone) relieved the condition for some time. Subsequently she suffered several fur-

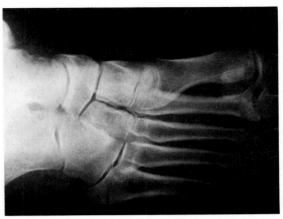

Fig. 12-8. Avulsion fracture of the base of the fifth metatarsal.

ther episodes, each following protracted periods of exercising on point.

CASE 2: A 19-year-old girl fell while skiing. Her bindings failed to unlock, and she twisted her foot severely. Despite physical therapy she did not recover and was left with, clinically, a spasmodic flatfoot; that is, a foot that showed valgus deformity on weight bearing.

Examination showed marked swelling and tenderness confined to the sheath of the tibialis anterior tendon. The tendon itself was not palpable. The passive range of motion of the foot was full (if painful), and a diagnosis of unbalanced paralysis of the foot due to loss of the tibialis anterior muscle was made. The tendon sheath was explored, revealing a florid inflammatory synovitis secondary to complete distal detachment of the tendon insertion into the navicular bone. The tendon was reattached with silk sutures inserted through drill holes in the bone. The patient recovered fully after plaster cast immobilization for 6 weeks, followed by mobilizing exercises.

CASE 3: A woman, aged 54 years, attended the orthopaedic clinic for renewal of the orthotic appliance which she had worn for 18 months to relieve the typical pain and swelling associated with an affection of the tibialis posterior tendon. Gradually her foot had developed a spasmodic pes planus; walking became increasingly painful. A double brace with T-strap overcame her problem to some extent, since it allowed her to walk without much pain, with her foot and ankle immobilized. She requested a replacement of the brace.

Since her symptoms were not adequately controlled by the device, the tendon sheath was explored surgically. It was found to be severely inflamed, with a thickened, polypoid appearance.

The cause of the condition was in the tendon itself, which was yellowish in color and somewhat translucent and had a fusiform swelling extending for about 3 inches at the level of the mesotendineum. In the center of this swollen region was a partial rupture of the fibers of the tendon. Apparently the synovial reaction was provoked by the abrasive effect of the ruptured fibers. The affected part was excised, and tenosynovectomy performed: then the fibrous sheath was sutured and the wound closed in layers. After some weeks the patient was able to walk comfortably and did not require the use of a brace again.

CONDITIONS OF THE PLANTAR FASCIA

Plantar Fasciitis and Calcaneal Spurs

One of the common syndromes that cause pain in the sole of the foot is plantar fasciitis. The patient, usually in his middle years, may develop pain beneath the heel for no apparent reason or after suffering a minor injury to the foot. This consists usually of a misstep or sudden twist of the foot. For some time there is no pain, but after a few weeks a painful heel develops. It rapidly worsens until great discomfort is experienced at every step. The condition may persist for months, or even years, fluctuating in severity every few weeks. It is self-limiting in most cases, even without treatment.

Trauma alone cannot be the whole cause of the lesion, not only because the injury may be trivial, but because it may affect both heels, either at the same time or in sequence.

It is significant that most patients are over forty, an age when other inflammatory conditions, affecting collagen fibers where they attach to bone, are common. Supraspinatus tendinitis, tennis- or golfer's elbow, even ruptured Achilles tendon, are similar collagen injuries occurring at the same time of life. In such conditions, usually requiring surgical exploration, the collagen fibers are macroscopically different from those in young adults. They are yellowish in color, which must represent a chemical change in the tissue.

The other significant factor is that the pain is so protracted, suggesting repeated trauma, or perhaps an exaggerated tissue reaction to such fiber breakdown. The tissue reaction is confirmed by the histological changes seen when biopsy is performed. These are usually diagnosed as nonspecific inflammatory changes, but they must represent a vascular reparative reaction to the original lesion.

Any general disease that adds to the inflammatory reaction may make the patient more vulnerable to plantar fasciitis. Rheumatoid arthritis, for example, or gout in particular, are important in this regard. The latter condition should always be considered, and a painful heel may lead to the diagnosis of hyperuricemia in some cases.

Obesity is also a potent initiating factor in plantar fasciitis and tends to make the lesion refractory to treatment. Most patients whose symptoms do not settle down spontaneously in a reasonable time or who suffer frequent recurrences are overweight. It may be necessary to institute an adequate regimen of dieting before the pain can be controlled adequately.

Examination of the foot confirms the diagnosis. Exquisite local tenderness can be palpated in the attachment of the plantar fascia to the under-surface of the heel bone, just distal to the calcaneal tubercle.

Treatment consists of local steroid injection in the tender spot. In the author's view the pain of the injection is so severe that injecting under local anesthesia is seldom justified. Instead, the patient is admitted to hospital as a day case and the procedure performed under intravenous anesthesia. The patient lies prone and receives 80 mg. of intraarticular methylprednisolone (Depomedrone) mixed with 2 ml. of 2-per-cent lidocaine (Lignocaine) in the tender spot in the plantar fascia, usually at the attachment to the medial and lateral tubercles of the calcaneus. The patient is usually comfortable when he awakes, but he should be warned that when the effect of the local anesthetic wears off, the pain may increase for 24 to 48 hours. Physiotherapy, in the form of Faradic footbaths and intrinsic foot muscle exercises, is given for 2 or 3 weeks.

If necessary a low-calorie diet is instituted and, in appropriate cases, serologic examination, including tests for rheumatoid arthritis and serum uric acid levels, is performed.

It will have been noted that no reference has been made to calcaneal spurs. Lateral radiographic examination of the heel shows the presence of a spur in many cases. This consists of an area of calcification in the plantar fascia in the exact site of the tenderness. The calcification may look fluffy and irregular at first, but later it is ossified, forming a bony projection with a well-developed cancellous structure. The presence of the spur does not always mean that the patient is suffering from a painful heel. Many middle-aged and older people have spurs without suffering, or ever having suffered, from the syndrome. The relation between pain and the spur is by no means a direct one. Presumably calcification leading to ossification occurs gradually in such cases, and the patient does not experience a painful heel.

The calcaneal spur is not the cause of pain: it is the result of an inflammation that may induce pain. Surgical excision of the spur is seldom justified, since in most cases the inflammation subsides when treated by conservative means. In any event, the operation succeeds by excising the inflammation rather than the spur.

Dupuytren's Contracture

Dupuytren's contracture of the sole resembles the palmar variety but is not as common and does not, as a rule, give rise to sufficient contracture to affect the toes.[9]

The condition occurs equally in men and women after the age of forty. Although direct injuries and lacerations of the palmar or plantar fascia may account for fibrosis and contractures, the pathogenesis is different in the two conditions.[10] Although Dupuytren's contracture used to be considered the result of multiple minor injuries, careful studies have failed to show an association with a previous history of heavy work or the use of such machines as those used to compress tarmac in road construction. Those with sedentary occupations seem equally liable to develop contractures. Ling has shown a definite familial tendency in the condition.[11] In a carefully studied series of 50 consecutive patients and their relatives, the figures suggested a Mendelian-dominant disease, not sex-linked, that manifested late in the second half of life, thus masking its genetic nature.

When the condition does arise in the plantar fascia, typical nodules form in the collagen fibers, followed by contraction of the fibrosed fibers. Nodules rarely form in the flexor aspect of the proximal phalanges of the toes (as they often do in the fingers). It is for this reason that flexion contracture of the toes seldom develops; nor does the condition necessarily give rise to pain.

One variant of Dupuytren's contracture, which occurs in younger patients, in the hand and foot equally, is of known etiology. Patients who have suffered from idiopathic epilepsy for many years, and who have taken Epanutin (sodium phenytoin) constantly to control attacks, are liable to get severe contracture of both the palmar and plantar fasciae. The drug seems to be the direct cause of the fibrosis.

In the foot the complaint is usually of pressure from the knobby masses, and may be relieved by appropriate pads or insoles. Excision of the disordered aponeurosis is seldom performed in the foot, but, when necessary, is not a complicated procedure.

Plantar Fibromatosis

Occasionally, a patient presents with a large, expanding, fibrous lump in the plantar aponeurosis. It is seldom tender and causes symptoms merely by its bulk. Contracture of the collagen fibers does not occur, but the lump continues to enlarge. The disorder behaves like a neoplasm, and there are few surgeons who would not excise the mass, if only for diagnostic purposes.

At operation, a greyish fibrous mass is found in the plantar fascia, which can be completely excised with the lump. Histologic examination reveals fibrous tissue only, with disordered collagen formation and apparently normal fibroblasts. It is usually reported as fibromatosis, but the nature of the pathologic process is not understood. The authors have seen recurrence of the condition in one patient after

---

Possible Causes of Pain in the Heel

Retrocalcaneal (sub-Achilles) bursitis
Subcutaneous adventitious bursa secondary to
  pressure from a shoe
The winter-heel syndrome
Achilles "tendinitis"
Sprain or incipient rupture of the Achilles tendon
Undiagnosed rupture of the tendon
Plantar fasciitis, with or without a cancaneal spur
Stress fractures of the calcaneus
Tibialis posterior tunnel syndrome

---

inadequate excision. A second excision was performed successfully.

PAIN IN THE HEEL

The painful heel is always significant because it is almost impossible to walk for any distance if the heel cannot be put to the ground. Walking on tiptoe is no solution, because so abnormal a gait soon tires the patient.

The condition merits early attention and careful diagnosis. The pain is always a manifestation of local pathology, and careful palpation of the anatomical features of the heel readily allows precision in diagnosis. It should not be forgotten that it may equally be a manifestation of a generalized disease condition—gout, rheumatoid arthritis, obesity, or the side effects of drugs.

DERMATOLOGIC CONDITIONS

The skin is an extraordinarily complex structure: apart from its function as a protective integument, it is the main organ of sensation, and plays a part as well in water metabolism and in the control of temperature. It is not surprising that, with so many physiological functions, it may manifest a wide variety of disorders, some of known, but many of unknown, etiology.

The Dermatoses

Eczema. Inflammatory conditions of the skin of the foot are common and occur for a number of reasons. Eczema is a term denoting a dry,

scaly, eruption of the skin. It may be familial, associated with other allergic conditions such as hay fever and asthma; or it may be a true contact dermatitis, the result of sensitivity to chemicals in shoe leather or the dyes used in stockings. The increasing use of chemicals such as synthetic rubber and adhesives in shoes has led to a rise in the number of such reactions. Many cases are of unknown etiology.

Treatment of the dermatitides is difficult and depends on careful investigation to find a cause and meticulous use of medications, both topical and systemic. Treatment should be undertaken only by a specialist.

Papulosquamous Conditions. These are a group of common dermatoses characterized by lumps (papules) and flat lesions (macules). They include lichen planus, a chronic, itching, red rash of the skin, the cause of which is unknown, and psoriasis, a common disorder of unknown cause which, in recent years, has been proved to have one remarkable feature. In normal people the epidermis is replaced constantly in about 28 to 30 days. In patients with psoriasis, the turnover time is reduced to about 3 or 4 days. This intense overactivity implies a severe metabolic hyperactivity. Treatment is difficult and should be left in the hands of experts.

Nodular Lesions on the Legs. A variety of conditions, many of unknown etiology, causes nodules on the leg. Some, for example erythema nodosum, are nonspecific reactions to infective agents. All require careful investigation, since they may be an indication of organic diseases, varying from tuberculosis to acute pancreatitis.

Ulcers. A break in the continuity of the skin that does not heal, that is, an ulcer, occurs much more commonly in the leg or foot than anywhere else in the body. The site of the ulcer often suggests the diagnosis. Varicose ulcers are usually confined to the anterolateral border of the leg on its lower third. Ulcer on the tip of a toe usually indicates severe arterial insufficiency, while skin loss over the heel is commonly caused by decubitus pressure in a severely debilitated old person, who must

Table 12-1   Classification of Ulcers of the Leg According to Causal Mechanism

External Causes

Primary
  Trauma
  Decubitus (trophic) ulcers
  Neurotic excoriations: factitious
Secondary to Predisposing Lesion
  Burns (thermal and chemical)
  Radiodermatitis
  Neoplasms

Internal Causes

Vascular Diseases
  Arterial
    Arteriosclerotic
    Hypertensive ischemic
    Thromboangiitis obliterans
    Livedo reticularis
  Venous
    Stasis
    Thrombophlebitis
Blood Dyscrasias
  Anemias (heritable)
    Sickle cell
    Thalassemia
    Congenital hemolytic
  Dysproteinemia
    Macroglobulinemia
    Cryoglobulinemia
Metabolic
  Diabetes mellitus
  Gout
Autoimmune Diseases
  Necrotizing angiitides
  Lupus erythematosus
  Scleroderma
  Rheumatoid arthritis
  Polyarteritis nodosa
  Pyoderma gangrenosum
Granulomas
  Microbiological
    Syphilis
    Erythema induratum
    Atypical mycobacterial
    Leprosy
    Deep fungal infections
Drugs
  Halides

Miscellaneous Causes

Acrodermatitis chronica atrophicans
Atrophie blanche

(Samitz, M. H., and Dana, A. S.: Cutaneous Lesions of the Lower Extremities. Philadelphia, J. B. Lippincott, 1971.)

remain in bed after a fractured neck of the femur, perhaps, or an attack of pneumonia.

All ulcers are significant, and their cause must be diligently sought. Most can be made to heal by correct treatment. Until epithelialization is complete, the patient is vulnerable to invasion by organisms. Samitz and Dana classified ulcers according to the cause: whether by an external mechanism, such as trauma or following a lesion on the skin, or internal diseases, which can vary from vascular deficiency to blood dyscrasias.[12] From Table 12-1 it can be seen that the diagnosis of a particular ulcer may require highly specialized investigation.

Viral Infections

A few viral conditions, such as herpes and some of the viruses of childhood, can affect the feet. Other rare viruses, such as some of the coxsackie species, have a predilection for the foot, as does that excessively rare condition in humans, foot-and-mouth disease. By far the most common viral conditions of the feet are warts.

Plantar Warts

Simple warts may occur on the toes, but in the foot, most warts are plantar in type. They are caused by a papovavirus, which probably enters the skin directly as a result of trauma. There is a long latent period before the characteristic lesion becomes visible.

Warts may be single or so numerous as to amount to a mosaic of warty excrescences on the sole of the foot. They vary in size from very small lesions to large lumps. There may be "mother-and-daughter" lesions.

Plantar warts differ from warts in other parts of the body because of their position. As a result of pressure on the wart, they grow inward, instead of outward, from the skin. Figure 12-9 shows the shape of a common verruca. It can be seen that it projects from the surface of the epidermis; plantar warts (Fig. 12-10) by being forced below the surface, have a horny wall around them, with a space between the wart and the horny layer. Callosities, on the other hand, have no such ring of

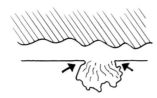

Fig. 12-9. Diagram of a common wart. The lesion can be seen to be growing out from the epidermis on its superficial aspect. The arrows show the edges of the verruca.

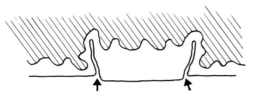

Fig. 12-10. A plantar wart is pushed into the epidermis by weight bearing. The arrows show the circumferential gap between wart and normal skin.

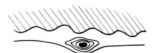

Fig. 12-11. A callosity, unlike a wart, is merely a thickening in the horny layer of the skin.

cornification (Fig. 12-11). They consist merely of a fusiform swelling of the skin as a result of the direct stimulus of constant pressure.

Plantar warts are tender and make walking difficult since they commonly grow beneath the heel or the metatarsal heads. They form hard lumps in the epidermis itself and soon project into the dermis. They can disappear spontaneously after a year or two. Occasionally, as a result of hypnosis or suggestion, they may disappear within a few days; otherwise they require treatment. Two physical methods exist: curettage and electrocoagulation. The procedure can be performed under local anesthesia or, in the case of large lesions, preferably under general anesthesia.

A fine-needle electrode is first inserted into the body of the wart to coagulate the central artery. Several such punctures can be made, but the needle should not pierce the base of the wart and should therefore not reach the dermis. A sharp curette of the right size is then inserted into the cornified wall around the wart, and the lesion is gently delivered onto the surface from its surrounding wall. When it has been freed circumferentially, the whole wart can be removed in one piece by the curette. Any bleeding from the central artery can be coagulated. Surgical excision is not recommended, as it may result in prolonged ulceration and a painful scar.

Castellani's solution, podophyllin, or acetic acid can be applied to warts when they are small, with some success, especially with an occlusive dressing.

Fungal Infections

Superficial fungal infection is discussed in Chapter 7. Fungal infection can occur at any age. The cause may have little to do with the exogenous etiological factors that exist for athletes and which are, in the main, environmental: shower room floors, locker rooms, inadequately cleaned swimming pools, and the practice of sharing towels have all been implicated.

The causes may be endogenous—in the skin itself. The presence of blisters on the skin has been held accountable in experiments.[13] Hypertrophic skin, for example between the toes, is more easily infected, as is moist skin. Meticulous attention to hygiene should be observed, including drying between the toes and removal of excess keratin.

There are two clinical varieties of tinea pedis: acute inflammatory infection with vesiculation followed by maceration and fissures in the skin leading to secondary infection; and chronic, hyperkeratotic tinea, causing asymptomatic thickening of the soles of the feet.

Diabetics are peculiarly liable to suffer from fungal infections. Treatment is both topical and internal. Powders or solutions are used during the day, and antifungal creams at night. The patient is instructed to apply the powder or solution twice a day, drying the feet afterward. Only cotton socks should be worn, and they should be changed twice a day. Wool socks may be necessary in cold climates, but nylon ones, which promote sweating, should certainly be avoided. Shoes should be changed frequently and aired well. Both socks and shoes should be powdered. In the evening, the feet should be washed and dried carefully, before the appropriate ointment is applied. The patient's towel should be kept separate from those of the rest of the household.

Fungal infections of the nail also occur and are particularly refractory. Internal treatment may be required, especially when the nails are infected. Griseofulvin is the drug of choice, but therapy may have to be prolonged.

DISEASES OF THE NAILS

The toenails may be affected in many conditions; from unusual congenital diseases, like the nail-patella syndrome, to the common thickening in toenails with advancing age. A few conditions have been chosen for discussion because they are common and amenable to treatment.

Subungual Hematoma

The hallux is susceptible to direct crush injury. Shearing strain causes separation of the nail from its bed. It is painful immediately, but the gradual collection of a subungual hematoma leads to increasing tension beneath the nail bed, so that the pain quickly becomes excruciating. Urgent decompression of the hematoma is required. Since the nail has been separated from its bed, it will probably stop growing and be replaced by a new nail. Removal of the injured nail, under local or general anesthesia, is a reasonable form of treatment, but it leaves the sensitive nail bed vulnerable to injury until the new nail grows. It is worthwhile leaving the nail in situ. It can be drilled to evacuate the hematoma. This is best performed without pressure being applied to the nail, since any increase in pressure adds to the pain. A large sailmaker's needle is employed. The blunt end is cleaned and heated in an open flame. It is held by the center in a pair of artery forceps, the blades of which have been covered by tube rubber to prevent the heat spreading

to the clamps and burning the operator. When the head of the needle is red hot it is withdrawn from the flame and applied, with a steady hand, to the surface of the nail at the center of the separated portion. It sinks into the nail, which smokes furiously. No pressure must be exerted. The needle cools very quickly and may have to be reheated and reapplied several times. Eventually it will sink right through the nail into the hematoma, which bursts out through the drill hole, decompressing itself and so relieving the pain. If care is taken, the needle sinks into the bloodclot and does not touch the nail bed, and so the treatment is painless. The nail will remain in position for months until a new nail pushes it off by its growth.

Onychogryphosis

Prolonged pressure on the nail bed leads to abnormal thickening of the nail. This is common in old age and can lead to gross thickening and irregularity of the nail. It may form a horn that causes pressure, and even ulceration, of the toe.

Once the tendency to develop onychogryphosis has begun, it cannot be overcome. Careful attention to cutting of the nail and meticulous, routine chiropody are needed. Occasionally it is necessary to use a bone cutter to trim the nail because of its hardness. In some cases, improvements may be obtained by avulsion of the nail under local or general anesthesia. This leaves the sensitive nail bed in need of protection until a new nail begins to form; but, provided the nail has been carefully removed, there should be no epithelial loss and, so, no ulceration. In rare instances, radical excision of the nail bed may be required to prevent further growth of the nail.

Ingrown Toenails

Pressure on the skin from sharp edges of a nail causes necrosis of tissue. The ulcer may become chronic, with secondary infection and granulation tissue. This leads to chronic pain and recurrent spreading infection, as well as local abscess formation.

Removal of the nail is followed by healing

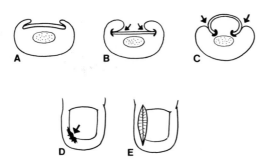

Fig. 12-12. Ingrown toenail. (*A*) Cross section of a normal hallux, showing the shape of the nail. (*B*) The infantile ingrown toenail is flat in cross-section. The skin flaps are hypertrophied. (*C*) The adult type of ingrown toenail. (*D*) Dorsal view of the ingrown toenail shows where ulceration occurs. (*E*) Wedge excision of the nail and bed.

of the ulcer. When the new nail is less deformed, it is not ingrowing; usually, however, the nail distortion recurs and so does the ulcer.

There are two varieties of ingrowing toenail affecting the Hallux.

The Infantile Type. The nail is flat, but the skin folds on either side of the nail are heaped up (Fig. 12-12A,B). This type of ingrown toenail is congenital in origin. It can be seen in children, but commonly requires attention in adolescence. It is more common in boys than in girls, perhaps because it is often associated with hyperhidrosis (see below) usually on both sides of the nail.

The adult variety of ingrown toenail is characterized by a curling deformity of the nail (Fig. 12-12C). The distal point of the lateral edge of the nail is the pressure point (Fig. 12-12D).

Treatment is surgical in most cases, except in a small number of the adult variety in which the points can be persuaded to grow over the skin flaps by lifting them daily with a nail file. Operation consists not only in excising the offending nail but in removing the whole or part of the nail bed from which it will regrow.

Zadek's Operation. Radical excision of the nailbed is best performed by this technique: The procedure should be carried out under general anesthesia, and certainly in a bloodless field. First, the nail is removed carefully by slipping one blade of a fine pair of artery

forceps (clamp) under the nail along its length to grasp it. If the instrument is then gently rocked from side to side and twisted, the nail will gradually loosen, without damage to the epithelium of the bed or any of the skin folds.

The growing portion of the nail bed, known as the *quick,* is now excised completely. It consists of the half-moon shaped, lighter portion of the nail bed which is visible. Figure 12-13A shows that the epithelium extends under the nail flap as a pocket of skin, lining the under-surface of the flap. It extends sideways under both medial and lateral nail flaps, to form pockets in both directions. All the pockets of epithelium must be excised totally if further growth of the nail is to be prevented (Fig. 12-13B).

The epithelium is firmly adherent to the periosteum of the distal phalanx and must be carefully dissected in one piece. Even a small fragment of white nail bed left behind contains a few epithelial cells, and a fragment of nail will grow again. (It is not without reason that the total extirpation of a nail bed has been likened to putting out a forest fire.) The prox-

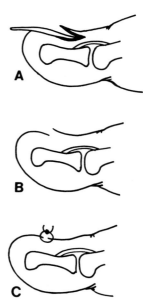

Fig. 12-13. Zadek's operation. (*A*) A diagram of a lateral view of the hallux. The nailbed is indicated by a thick black line. (*B*) After removal of the nail and excision of the pocket of epidermis that constitutes the nail bed. (*C*) The skin edges are sutured.

Fig. 12-14. Amputation of the distal end of the terminal phalanx. (*A*) The arrow indicates the amount of tissue to be excised. (*B*) A flap of the pulp is turned to cover the end of the stump.

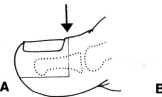
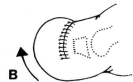

imal and side flaps of skin can now be sutured to the distal part of the nail bed (Fig. 12-13C).

Wedge Excision of the Nail Bed. On occasion, excision of a medial or lateral wedge of nail bed leaves a narrow nail without further ingrowth. It is even possible to excise both medial and lateral wedges. This operation is usually more appropriate in the infantile type of ingrown toenail, where the medial and lateral skin flaps are at fault rather than the nail itself.

The operation is performed under bloodless field. The nail itself is not removed. A vertical incision is made along the nail with a fine scalpel, from distal to proximal. The excision is made right down to bone. A second, elliptical, incision is made through the skin flap, also down to bone, so that the two incisions meet proximally and distally (Fig. 12-12E). All the tissue in the slice is removed, including the nail, excess skin, and the lateral pocket of the nail bed. The skin of the flap is now sutured to the nail itself. If the operation is performed carefully, the wound heals by first intention, leaving a narrower nail and just enough skin for comfort.

Amputation of the Tip of the Distal Phalanx. This operation, once popular for ingrown toenail, is seldom carried out today, since carefully performed, radical excision of the nailbed has replaced it. Skillfully executed, it gives a good result, provided an adequate plantar skin flap is turned from the pulp of the hallux (Fig. 12-14) to give a soft, sensitive stump to the toe.

Subungual Exostosis

In children, and occasionally in adolescents, a bony lump may grow from the tip of the distal phalanx. It is usually not in the midline of the bone but on the lateral side and is usually seen radiographically. The architecture

of bone within it is mature, and it is difficult to be sure whether it represents a benign tumor or a reaction to pressure on the growing phalanx.

Whatever the cause of the exostosis, it soon forms a hard lump under the skin of the distal part of the nail bed. The overlying portion of the nail becomes detached and is then worn away by the pressure of the shoe. The lesion simulates an ingrown toenail, but ulceration does not occur until later. Diagnosis is by radiographs, which confirm the existence of the underlying bony exostosis.

Treatment is surgical. Under general anesthesia and in a bloodless field, an incision is made transversely across the toe at the level of the end of the nail. The exostosis is dissected free of its soft-tissue attachments and excised. Care is taken to remove all the projecting bone from the phalanx; any residual bony spike could recreate an exostosis. Results are good if the operation is performed with care.

HYPERHIDROSIS

In late adolescence, young boys especially are vulnerable to overactivity of the sweat glands in the feet. Whether this is an abnormal reaction, or a normal response to hormonal change that occurs at this time, is unknown. In those cultures where shoes are not worn it has no significance, but in cold climates it may cause quite a severe problem for a sensitive young person.

When a patient with this condition has a toe operation, there is a greater likelihood of wound infection, probably because organisms grow more easily on the surface of a soggy foot. In particular, infection after operation for ingrown toenails is common. Patients with hyperhidrosis are best treated without a great deal of bandaging; incisions left open to the air heal better.

In some people the amount of sweating may be so severe as to constitute a pathological entity, and occasionally sympathectomy is required. There is some evidence to suggest that patients with hyperhidrosis are more likely to develop Sudek's atrophy, since both conditions are manifestations of sympathetic overactivity. Most people find that as they get older the excessive sweating subsides.

REFERENCES

1. Thompson, T. C., and Doherty, J. H.: Spontaneous rupture of tendo achilles. A new clinical diagnostic text. J. Trauma, *2:*126, 1962.
2. Simmonds, F. A.: Diagnosis of the ruptured Achilles tendon. Practitioner, *179:*56, 1957.
3. Forste, R. L., Ritter, M. A., and Young, R.: Rerupture of conservatively treated Achilles tendon rupture. J. Bone Joint Surg., *56A:*174, 1974.
4. Bunnell, S.: Surgery of the Hand. ed. 3. Philadelphia, J. B. Lippincott, 1956.
5. Watson-Jones, R.: Fractures and Joint Injuries. vol. 1. Baltimore, Williams & Wilkins, 1951.
6. Devas, M.: Stress Fractures. Edinburgh, Churchill Livingstone, 1975.
7. Jansen, M.: March foot. J. Bone Joint Surg., *8:*262, 1926.
8. Bernstein, A., and Stone, J. B.: March fractures—a report of 307 cases and a new method of treatment. J. Bone Joint Surg., *26:*743, 1944.
9. Stoyle, T. F.: Dupuytren's contracture in the foot. J. Bone Joint Surg., *46B:*218, 1964.
10. Burch, P. R. J.: Dupuytren's contracture: an autoimmune disease. J. Bone Joint Surg., *48B:*312, 1966.
11. Ling, R. S. M.: The genetic factor in Dupuytren's disease. J. Bone Joint Surg., *45B:*593, 1963.
12. Samitz, M. H., and Dana, A. S.: Cutaneous Lesions of the Lower Extremities. Philadelphia, J. B. Lippincott, 1971.
13. Strauss, J. S., and Kligman, A. M.: An experimental study of tinea pedis and onychomycosis of the foot. Arch. Dermatol., *76:*70, 1957.

13 The Manifestations of Rheumatoid Disease in the Foot

Of all the conditions that afflict the foot, the manifestations of rheumatoid arthritis are the most protean. Almost all the disorders that are discussed elsewhere in this book, whether of soft tissue, joint, or bone, are reflected by the disease. The surgeon taking part in a combined rheumatoid/orthopaedic clinic may neglect to ask the patient to remove his or her shoes at the time of the examination. Interested as he is nowadays in the replacement of the large joints of the lower limb, he can easily overlook the fact that some 70 per cent of all patients with rheumatoid arthritis have foot trouble. In a few cases, a single joint may be swollen, with consequent pain and a limp; at the other end of the scale, there are feet so deformed that the patient is severely disabled or unable to walk at all.

THE DIAGNOSIS OF RHEUMATOID ARTHRITIS

Over the past twenty years or so the ability to diagnose rheumatoid arthritis, as well as the definition of the condition, has changed gradually. The increasing tide of research has defined and differentiated, one by one, a series of syndromes of known etiology from the ragbag of elusive signs and symptoms we continue to call rheumatoid arthritis. Lord Ritchie Calder has said that scientific advance is concerned with making increasingly fine distinctions, and the growing list of exclusions from the diagnosis of rheumatoid disease confirms such a view. Rheumatoid arthritis itself is in quite another category. Not only has it proved impossible to find a cause for the condition, but it seems likely that the very concept of one cause is illusory. At present the disease, if one disease it is, can only be called idiopathic.

This vagueness in describing the condition has made diagnosis difficult. The criteria adopted by Ropes et al.,[1] as revised in 1958, remain the most practical method of identifying rheumatoid arthritis, consisting as they do of an empirical list of clinical signs and symptoms and radiographic and histological features. They are worth considering, not only because of the importance of diagnosing the disease as early as possible to begin treatment, but also because the apparently random list of signs, symptoms, and other observations is a good indication of our present knowledge of what comprises the condition. The list is as follows:

1. Morning stiffness
2. Pain on movement, or tenderness, in at least one joint, as noted by a competent observer such as a doctor
3. Swelling of the soft tissues of at least one joint, with or without an effusion, observed by a doctor
4. A competent history of swelling of at least one other joint, provided it occurred no more than three months before the second joint was affected

159

5. Symmetrical swelling of joints occurring simultaneously on both sides of the body

6. The presence of subcutaneous nodules anywhere in the body

7. Roentgenographic changes typical of rheumatoid arthritis: these must include bony decalcification localized to, or greatest around, the involved joints, and not just degenerative changes in the joints. Such changes may have nothing to do with the synovitis, having preceded it. They do not exclude a diagnosis of rheumatoid arthritis.

8. Positive serum agglutination tests: any method used to demonstrate the presence of "rheumatoid factor" in the serum is acceptable, provided two independent laboratories have shown positive results in no more than 5 per cent of normal controls.

9. Poor mucin precipitate from synovial fluid, with shreds in a cloudy solution

10. Characteristic histological changes in the affected synovium, including three or more of the following features: marked villous hypertrophy; proliferation of superficial synovial cells, often with palisading; marked infiltration with chronic inflammatory cells (lymphocytes or plasma cells predominating), with a tendency to form "lymphoid nodules"; deposition of compact fibrin, either on the surface of the joint or interstitially; foci of cell necrosis

11. Characteristic histological changes in the rheumatoid nodules, including granulomatous foci with central zones of cell necrosis, surrounded by proliferating fixed cells, and finally, peripheral fibrosis with chronic inflammatory cellular infiltration, predominantly perivascular

A definite diagnosis of rheumatoid arthritis can be made if five of the above criteria are present in a particular case. The joint signs enumerated in criteria 1 to 5 must have been present continuously for at least six weeks.

A probable diagnosis of rheumatoid arthritis requires three of the above criteria. At least one of the first five must have been present for no less than six weeks.

Possible rheumatoid arthritis may be diagnosed if two of the above criteria are present, provided that they have been so for at least three weeks.

DIFFERENTIAL DIAGNOSIS

Ropes[1] enumerated seventeen differential diagnostic criteria. They add up to a formidable list of other serious conditions that must be excluded.

Exclusions

1. Disseminated lupus erythematosus, characterized by a distinctive butterfly rash on the face, with plugging of epidermal follicles and skin atrophy

2. The presence of four or more so-called lupus erythematosus cells in smears prepared from heparinized blood incubated for not more than two hours

3. Histological evidence of periarteritis nodosa, including segmental arterial necrosis and nodular eosinophilic infiltration extending perivascularly

4. Weakness of the neck, trunk, and pharyngeal muscles, or persistent muscle swelling, indicative of dermatomyositis

5. Definite scleroderma, provided it is not limited to the fingers

6. A clinical picture characteristic of rheumatic fever, including a migratory pattern of joint involvement; evidence of endocarditis; subcutaneous nodules and chorea

7. Signs of gout: these include a history of acute attacks of pain, redness, and swelling in one or more joints, especially if relieved by colchicine. The presence of tophi is pathognomonic.

8. A clinical picture of acute infective arthritis, whether bacterial or viral: this includes signs of infection elsewhere, rigors, and pyrexia.

9. The presence of the tubercle bacilli

10. A clinical picture of Reiter's syndrome, with urethritis, conjuctivitis, and acute joint involvement which tends to flit from joint to joint in the early stages

11. Hypertrophic pulmonary osteoarthropathy may mimic rheumatoid arthritis: clubbing of fingers and toes accompanied by hypertrophic periostitis along the shafts of the long bones, including metatarsals. An intrapulmonary lesion will be found.

12. A clinical picture of a neuropathic joint, with condensation and destruction of surrounding bone and neurologic findings

13. Sarcoidosis, diagnosed histologically or by a positive Kveim test

14. Multiple myeloma, distinguished by a marked increase of plasma cells within the bone marrow and the presence of Bence Jones protein in the urine

15. Skin lesions characteristic of erythema nodosum

16. A diagnosis of leukemia or lymphoma

17. The presence of agammaglobulinemia

Some features of the eleven diagnostic criteria deserve further consideration.

Morning Stiffness. Of all the symptoms arising from a rheumatoid joint, morning stiffness is so common as to be almost pathognomonic of the condition. The fluid secreted by inflamed synovium, while copious, is not normal in biochemical makeup or rheological characteristics (as described in criterion 9). The abnormal synovial fluid has poor lubricating qualities, especially when the patient first wakes up. It is probable that this is an effect of the type of fluid secreted in an immobile joint. As a result, when the patient first rises after being immobile, movements of the affected joints can be made only slowly and with difficulty. Repeated movements over the succeeding half hour result in the secretion of fluid of a more normal consistency, so that movement becomes progressively easier.

Joint Involvement. The problem has always been to know whether or not a patient with constant pain and swelling of one joint is suffering from rheumatoid arthritis, with all that that diagnosis implies, because, by definition, rheumatoid disease is a polyarthritis. It is surprising how often the clinician is presented with this problem. The criteria concerned with the occurrence of joint involvement, both in regard to the number of joints involved and the period of time that such an inflammation has lasted, are an attempt to find a way out of this quandary. These criteria are also a clear indication of one of the basic facts about rheumatoid arthritis: it consists of a whole series of clinical syndromes of differing severity. There is a marked distinction between the young patient with symmetrical effusions (so-called ''hydrops'') in the knees without much synovial thickening and the woman in her late thirties with generalized florid synovial swelling, collapsing joints, subcutaneous nodules, and positive serologic tests. The prognosis may be very different.

To describe a particular case of rheumatoid arthritis, the use of qualifying adjectives to define some of its features is desirable from the point of view of both prognosis and treatment. Such terms as *seropositive* or *seronegative, erosive* or *nonerosive, nodular* or *anodular, poly-* or *oligoarthritis* (or, recently, even *pauciarthritis*) are in common use. Provided they have been properly defined, they may aid communication between experts, even if they are jargon.

ETIOLOGY

Currey,[2] in his comprehensive review of the etiology of rheumatoid arthritis, commented that the ultimate cause of the condition remains elusive. Many features are, however, well recognized. Although rheumatoid arthritis may begin at any age, it is most common between the ages of thirty and sixty years. That women are more often afflicted than men is well documented. Statistically, there is a modest familial clustering with regard to both the clinical disease and the presence of serum rheumatoid factor in the blood of affected people.

Rheumatoid arthritis usually runs a protracted course, with fluctuating remissions. This must always be borne in mind when the results of a particular treatment are being assessed. Pregnancy may induce a remission, as may an attack of hepatitis.

Some features of the disease have hinted at a cause or combination of causes. The simultaneous occurrence of widespread inflammatory lesions, often symmetrical, suggests a generalized reaction of the body to some agent rather than a local cause. Climatic differences in the incidence and severity of the disease exist, and must have an etiological significance. There has been a suggestion that the disease is historically of relatively recent onset; a fascinating observation if true. Since bone and joint changes are so important in the condition, an examination of bones of known date from earlier ages ought to clear up this point.

What is surprising is that most etiological hypotheses that have been tested have yielded negative results. For example, no nutritional relationship has been found. So far, investigation of the autonomic nervous system has shown no signs of imbalance, nor has any feature of endocrine abnormality been found. Occupational factors do not seem to play a major role in the onset of the condition.

Currey quoted Burch[3] as suggesting that the epidemiology of the disease pointed to a somatic mutation as the trigger mechanism. In such an event, an investigation of victims of radiation ought to have shown an association, but an examination of atomic bomb survivors failed to reveal the expected statistical link.

Attempts to transmit the disease, and thus prove an infective cause by adhering to Koch's postulates, failed. Focal sepsis as a trigger of rheumatoid arthritis had its protagonists, so that past generations of sufferers were subjected to removal of teeth and tonsils, all to no avail.

Even psychosomatic mechanisms were thought at one time to be implicated. Most clinicians have seen cases in which erosive, seropositive rheumatoid arthritis seems to have been started by a severe psychological shock such as the unexpected death of a close relative. These theories have proved difficult to assess statistically and appear to be a blind alley.

The early reports of a good response to corticosteroid extracts, now known to be a nonspecific reaction, inspired a premature hope that the cause of rheumatoid arthritis had been found; that it was a disease of adaptation[4] as a result of stress of one sort or another on the adrenal cortex.

Later, the presence of "fibrinoid necrosis" within the lesions of rheumatoid arthritis was responsible for the classification of the condition as a "collagen disease," but this did not prove helpful in understanding its etiology.

In recent years, investigation of the newly discovered genetic markers such as the histocompatability antigens has failed to prove a direct hereditary cause for the disease, unlike the circumstances in some of the spondyloarthropathies[5] in which HL-A 27 antigen is highly significant. Recent work suggests that further research in this direction may be productive.[6] Were it to be so, there would be a certain irony in the fact. After a hundred years of medical advance, based on the work of Pasteur and Koch, during which an extrinsic cause has been found for most of the major diseases, we find ourselves in the position of having to postulate a disease that depends upon the chemical nature of the patient and not on some foreign invasion. This theory sounds suspiciously like the old concept of humors as the cause of disease, a theory that reigned for hundreds of years until Koch overthrew it!

The general notion of autoimmune disease has led to advances in our knowledge. Burnet's hypothesis[7] or "self" and "nonself" antigens implied that the trigger was an abnormal immune reaction aganist one of the normal tissues in the body. It seems logical to presume that certain individuals are vulnerable to such a pathologic autoimmune reaction as a result of their inherited biochemical structure, although something would have to trigger off such a reaction, even in a susceptible individual.

PATHOGENESIS

Biochemical Factors. Immunologic processes almost certainly play an important part in triggering the basic lesion of rheumatoid arthritis. Whether within the synovium or in connective tissue elsewhere in which nodules occur, a reaction more complex than the straightforward autoimmune reaction initiates the process. Currey described it in the following way: immune complexes consisting of antigen/antibody protein activate the complement system, thus causing a migration of polymorphonuclear leukocytes into the area of the developing lesion. These scavenger cells absorb the protein and, in so doing, release lysosomal enzymes. The enzymes are the chemical mediators of inflammation and are the immediate cause of the synovitis.

Chronic synovitis leads to the formation of granulation tissue. The effect of rheumatoid arthritis depends upon whether articular cartilage erosion takes place. This erosion follows upon invasion of the articular cartilage by the granulation tissue (pannus), and is due to local release of degradative enzymes that directly erode articular cartilage and subchondral bone. No wonder the adjective "invasive" has been applied to such synovium.

Patterns of Cartilage Erosion. In the articular cartilage of an affected joint, three regions of differing erosion occur (Fig. 13-1 A and B). This pattern of cartilage loss depends on the anatomical features of the joint.

The central area, which is constantly opposed to the other cartilage surface, is protected from erosion: whatever the severity of the disease, this region of the cartilage is spared to some extent.

Around this protected area is one in which the synovium lining the inner surface of the capsule of the joint is applied to the surface of the articular cartilage, at least in some positions of movement of the joint. Despite, or perhaps because of, the thin layer of synovial fluid separating the two surfaces, erosion occurs. The pattern of erosion in this area is typical, with progressive loss of cartilage extending from the surface inward. It tends to be regular.

At the edges of the joint the position is very different. The fold of synovium in this region, lining the edges of the joint, often has the most florid inflammatory reaction with marked thickening and even villus formation. Here, the reaction is the most aggressive, and erosion in this area is generally severe; in some cases so extreme as to undermine the articular cartilage completely, by invasion of underlying bone from the edges. In small joints, such as the metatarsophalangeal joints, the excavation of bone may be total, until the metatarsal head is left completely free within the joint, the synovium having met deep to it. Radiographic changes of rheumatoid arthritis appear first, and are usually most severe, in this region. The presence on a film of lateral erosions in a joint may be helpful in the diagnosis of the condition.

Finally, from the peripheral synovium, "fingers" of pannus grow directly across the cartilage surface, eating through to subchondral bone. Deep irregular grooves are seen to be etched into the surface of the joint when the pannus is pulled off during surgery. Soft tissue changes are not confined to the joint itself. Rheumatoid arthritis is a general condition of connective tissue and collagen is involved throughout the body.

Joint Capsule and Ligaments. Synovial erosion affects the capsule and ligaments of the joint by direct invasion, with resulting stretching and subluxation. The synovium may break

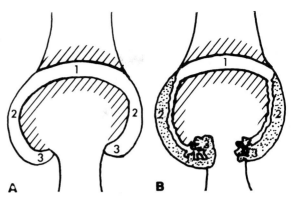

Fig. 13-1. (*A*) Diagrammatic representation of the three regions of articular cartilage in a typical joint. Area 1 is that part of the cartilage which is opposed to the cartilage on the other surface of the joint. Area 2 is that part of the cartilage usually covered by synovium. Area 3 is the reflected layer of synovium at the edge of the joint. (*B*) Diagram of the same joint, in which rheumatoid erosion has occurred. Area 1 shows the least and area 3 shows the most erosion.

completely through the capsule and extend via the periarticular tissues toward the surface of the body. In some patients, large masses of invasive synovium may be felt. Rupture of the joint can occur spontaneously, with sudden wide dissemination of synovial fluid through the tissues of the body, in the region of the joint. Posterior rupture of the knee results in synovial fluid running down the calf between the soleus and gastrocnemius muscle bellies, a condition often misdiagnosed as deep vein thrombosis in the calf, and unwisely treated with anticoagulants.

Spreading extraarticular synovium may erode bone at some distance from the joint itself, causing severe disruption.

It is to be remembered that the collagen forming the capsule and ligaments may have been weakened by the generalized protein loss that accompanies rheumatoid arthritis, and may be more vulnerable to synovial erosion than normal tissues.

Nonarticular Synovitis. The synovium of the tendon sheaths and bursae is also affected, leading to large masses of soft tissue swelling which, in the tendon sheaths, obstructs the movements of the tendons, causes pain in its own right, and, in some cases, erodes the tendons until they rupture spontaneously. Local tenderness may be extreme, and its anatomical distribution allows the diagnosis to be made. In the foot it is usually the peroneal and tibialis anterior and posterior sheaths that are affected, but when the extensors are involved, rupture occurs by attrition, leading to drop toes. Swelling within the flexor tendon sheaths is more insidious, giving rise to deep pain extending from the back of the ankle medially into the sole of the foot and causing difficulty in walking. The synovial bulk may give rise to tarsal tunnel syndrome due to nerve compression.

Muscle Contracture. There has been controversy in the past about whether muscles are involved in the rheumatoid process. They are certainly affected; some more than others, perhaps reflecting a difference in their chemical constitution. In particular, the small muscles of the hands and feet are commonly affected. The collagen between muscle fibers is attacked, and the resulting fibrosis, together with the atrophy of the muscles themselves, leads to contracture which may be severe. In the feet the intrinsic muscle contracture is one of the main deforming forces on the knuckle joints as well as the toes. Together with the bulk of synovium surrounding and spreading the metatarsal heads apart, the abnormal muscle pull may cause not only clawing of the toes and dislocation of the metatarsophalangeal joints, but in some cases might even produce inversion of the whole transverse arch, so that the second, third, and fourth metatarsal heads are the most prominent; callosity formation in the underlying skin is intense and the patient soon experiences the pain of "walking on pebbles."

Bone Changes. Generalized rheumatoid arthritis is almost always accompanied by softening of bone. There are several reasons for this. As part of the general loss of collagen the main protein matrix of bone is reduced. Less calcium can be laid on the reduced matrix, and calcium turnover in this situation leads to a condition of demineralization. Loss of protein and mineral from bone is, by definition, *osteoporosis.* Pain and increasing joint stiffness lead

to typical periarticular *disuse atrophy* of the bone. In many such severe cases, the patient requires steroid administration in an attempt to dampen down the severity of the inflammatory disease. This has the unfortunate side effect of causing *endocrine osteoporosis.* The result may be catastrophic collapse of bone, leading to severe deformity.

Even in less serious instances, osteoporosis may lead to repeated march fractures, resulting in recurring episodes of pain and edema in the foot.

Vasculitis. In seropositive rheumatoid arthritis, perivascular infiltration commonly occurs, and this frequently leads to generalized vasculitis. It is often clinically silent and may easily be overlooked, but the surgeon does so at his patient's peril. The injudicious use of tourniquets for bloodless field operations may result in unexpected skin necrosis.

Digital arteries in the hands and feet are often involved and roentgenograms may show calcification in such vessels. The condition may be asymptomatic, but spasm may occur with repeated Raynaud's phenomenon. There may be associated vascular lesions in the nail folds.

Extensive arterial and arteriolar involvement may be associated with systemic illness, including pyrexia, subcutaneous nodules, and even pleural and pericardial involvement with inflammatory signs and effusion. Sometimes there is patchy or even extensive dermal infarction, leading to scattered ulcers which are usually most obvious in the shins, ankle regions, and on the dorsum of the feet. They do not conform to the typical shape and position of varicose ulcers and differ from them in being due to loss of arterial blood supply rather than to venous engorgement and extracapillary hemosiderin deposition. The intervening skin appears atrophic and avascular. Occasionally the areas of skin necrosis may be widespread, owing to the extent of vascular involvement. Such a condition has been called "malignant" and may lead to the loss of one or more limbs, or even to gangrene of bowel or myocardial infarction and the death of the patient.

Vasculitis may respond to antiinflammatory

drugs. The author has seen severe cases respond remarkably to penicillamine, with healing of extensive ulcers on the legs, allowing major surgery to be performed.

Peripheral Neuropathy. Rheumatoid arthritis may cause peripheral neuropathy, especially in severe seropositive, nodular disease. It is more common in men than in women. If mild it leads to distal sensory loss, especially in the feet, with typical "stocking" anesthesia. Amidst the patient's many other problems, it may easily be missed. The often associated autonomic neuropathy, with loss of sweating, may suggest the diagnosis.

Involvement of peripheral nerves may be fulminating, with motor as well as sensory loss leading to paralysis and foot drop. This has a poor prognosis; many patients develop necrotizing vasculitis with all its hazards to life and limb.

CLINICAL SYNDROMES IN THE FOOT

Metatarsalgia

Unless the synovitis in the metatarsophalangeal joints is transient, stiffness usually intervenes, aided by intrinsic muscle contracture. The bulk of synovial tissue (as described in the previous section) tends to spread the metatarsal rays apart, while clawing of the toes forces the transverse arch to the ground. Wasting of the intrinsic muscle layers in the sole makes the metatarsal heads increasingly vulnerable to weight-bearing pressure. So-called protective callosities increase in thickness, adding, in the end, to the pain beneath the metatarsal heads. Similar pressure effects occur in the prominent bony projections of the stiff, clawed toes. Habitual hyperextension of the metatarsophalangeal joints leads finally to dislocation. Vasculitis may cause necrosis of skin with chronic sinus formation in the affected joints. Occasionally, the metatarsal heads may come "shining through" the skin on the soles of such feet.

Into this situation the specific pathologic changes of rheumatoid disease intrude, causing joint disruption as erosion takes place.

At first, metatarsalgia is very similar to the condition that occurs in old age, with atrophy and stiffening, but the onset of destructive changes in the joints turns the forefoot into a parody of the normal collapsing situation. Gross deformities of the transverse arch and toes follow. The result can be very disabling, especially since such patients are often young and actively engaged in a fulltime career or the rigors of bringing up a young family. Treatment becomes essential.

The Hindfoot

Erosive arthritis commonly extends from the metatarsophalangeal joints or begins primarily in the hindfoot. In some cases all the joints of the tarsus and those surrounding it are affected equally and progressively, so that the increasing stiffness of the foot is balanced and the extremity maintains a more or less normal shape. Although the muscle wasting and stiffness give rise to prominent bony points which may be pressed upon during weight bearing, such a foot can usually be fitted into a normal shoe.

If only part of the tarsus is involved, especially if it includes a major weight-bearing joint, there is early distortion of the foot and the orthotic problem is more difficult. In particular, subtalar joint involvement may lead to a spasmodic flatfoot very similar to that found in adolescence associated with injury to a congenital tarsal bar. The result is the severely stiff, painful planovalgus foot so typical of the latter condition, but again modified by the collapse that takes place in rheumatoid bone and joint surfaces. Since the subtalar joints with erosive disease will never return to normal, most cannot recover without operation.

As far as symptoms from the hindfoot are concerned, tenosynovitis often plays a large part, especially peroneal and posterior tibial tenosynovitis. If recognized and treated adequately, whether by the injection of local steroids, antiinflammatory drugs and correct splintage, or by synovectomy of the sheath, the prognosis may prove better than expected.

The Ankle Joint

The ankle joint is less often involved than

the knee or hip, perhaps because it contains less synovium. Furthermore, the functional position of the ankle is in the middle of its range of movement, again in contradistinction to the hip and knee, which are held at the extremes of extension during standing. As a result, a fair amount of ankle involvement can occur before the patient begins to get symptoms from the joint. In the hip and knee, stretching of the fibrosed capsule causes early pain.

It is only when collapse of the talar condyles leads to complete loss of movement, or when increasing stiffness in the subtalar and midtarsal joints reveals an underlying unexpected stiffness of the ankle, that the patient develops symptoms. At this stage there is already stiffness of the whole foot and ankle. Such a situation is comfortable provided all the elements of the foot, heel, and ankle are in a correct relationship for weight bearing. Any deformity, for example inversion or eversion of the heel, immediately throws abnormal load bearing onto a fibrosed joint, causing pain. Stiffness of the tarsal joints with deformity, if accompanied by fibrous ankylosis of the ankle, is very likely to bring the patient to a surgeon for help.

Complex Patterns of Deformity

Collapse of joints in the foot has been described in isolation. Whereas in some cases such consideration of the foot alone is adequate, many patients with severe large joint polyarthritis suffer from complex patterns of deformity in the upper and lower limbs that may be difficult to understand if the joints are viewed in isolation. If the limb as a whole is inspected, the reason for a particular deformity may become obvious.

In other words, synovitis resulting in erosive collapse of cartilage, capsular fibrosis, and intrinsic muscular contracture is not the whole story as far as the foot is concerned. There is another factor in the development of deformity. That factor is the habitual load bearing applied to the limb and the habitual posture of the joints of that limb. The former causes characteristic bone collapse and the latter stiffens the joints in the position in which they are held. For example, it is not unusual to see a patient with two stiff wrists, the one fixed in flexion and the other in extension. This may seem difficult to explain, but if the patient is observed as a whole it will be seen that the characteristic posture of the two limbs is different, perhaps because on one side the patient has a stiff shoulder and consequently holds the arm to the side, while on the other side stiffness of the elbow causes the wrist to be dropped. Sometimes it is the position of the arms that the patient adopts to perform his usual work that is responsible for this situation.

In the foot it is the standing posture that usually regulates the developing pattern of deformity, but the patient confined to a wheelchair will show a very different picture. Such a patient may sit eccentrically in his chair, with his two knees together but his legs tilted to one side. He will develop fixed flexion and abduction contracture of one hip, accompanied by fixed flexion and adduction of the knee and valgus deformity of the foot on the same side. The other leg will have an opposite pattern, with adduction of the hip, abduction of the knee, and an inverted foot. Such contrasting deformities occur in ambulatory patients as well, resulting in zigzag but parallel limbs, the appearance of which has been described as "windswept."

Abnormalities of shape are always three-dimensional, but they may be resolved, for ease of understanding, into deformities in two planes: side-to-side or *transverse,* and anteroposterior or *sagittal.*

Deformities in the Sagittal Plane. Rheumatoid collapse of the hip joint occurs in a way similar to osteoarthritis, with the obvious differences of emphasis that depend upon the dissimilarities in pathogenesis. Of these, the texture of the bone is the most significant. Osteoarthritis is associated with increased blood supply and bone density, while rheumatoid bone is soft and avascular. Eventual segmental necrosis is common, converting a stiff joint into a dislocating, unstable one.

The first phase of increasing stiffness leads to fixed flexion of the hip. The patient tends to walk with the trunk bent forward and the weight partially borne by a stick held in the opposite hand, or with excessive lumbar lordosis. As a result, the knee comes to be held in a position of slight flexion and, in a third stage of accomodation to the situation, the patient has to walk with a dorsiflexed ankle so that the heel can be conveniently brought to the ground.

Unfortunately, continuous dorsiflexion of the ankle is not in the patient's long-term interest. Should erosive changes be taking place within the ankle, this posture is converted into a permanent shape by collapse of the dome-shaped talar condyles, the "flat top talus." If the hip and knee are straightened, whether by natural resolution, splintage, and physiotherapy, or by operative means, the patient will be left with a foot in which all the weight is borne on the heel; a situation that makes for poor gait. In this condition, the presence of a heel on the sole of a shoe makes walking impossible. On the other hand, if stiffness of the ankle was present before the onset of fixed flexion in the hip and knee, dorsiflexion cannot take place, and the patient's heel soon leaves the ground, forcing the load onto the contracted anterior capsule of the ankle joint. At the same time, the metatarsal heads are forced to bear the full load of walking. Such constant loading, especially with toes dorsiflexed, leads to early collapse of the transverse arch, with all that implies; a situation not conducive to normal walking.

It will be seen that sagittal deformities in the leg transfer abnormal load bearing to those joints normally capable of movement within the sagittal or anteroposterior plane. The joints of the hindfoot are not included with these, but at the junction of the fore- and hindfoot the joints have an element, although a minor one, of extension and flexion. The proximal row of joints in this region, the talonavicular and calcaneocuboid, as well as the more distal tarsometatarsal joints, if subjected to such dorsiflexion loading, undergo some degree of subluxation. If they are subject to inflammatory disease, the amount of stiffness, capsular stretching, and dorsal subluxation may be severe enough to prevent normal walking without special shoes. If tiptoe walking is necessary because of loss of ankle dorsiflexion, load bearing is taken at right angles to the joints and dorsal subluxation does not occur. On the other hand, the softened bone may not be able to withstand body weight and the longitudinal arch may undergo axial collapse, leading to shortening and distortion of the foot as a whole.

Deformities in the Transverse Plane. Valgus or varus deformity, whether in the hip, knee, or foot, gives rise to a similar balanced, complex pattern of deformity throughout the limb. When the disease starts in the hip, the transverse component of the deformity is nearly always one of varus, causing increasing valgus strain on the knee. In particular, if rheumatoid disease coexists in the knee, the affected ligaments cannot long withstand the strain of valgus load bearing. The medial collateral ligament becomes stretched, with widening of the medial joint line and lateral subluxation of the tibia, while the lateral compartment of the joint undergoes cartilaginous and bony collapse.

At the same time, the valgus deformity of the knee forces abnormal load bearing onto the medial side of the foot. Although such abnormal load bearing has been analyzed into two planes, the reality is, of course, three-dimensional. In the foot particularly, it shows up as a rotational deformity, rolling into valgus for walking. Such pes planovalgus, habitually adopted, leads to collapse of the anterior and posterior subtalar joints in the first instance. These never function in isolation. Normal inversion and eversion take place around an axis of rotation extending more or less longitudinally through the hindfoot. Synchronous movements occur in all the joints in this region. Not only the subtalar but the talonavicular, naviculocuneiform, and calcaneocuboid joints become equally involved. All are likely to collapse. The critical areas are usually the heel bone, which is forced into an extreme valgus position, and the talonavicular joint. The former impinges on the tip of the lateral malleolus, giving rise to local pain that may be severe.

The valgus heel also throws the weight onto the medial longitudinal arch, so that lateral strain is placed upon the talonavicular joint in particular. Subluxation can affect the whole forefoot, leading in the worst cases to complete talonavicular dislocation. An example of such a dislocated forefoot is illustrated in the chapter on the stiff flatfoot (Chap. 6). In that case, the cause was rheumatoid arthritis, and the foot was capable of only the most modest function.

THE MANAGEMENT OF THE RHEUMATOID FOOT

Careful assessment of the patterns of deformity is necessary to avoid dealing inadvisably with one element of a deformed limb and unbalancing one or more of the others. Treatment requires careful planning in the choice of operations, the best position for a joint that has to be stiffened, and the correct order of procedure. The treatment of the rheumatoid foot must rest basically in the hands of the rheumatologist, but the surgeon plays an increasing part in the treatment.

Stabilization of the hindfoot, and the ankle if necessary (by means of arthrodesis), and the removal of dislocated metatarsophalangeal joints by excision arthroplasty, as described by Fowler[8] or by Kessel in Chapter 14, can do a great deal to get a patient functioning normally both at home and at work. The most common arthrodesis, triple fusion of the hindfoot (Fig. 13-2A and B), has particularly good results in rheumatoid arthritis, because the soft bone fuses easily. Excision arthroplasty of the knuckle joints gives remarkably good results, with a surprisingly short recovery time to full walking, until one remembers the state of the foot before operation, to which the patient has become adapted. In the latter the author has abandoned the use of a tourniquet because of the possibility of vasculitis. In a personal series of 24 operations performed in this manner, he has had no example of wound breakdown.

In many cases in which a large joint of the lower limb as well as the feet are involved, it

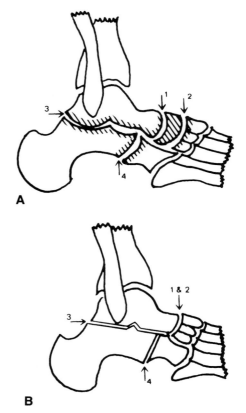

Fig. 13-2. (*A*) Diagrammatic representation of the bones and joints of the hindfoot: (1) the talonavicular joint; (2) naviculocuneiform joints; (3) posterior and anterior subtalar joints; (4) calcaneocuboid joint. (*B*) After triple arthrodesis the navicular bone has been excised entirely and the talocuboid articulation has been denuded of cartilage (1 and 2), as have the two subtalar joints (3) and the calcaneocuboid joint. When fusion is complete, the talus, calcaneus, cuboid, and cuneiforms will constitute one bone.

is often advisable to operate on the feet first so that the patient can gain the full benefit of total hip or knee replacement by early walking. Such planning aids rehabilitation.

The administration of drugs to the rheumatoid patient requires careful control and is usually best left to the rheumatologist. Adequate footwear is essential. Properly made leather-soled shoes, measured for the patient's feet, are indispensible. Molded insoles can be of great benefit. Occasionally boots are required to control the hindfoot. Calipers may be needed to control a drop foot, or even to fix a heel in a good position, but such feet are usually better treated by surgery. Vascular problems may prevent operation and the orthotist is presented with a formidable problem. Some patients are helped by one of the varieties of "space shoes."

During acute episodes, correct splintage in a functional position for each joint of a limb is very important, either by the use of plastic or plaster-of-Paris splints. Physiotherapy is vital, both in the acute and the chronic case, to maintain movement in joints and so minimize contracture as well as to prevent muscle wasting.

Finally, patients with juvenile arthritis require special attention to splintage to prevent deformity occurring from the abnormal growth of part of the epiphyses (see below). Calipers may well be necessary.

For adequate management of the rheumatoid patient, a team is essential. The use of teams in the treatment of many conditions, while increasingly fashionable, is not always necessary and may actually lead to a deterioration in management if there is no clear chain of command. One clinician should always bear the ultimate responsibility for a case. Patients who are treated by a committee do not do well. Within these limits, a combined team, including rheumatologist, orthopaedic surgeon, physiotherapist, occupational therapist, rehabilitation officer, chiropodist, and orthotist can supply overall care. Usually it is wise for the rheumatologist to be in charge, except while the patient is undergoing surgery.

OTHER RHEUMATOID CONDITIONS IN THE FEET

Significant differences are seen in some of the other rheumatoid conditions that commonly affect the feet. Although any of the rheumatoid arthropathies may affect the distal parts of the limbs rather than the trunk and proximal joints, the following diseases deserve particular mention.

Juvenile Chronic Polyarthritis

The above term is advocated by Ansell and Bywaters[9] to describe any of the variants of rheumatoid disease in childhood. Their so-called Taplow (from the Canadian Hospital for Rheumatic Diseases on the Thames) criteria for diagnosis are simple and useful. They define juvenile chronic arthritis as "arthritis starting before the age of sixteen, manifesting with two of the following: pain; swelling; limitation of movement in four or more joints, reliably observed for at least three months; or affection of one joint for three months, accompanied by histological biopsy confirmation."

There are many causes of juvenile chronic arthritis, of which Still's disease is the best known. In 1897 Still[10] described 22 cases of juvenile arthritis, almost all of which had the classic signs: fever, rash, lymphadenopathy; and arthritis. Eighty years later the condition remains a separate entity, easily differentiated from rheumatoid arthritis by serologic testing. It can occur in adult life[11] but is most common in children. In contradistinction, rheumatoid arthritis, while much more common in adult life, can also occur in children. It can be distinguished from Still's disease both by serology and by the clinical differences.

Three variants of Still's disease are seen: polyarticular; systemic manifestations; and cases with only a few joints involved, with or without inflammatory iridocyclitis.

Of the other causes of juvenile chronic arthritis, psoriasis, ulcerative colitis, lupus erythematosus, and ankylosing spondylitis can all occur in childhood and give rise to arthropathy.

Arthritis in children causes similar problems to those in adult life, with slight variations. Capsular fibrosis may be severe, but articular cartilage erosion is overcome to some extent by further growth of cartilage. There is usually little true osteoporosis, but disuse demineralization may occur, especially in the juxta-articular bone.

The essential difference between child and adult is that the epiphyseal cartilage continues to grow in the child during the disease. The increased blood supply that accompanies synovitis causes increased growth of the epiphysis. This may be so obvious as to be visible on roentgenograms. It causes distortion of joints, and, in particular, any joint held in a contracted position runs the risk of that portion of epiphysis lying against the opposing cartilage being held in check, while those parts unopposed growing too much. The dome of the talus, for example, may be held in check by the tibial surface, while the anterior and posterior parts of the talar condyles hypertrophy. A foot held in plantarflexion by the bedrest imposed on a child with a painful ankle joint may result in such distortion of the talus by abnormal epiphyseal growth that the ankle can never again be brought back into a position of function without operation.

In juvenile chronic arthritis, therefore, splintage in the position of function and competent physiotherapy are essential during acute phases of the condition if deformity is to be prevented.

Psoriatic Arthropathy

Patients with psoriasis may develop arthritis. This is especially common in familial psoriasis, with some families alternating generations with skin pathology and inflammations in joints.

Synovitis is often limited to the distal joints of the limbs, especially the fingers and toes. In the feet, characteristic square-shaped toes are seen, because the proximal and distal interphalangeal as well as the metatarsophalangeal joints are involved. This differentiates the condition from rheumatoid arthritis, as do the characteristic lesions that occur in the finger- and toenails. These lesions consist of pitting of the surface of the nails, longitudinal ridging, distal discoloration, and hyperkeratosis of the surrounding skin.

Erosion of the joints may be very severe in psoriatic arthropathy in both hands and feet. Sometimes the joint contractures are severe, with marked disability from stiff, painful toes. Large joints may be affected. Many patients with psoriatic arthropathy require operations on the forefeet, and an interesting characteristic of such surgery is that incisions tend to heal in a much shorter time than normal. This is an indication of the basic characteristic of

psoriatic skin: its cellular turnover is much faster than the average; in some cases, almost twice that of the rest of the population.

Arthritis in Patients With Congenital Hypermobility

Congenital hypermobility is not really a disease,[12] but rather a normal variant. It may be generalized or more marked in the distal joints of the limbs.

In rare instances, patients with distal hypermobility develop erosive synovitis in the joints of the hands and feet. This is probably small-joint rheumatoid arthritis and it is not suggested that the condition is unusual in any way so far as etiology is concerned. The erosions that develop are distinguished by their severity: the joints become markedly excavated, almost like neuropathic ones. It is probable that this is the effect of erosive synovitis on lax joints. The significance of the condition is that since stiffness is not a feature, there is surprisingly little disability from the dislocated joints and no treatment may be required.

Gout[13]

Gout is a disease caused by an excess of urates in the blood and other tissues. Such hyperuricemia is a disease with a strong familial tendency, and it is more common in men than in women.

Acute Gout. The patient may have hyperuricemia without any symptoms, but sooner or later develops an acute episode of pain in a joint. The process is one of acute chemical or irritative arthritis. It may occur in any joint, but by far the most common (70% of cases) joint involved is the metatarsophalangeal joint of a big toe. The patient develops a sensation of throbbing that develops into pain over the affected joint. It often starts at night and may wake the patient. Within a few hours the joint becomes red, swollen, and exquisitely tender. Venous engorgement is present, with a hot, shiny skin. Walking becomes impossible. Without treatment the attack may last several days or weeks, but it eventually subsides and the joint returns to normal. An irritating desquamation of the overlying skin is sometimes seen during resolution.

Chronic Tophaceous Gout. Chronic inflammation is found in the fingers, toes, and ears, and is due to the deposition of insoluble urates into the tissues to form palpable lumps of chalky crystals known as tophi. They usually follow repeated untreated acute attacks, but they can also occur insidiously with previous acute episodes. Tophi lead to destructive arthropathy and secondary degenerative changes.

In time, as the tophi become larger, they become visible through the atrophic skin overlying the joint and may eventually cause skin necrosis, so that the crystalline material is discarded like a foreign body. The ulcer may then heal or reopen several times.

Gout may be considered as having several etiological factors. Primarily, there is an inherited metabolic disorder causing hyperuricemia, due either to deficient breakdown or excessive formation of urates. Secondarily, some environmental factor, for example cold (in the ears) or local injury (in the hallux), causes crystallization of urates, which may give rise to acute inflammation.

Treatment. In acute gout, the time-honored treatment has been the administration of colchicine. The drug is used as a diagnostic test and is prescribed orally as soon as the pain begins. A dose of 1.0 mg. is given immediately, followed by 0.5 mg. every 2 hours until the attack subsides. The effect of the drug varies and may cause severe gastrointestinal problems.

Phenylbutazone, in doses of 200 mg. 4 times daily, is equally effective but it is important to limit the use of this drug to the acute attack because of the possible side effects. Indomethacin, in doses of 50 mg. 4 times daily, is just as effective.

Long-term treatment of hyperuricemia consists of the use of uricosuric drugs to increase urate excretion in the urine by preventing renal reabsorption and to reduce the plasma level of uric acid to normal and keep it there. The drug most often used is probenecid, in doses of 0.5 to 1.0 gm. daily by mouth. Surgery is indicated in gout mainly to remove tophi that are causing symptoms.

Pseudogout is a condition similar to gout in some of its manifestations, but it is caused by crystals of calcium pyrophosphate dihydrate. Unlike gout, it rarely affects the feet.

REFERENCES

1. Ropes, M. W., Bennet, G. A., Cobb, S., Jacox, R., and Jessar, R. A.: Diagnostic criteria for rheumatoid arthritis, 1958 revision. Ann. Rheum. Dis., *18:*49, 1959.
2. Currey, H. L. F.: Aetiology and pathogenesis of rheumatoid arthritis. *In* Scott, J. T. (ed.): Copeman's Textbook of the Rheumatic Diseases. ed. 5. New York, Churchill Livingstone, 1978.
3. Burch, P. R. J.: Autoimmunity: some etiological aspects. Lancet, *i:*1253, 1963.
4. Selye, H.: The general adaption syndrome and the disease of adaption. J. Clin. Endocrinol., *6:*117, 1946.
5. Solomon, L., and Berman, L.: Rheumatoid disorders of the lumbar spine. *In* Helfet, A., and Gruebel-Lee, D. M. (eds.): Disorders of the Lumbar Spine. Philadelphia, Lippincott, 1978.
6. Panayi, G. S., and Wooley, P. H.: HLA antigens in rheumatoid arthritis. Ann. Rheum. Dis., *36:*365, 1977.
7. Burnet, F. M.: The Clonal Selection Theory of Acquired Immunity. Cambridge, Cambridge University Press, 1959.
8. Fowler, A. W.: A method of forefoot reconstruction. J. Bone Joint Surg. *41B:*507, 1959.
9. Ansell, B. M., and Bywaters, E. G. L.: Prognosis in Still's disease. Bull. Rheum. Dis., *9:*189, 1959.
10. Still, G. F.: On a form of chronic joint disease in children. Medico-Chirurgical Transactions, *80:*47, 1897.
11. Bywaters, E. G. L.: Still's disease in the adult. Ann. Rheum. Dis., *30:*121, 1971.
12. Grahame, R.: Joint mobility—clinical aspects. Proceedings of the Royal Society of Medicine, *64:*693, 1971.
13. Scott, J. T.: Gout. *In* Scott, J. T. (ed.): Copeman's Textbook of the Rheumatic Diseases. ed. 5. pp. 647–691. New York, Churchill Livingstone, 1978.

14 Arthroplasty of the Forefoot

LIPMANN KESSEL

This operation is intended for patients who have severe disability due to fixed clawing of the toes with associated subluxation or dislocation of the metatarsophalangeal joints. It is indicated only for severely afflicted feet; indeed, the worse the foot, the less difficult the operation and the more pleasing the end result. Such deformity is encountered mostly in cases of rheumatoid arthritis, rarely in cases of severe pes cavus. The operation is recommended when all conservative measures and minor surgical procedures have failed to relieve symptoms, and as an alternative to amputation of all the toes. It is a modification of the procedure described by Hoffman and by Fowler.[1-3]

The essential pathological anatomy which the operation is designed to overcome, is *forward subluxation of the metatarsal fat pad* (Fig. 14-1) in order to restore it to its normal weight-bearing function.[4]

OPERATIVE PROCEDURE

The operation is performed entirely from the *plantar* surface of the foot. The patient lies prone and a flat curved convex incision is made proximally from the neck of the first metatarsal to the neck of the fifth metatarsal (Fig. 14-2). The skin, including the entire depth of subcutaneous fat, is carefully dissected from the underlying tissues, often directly off the depressed metatarsal heads. The most prominent metatarsal head, generally the second or third, is removed first. The remaining metatarsal heads are then removed, a separate deep exposure being made in the line of each metatarsal to avoid damage to the neurovascular bundles. If the sesamoid bones are adherent, as they generally are, they are removed before the first metatarsal head is excised (Fig. 14-3A). Neat division of the bone is facilitated by a motor-driven power saw. After the metatarsal heads have been excised, the metatarsal stumps should form a flat arc (Fig. 14-3B). An anteroposterior radiograph taken at this stage is often helpful to determine whether one or another metatarsal stump is too prominent (Fig. 14-4). A Kirschner wire run through the proximal ray (Fig. 14-5) will maintain general alignment of the forefoot.

The distal flap of the skin is now drawn proximally with tissue forceps, and the overlap is marked. The redundant skin from the distal flap is excised (see Fig. 14-2). Vacuum drainage tubes are inserted, and the wound is sutured. Sutures are required for the subcutaneous fat and skin only. Because of the resected skin, the distal flap is pulled proximally, thus replacing the metatarsal fat pad. When the flap is pulled proximally the toes take up an improved physiological position and may now be seen more clearly in outline from the plantar surface (Fig. 14-6). A fully padded plaster cast is applied. The patient is allowed to be up and to walk with crutches (but bearing no weight) after about 1 week. The original plaster is retained for 4 weeks, after which full weight bearing is allowed, generally without any protection other than simple elastic bandaging.

RESULTS

The results of this forefoot arthroplasty have been fully reported,[4] and experience in the subsequent decade, notably by my colleague Mr. Alexander Kates, amply confirms the original impression that the vast majority of patients are extremely satisfied with the results of the operation by the criteria of appearance, freedom from pain, and the ability to wear socially acceptable footwear (Fig. 14-7). The restoration of effective weight bearing on the forefoot is well illustrated by footprints taken before and after operation (Fig. 14-8). Dramatic results are often achieved, as shown in the pre- and 2-year-postoperative photographs of the feet of patients who underwent this operation (Figs. 14-9 and 14-10).

SELECTION OF PATIENTS, CONTRAINDICATIONS AND HAZARDS

The selection of patients for forefoot arthroplasty is essentially the same as for all patients suffering from generalized inflammatory joint disease. It takes place at a joint orthopaedic and rheumatology clinic after careful general and local preoperative assessment. Very rarely the presence of rheumatoid arteritis has proved a hazard and portions of one or two toes may be lost owing to inadequate blood supply. In doubtful cases—certainly in patients of advanced years—it is probably better to do the operation without a tourniquet, relying entirely on a high Trendelenburg position to provide an acceptably bloodless field in the course of operation.

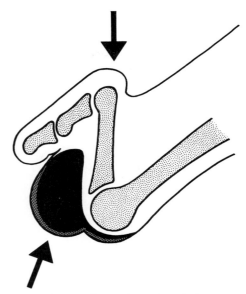

Fig. 14-1. Destructive arthropathy of the metatarsophalangeal joints leads to forefoot collapse (anterior pes planus), subluxation and then dislocation of one of more metatarsophalangeal joints, complete loss of intrinsic muscle action, and, eventually, forward dislocation of the metatarsal fat pad. The arrows indicate the vertical compression that leads to dislocation of the fat pad.

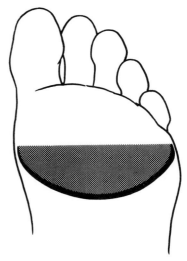

Fig. 14.2 Note that the incision is placed well proximal to the metatarsal heads. After excision of the bone, a varying amount of the skin (*shaded area*) is removed in order to pull the toes into plantar flexion and relocate the metatarsal fat pad.

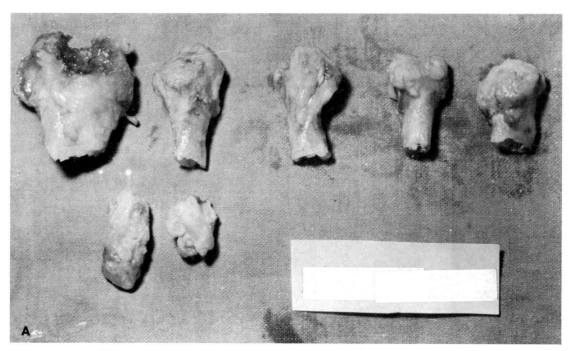

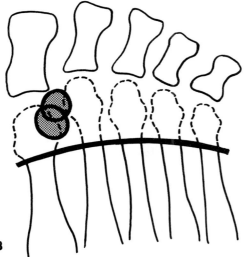

Fig. 14-3. (A) A generous length of each metatarsal is removed from the neck onward, and both sesamoids are usually excised, so that the stumps form a flat arc. (B) Diagram of the amount of bone removed.

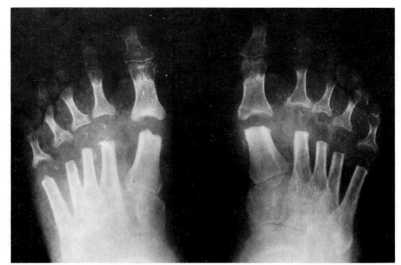

Fig. 14-4. It is often helpful to have an anteroposterior radiograph taken of the foot in the course of the operation, in order to insure that no metatarsal stump is too prominent.

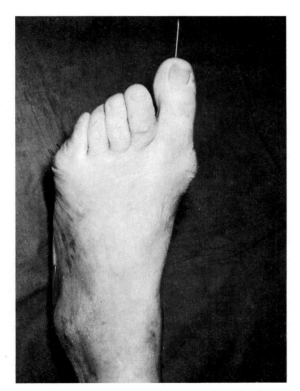

Fig. 14-5. A Kirschner wire inserted in a retrograde manner from toe to metatarsal stump insures good alignment. Occasionally, for severe instability, two or more Kirschner wires may be employed.

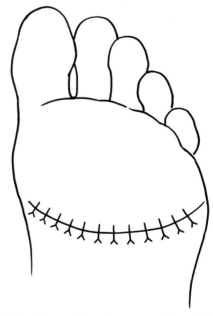

Fig. 14-6. After excision of an appropriate width of skin from the distal flap, suture of the wound brings the toes down into improved plantigrade alignment.

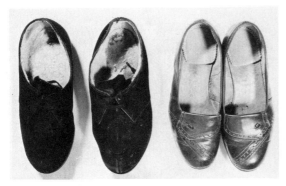

Fig. 14-7. The vast majority of patients have worn surgical footwear prior to operation, and about 1 year thereafter can wear normal shoes.

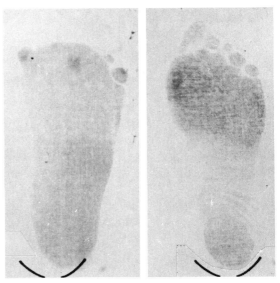

Fig. 14-8. An imprint of the sole of the foot provides a good record of its weight-bearing pattern prior to operation, and shows the improved weight-bearing function of the metatarsal fat pad and toes following operation.

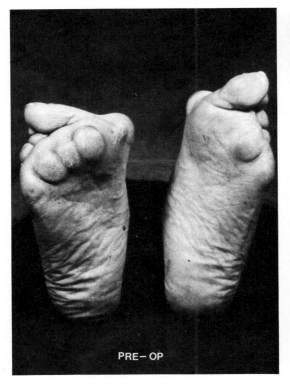
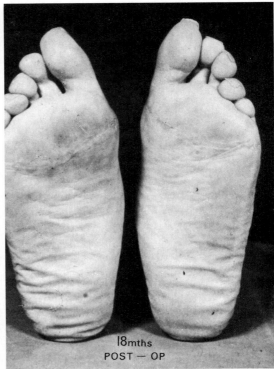

Fig. 14-9. Pre- and postoperative photographs of this patient's feet speak for themselves.

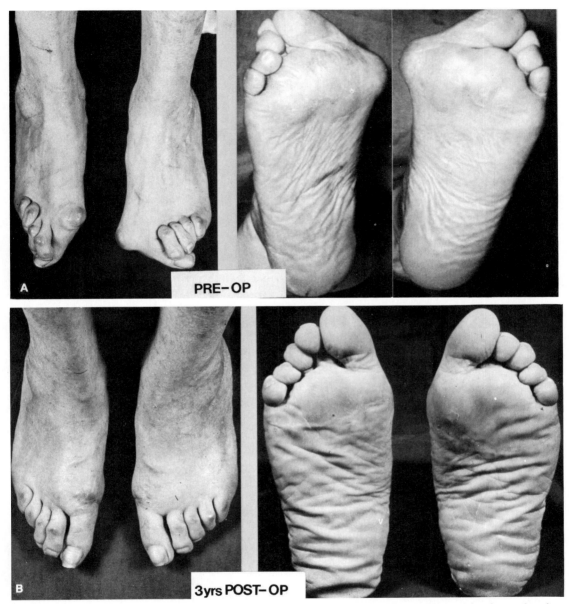

Fig. 14-10. (*A*) Dorsal and plantar views of the feet of a patient who later underwent bilateral forefoot arthroplasty for gross disfigurement and pain. (*B*) After operation, note not only the considerable improvement in the shape of the foot, especially the weight-bearing surfaces, but also the fact that plantar skin wounds usually heal extremely well and ultimately leave a scar that is barely visible.

REFERENCES

1. Fowler, A. W.: The surgery of fixed claw toes. J. Bone Joint Surg., *39B:*585, 1957.
2. Fowler, A. W.: The method of forefoot reconstruction. J. Bone Joint Surg., *41B:*507, 1959.
3. Hoffman, P.: An operation for severe grades of contracted or clawed toes. Am. J. Orthop. Surg., *9:*441, 1912.
4. Kates, A., Kessel, L., and Kay, A.: Arthroplasty of the forefoot. J. Bone Joint Surg., *49B:*552, 1967.

15 The Role of the Podiatrist

GLENN S. QUITTELL

The foot is possibly the most used and the most neglected part of the human body. The average person walks approximately 8 miles a day. With each step the foot is subjected to a minimal degree of trauma. In spite of this, the foot endures remarkably well for most people; for the rest, the feet often become a constant source of annoyance or disability.

Podiatry, known as *chiropody* in England and in Canada, has developed as a profession to help meet the needs of those with foot disorders. There appears to be confusion among the medical profession and the general public about what a podiatrist is and what he does. In this chapter we shall define the scope and practice of podiatry in the United States.

The podiatrist is one who engages in the specialty that includes the diagnosis and treatment—medical, surgical, mechanical, physical, and adjunctive—of diseases, injuries, and defects of the human foot.

Today's podiatry student is required to complete a minimum of 2 years of accredited undergraduate study prior to admission to a college of podiatry. The majority of entering students have received baccalaureate degrees, and the same MCAT examination used by American medical colleges is also required of all podiatry applicants.

Following admission to a college of podiatry, a student will undertake four years of professional study. The curriculum includes all those subjects incorporated in the study of medicine. Considerable time is spent in clinical practice and hospital training. The degree of Doctor of Podiatric Medicine (D.P.M.) is conferred upon the student following satisfactory completion of his studies. A license to practice is contingent on success in national and/or state examinations.

Postdoctoral study, in the form of accredited internships, residencies, fellowships and preceptorships, is available and the number of these is rapidly expanding. At present, more than 50 per cent of all graduating students continue their education in this manner before entering practice.

The modern podiatrist is concerned with all aspects of the human foot and ankle and is responsible for the examination, diagnosis, and treatment of conditions affecting this organ. Consultation or referral to other medical specialists may also be indicated.

Deformities may be congenital, hereditary, or acquired, but trauma and prolonged use of improper footwear will have an impact on the severity and the degree of disability associated with these disorders.

Most foot surgery is elective in nature and is performed to correct deformity, relieve pain, improve function, or prevent future disability. The conditions most frequently encountered for which surgery is indicated are hammer toes, corns, contracted toes, overlapping or underlapping toes, bunions, bone spurs, enlarged bursas, ganglions, cysts, tumors, and disfigurements of the feet and toenails.

The podiatric surgeon may choose to perform surgery in the hospital or in the office operatory. Laboratory testing, radiographic examination, biomechanical evaluation, and hemorheographic study should be conducted preoperatively.

Forefoot surgery is the type most often performed. Arthroplastic techniques associated with tenotomy or tenectomy are the most frequently selected procedures for the correction of hammer toes and corns. Historically, this condition has been treated by surgical debridement of the hyperkeratotic tissue and padding of the lesion with felt or moleskin to protect the area from further insult. Shoe modification, orthodigital appliances such as polyurethane molds, latex toe shields, moldable silicone, and splinting devices, have been used to protect or remove the area from chronic irritation. Injection of a steroid into an inflamed bursa is often recommended when pain is acute. Surgical correction of hammer toes by excision of the proximal phalangeal head with tenotomy or tenectomy of the extensor tendon is necessary in the more severe and chronic hammer toe. More recently, minimal-incision surgical techniques have been developed.

This procedure appears to be less debilitating and less traumatic for many patients. It involves the removal of the phalangeal exostosis which lies beneath the painful corn on the hammer toe. This is effected by making a small incision just proximal or distal to the lesion, undermining the skin, and denuding the exostosis of all attachments; a power-driven surgical burr or reciprocating rasp is then inserted through the incision, and the exostosis is reduced with light, sweeping motions. One must then extrude the "bone paste" created by rasping, and flush the area well with sterile saline. Contraction of the toe is reduced by a stab incision of the plantar interphalangeal capsule. Closure is by butterfly or one simple, interrupted suture. The patient is usually able to walk the same day and requires little or no postoperative analgesics. The decision to perform minimal incision surgery should not be made precipitously: although the method may appear to be technically simple, it entails the usual surgical risks and complications.

Hallux valgus and hallux abductovalgus may present with bursal inflammation of the first metatarsophalangeal joint, arthritic degeneration, and limitation or absence of motion. Conservative treatment includes use of "bunion last" or molded shoes, protective padding, and splinting to relieve irritation. When arthritis is present, analgesics and steroidal or nonsteroidal antiinflammatory agents are indicated. Range-of-motion exercises and physical therapy are also useful.

Operations for bunion deformity include a Silver or McBride type of bunionectomy if the condition is minimal; Keller's procedure coupled with a great toe implant when hallux valgus is associated with arthritis; and wedge osteotomy (opening or closing) in metatarsus primus adductus. An Aiken type of osteotomy of the proximal phalanx can be used to correct the hallux abductus associated with hallux valgus.

Hindfoot surgery is less frequently performed by podiatrists. Procedures for correction of heel spurs and removal of exostoses are the most common. Extensive procedures, including flatfoot surgery, ankle stabilization, and total ankle replacement can also be performed by the podiatric surgeon.

The advent of hard, unyielding walking surfaces, and the wearing of shoes, has hindered the foot's ability to function naturally. The podiatrist, therefore, must perform a biomechanical and gait evaluation of each patient to determine the factors predisposing to callosities, foot strain, plantar fasciitis, or other foot pain. Examination consists of measuring the range of inversion and eversion of the hindfoot. From this, the neutral subtalar position can also be ascertained by the formula: neutral position = eversion $- \frac{1}{3}$ total range of motion. Whether forefoot varus or valgus, tibial varus or valgus, or tibial torsion is present must also be decided. The goal of good management is to maintain the foot as near as possible to the neutral position. This will diminish the abnormal pronatory or supinatory forces which lead to deformity.

Biomechanical treatment consists of the fabrication of an orthotic device which will maintain the foot in a sound functional position during walking. This device is made by taking a negative cast of the foot in its neutral position. From this, a positive cast is made, over which the orthosis is molded. The device is then balanced with wedges (called *posts*) in the forefoot and/or hindfoot, to prevent abnormal motion. This is a very specialized and technical device and must not be likened to prefabricated arch supports.

The current popularity of running has created a sudden surge of complaints of foot and knee pain among runners. The podiatrist and orthopaedist must work in close harmony to provide the athlete with the best care.

Most injuries to runners fall into two categories: overuse and impact shock. The overuse syndrome is most commonly observed in the flexible foot, where excessive pronatory forces are present. The problems most often presented are medial arch pain, heel spurs, and plantar fasciitis. In the knee one finds chondromalacia, strains of the vastus medialis and pes anserinus, and pain referable to the medial aspect of the knee. Impact shock injuries occur primarily in the supinated or rigid foot. These include "painful jogger's heel," Achilles tendinitis, lateral knee pain, stress fractures, and shin splints.

It must be determined whether the runner's complaint is caused by foot imbalance, muscle weakness or osseous or articular derangement. The podiatrist may then advise the patient on proper shoe type, make an orthosis, or institute a muscle-stretching and -strengthening program. When injury to the leg or the knee has occurred or is suspected, orthopaedic consultation and treatment become mandatory.

Disorders of the toenails are probably diagnosed and treated more often by podiatrists than by any other medical specialty. Hyperkeratotic and dystrophic nails are commonly encountered in the elderly, in diabetics, and in patients with peripheral vascular disease.

These conditions may result from injury, subungual exostosis, impaired circulation, or mycotic involvement. Hematoma formation below the nail, resulting from constant jamming of the toe against the shoe, is often seen in the athlete. Infected, ingrown toenails usually result from improper cutting of the nails, or from injury. Treatment by the podiatrist consists of mechanical debridement of the nail, use of antifungal agents, or excision of the exostosis when present. Infected ingrown toenails are treated with antibiotics and surgical excision of the offending portion of the nail, nail bed, and nail matrix, where necessary.

It is well known that diabetics have an increased tendency towards serious foot pathology. Peripheral vascular disease, especially in the form of small vessel disease, is common. This circulatory involvement, coupled with neuropathy, greatly increases the risk of trophic changes, ulceration, and gangrene.

Management of the diabetic must include regular care by the podiatrist, who should be responsible for the care of the toenails and debridement of corns and calluses which may become infected or ulcerated. Regular evaluation of the patient's peripheral vascular status is also indicated. It should be noted that in hospitals and in nursing homes where podiatric care is regularly rendered the rate of amputation of the lower extremities in patients with diabetes is significantly lower than in other institutions.

All forms of arthritis commonly affect the lower extrimities. Practitioners are regularly confronted with complaints of foot pain and deformity that stem from rheumatic involvement. Osteoarthritis, rheumatoid arthritis, gout and pseudogout, psoriatic arthritis, and traumatic arthritis are often encountered. Less frequently seen are pyogenic arthritis, Reiter's syndrome, and arthritis associated with rheumatic fever, lupus erythematosus, and sarcoid.

Treatment is given for the total range of pedal manifestations. Depending upon the severity of symptoms and the deformity, this treatment might include analgesics, intraarticular injection of steroidal agents, orthotics, or surgical intervention. Management of the patient with arthritis would include referral to, and cooperation with, the rheumatologist or orthopaedic surgeon.

It cannot be overemphasized that the foot is but one part of a whole. Any condition affecting the foot may have manifestations elsewhere, and vice versa. To examine and treat disorders of the foot adequately, one must consider the rest of the body.

The podiatrist and the physician share a common goal in the care of the feet. Each is a highly trained specialist with skills capable of augmenting the other. It is through interdisciplinary cooperation that disorders affecting the foot are most effectively treated.

REFERENCES

1. Fielding, M. D. (ed.): The Surgical Treatment of the Hallux Abducto-Valgus and Allied Deformities. Mt. Kisco, N.Y., Futura Publishing Co., 1973.
2. Rinalde, R. R., and Sabia, M. L., Jr. (eds.): Sports Medicine '78. Mt. Kisko, N.Y., Futura Publishing Co., 1978.
3. Stedman's Medical Dictionary. Baltimore, Williams & Wilkins, 1966.

16 The Paralyzed Foot

Normal function of the foot depends upon an intact nervous system. The nerve pathways consist of afferent fibers carrying sensory impulses from the limb, via the posterior nerve root with the cell body within the sensory ganglion, to the spinal cord. Synapse occurs in the posterior horn of grey matter within the cord. Impulses then run to the anterior horn, where the motor cell body is situated, passing through one or more internuncial cells. The axon of the motor cell runs from the anterior horn, via the anterior nerve root, to the peripheral nerve, and terminates at the motor end-plate of the muscle fibers. The cerebral cortex is similarly connected from above to the anterior horn cell, which is thus the final common pathway for electrical impulses either from the sensory side of the reflex pathway or from higher centers.

Paralysis is the condition of loss of control of some or all the muscles of a limb, owing to loss of nerve control. There are two types, depending upon the tone within the affected muscle.

Definition of Flaccid Paralysis

When the loss of voluntary movement is accompanied by complete loss of tone within the muscles, the paralysis is well described as flaccid (Fig. 16-1). The term implies loss of the final common neural pathway, due either to damage to the anterior horn cell itself, as occurs in poliomyelitis, or to trauma to the axon; that is, to the peripheral nerve. Depending upon the cause, flaccid paralysis may be temporary or permanent.

Definition of Spastic Paralysis

Impulses from higher centers in the brain have the effect of controlling the simple spinal segmental reflex. This control includes coordination of muscles and inhibition of tone. When the anterior horn cell is cut off from cerebral control, for example by a vascular catastrophe within the brain resulting in a stroke, the cerebral inhibition is lost and the tone of the muscle is increased. Clinically, spasticity is present.

Interestingly enough, part of the trouble is that not enough impulses reach the anterior horn cell because communication with the cerebral cortex is cut off. This fact has a clinical significance in treatment, and will be discussed.

Spastic paralysis (Fig. 16-2) has also been called upper motor neuron paralysis, implying loss of the nerve cell connecting the cerebrum to the anterior horn cell, that is, the upper motor neuron. Flaccid paralysis may be called a lower motor neuron lesion, another name for the motor cell in the anterior horn, or its axon. Table 16-1 compares the difference in clinical features between upper- and lower motor neuron lesions.

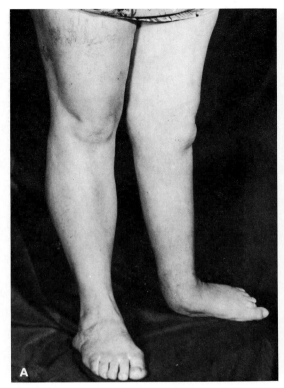 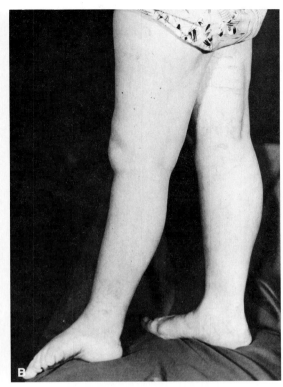

Fig. 16-1. Anterior (*A*) and lateral (*B*) views of flaccid valgus paralysis of the left foot following anterior poliomyelitis.

Children with flaccid or spastic paralysis may overcome their disability to a greater or lesser degree. Lord Byron, generally supposed to have suffered from a clubfoot, is more likely to have been the victim of a dysplasia or one of the neurogenic varieties of foot deformity associated with spinal dysraphism. His gait

was described as halting and sliding; a description consistent with either condition. John Hunter, examining the newborn infant, said of the foot, "It will do very well." Byron himself, abnormally sensitive about his infirmity, would not have agreed. It is interesting to compare his situation with that of Sir Walter Scott, whose lameness is known to have followed an attack of infantile paralysis at the age of 18 months, whose degree of disability was comparable, but whose view of himself was not affected to the same extent.

Table 16-1. **Clinical Features of Flaccid and Spastic Paralysis**

Clinical Sign	Upper Motor Neuron Lesion	Lower Motor Neuron Lesion
Muscle tone	Increased	Decreased
End result	Spasticity	Flaccidity
Power	Reduced or absent	Reduced or absent
Coordination	Reduced	Reduced
Reflexes	Increased	Absent
Babinski response to scratching sole	Upward (i.e. positive)	Absent

THE MECHANISMS OF DEFORMITY IN PARALYSIS

The deforming forces in upper- and lower motor neuron lesions are basically different and must be considered separately.

Spasticity

Associated with the paralysis is increased muscle tone, the result of loss of cortical

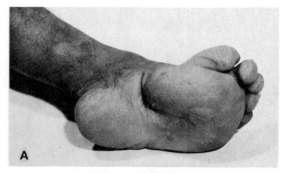

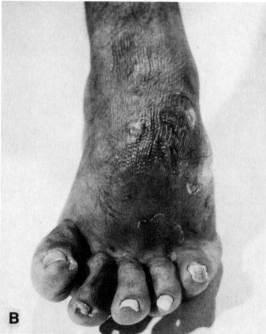

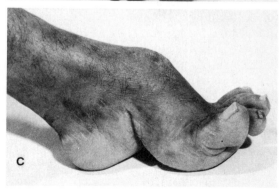

Fig. 16-2. Severe spastic equinovalgus deformity due to an upper motor neuron lesion. (*A*) The sole of the foot. (*B*) Front view. (*C*) Side view.

inhibition. Spasticity, or reflex increase in tone, is a consequence. The pattern of deformity adopted by the foot depends on the balance of spasticity of the muscles; the greater the tone in a particular muscle, the greater will be its deforming effect. It is the paralyzed muscle that causes the deformity in upper motor neuron lesions in both child and adult.

The Test for Infantile Cerebral Palsy. Cerebral palsy is not always easy to diagnose in the infant, especially in mild cases. The increase in tone may be used as an early and accurate test for cerebral palsy.

If one lifts a normal infant by placing the hands under the child's armpits, the legs hang relaxed and straight. In a baby with cerebral palsy, the increased tone and lack of coordination cause the legs to scissor.

The Treatment of Stroke. Tone depends upon reflex impulses. If these are abolished, for example by deep general anesthesia, the spasticity disappears, and with it the deformity. As the patient wakes, it recurs. It appears, furthermore, that the lack of inhibition on the anterior horn cell can be overcome to some extent by bombarding it with sensory stimuli. This facilitated sensory feedback may reduce spasticity. The deliberate addition of weight to a shoe may improve the gait by increasing sensory stimuli and reducing the tone in the foot. In a similar way, the use of a light brace may increase the channels of central nervous system awareness.

Some patients may gain communication between the unaffected motor cortex in the opposite cerebral hemisphere after damage to one side of the brain. The factors that lead to such linkage are unknown, but undoubtedly the patient has to work hard to achieve such recovery. It is almost as though exertion of will power were required to create new synapses between the higher centers and the anterior horn cell. This is not always possible, and there is a time limit in which this can occur following a cerebrovascular accident or cortical injury.

In the end, muscle atrophy is followed by intramuscular fibrosis, and the deformity cannot be overcome even under deep general or regional anesthesia.

Early physiotherapy and bracing are essential, as is the judicious use of soft-tissue surgical procedures to rebalance the foot for walking. Occasionally bone stabilization is required.

Flaccid Paralysis

In lower motor neuron lesions the spinal reflex pathway is interrupted either at the level of the anterior horn cell, as in poliomyelitis; in the nerve root, as in disc prolapse and cauda equina expanding lesions; or in the peripheral motor nerve, as in injury to the limb itself.

Throughout the body, every functioning group of muscles has an antagonistic group. As the former contracts or increases in tone, the latter relaxes due to reflex inhibition. Since each of the opposing muscles is supplied by a different motor nerve or group of anterior horn cells, damage to the one usually occurs independently of the other. The result is unopposed tonic contraction of the normally enervated muscles. In the adult, this unopposed tone of one muscle group seldom results in fixed deformity, because the tone is normal. It is usually gravity, or some other external force, that causes a flaccid condition, such as a drop-foot, on walking. It is not fixed and can be overcome by passive movements of the examiner.

Lower motor neuron lesions can, and frequently do, cause fixed deformity in children. Sharrard, by the careful application of physiological principles, has explained the mechanism of such disfigurement.[1] He pointed out that when a limb grows in length, the primary growing tissue is the epiphyseal cartilage at either end of each long bone. The pressure of such growth is surprisingly strong; sufficient, in some cases, to snap wires that have been inserted through the epiphyseal ossification centers and the metaphysis and tied externally; whether for experimental purposes in animals or in children requiring epiphyseal arrest for limb inequality. If the epiphysis is prevented from growing, the other surrounding soft tis-

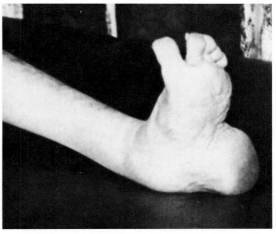

Fig. 16-3. Flaccid paralysis of the calf muscles in childhood has led to extreme imbalance by the normally innervated extensor muscles. An extreme calcaneus deformity has resulted.

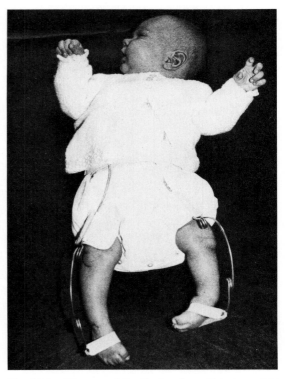

Fig. 16-4. The use of the lively-wire splints in a child with anesthetic, paralyzed feet.

sues, such as tendons, nerves, blood vessels, or even skin, do not grow excessively. It is logical to assume that the primary stimulus to growth of the soft tissues is the pressure of the growing bone.

How does this apply to the antagonistic groups of muscles causing opposing movements at each joint? The two groups of muscles may be likened to a balance, in which the tone of each group is perfectly counterpoised by its opposing muscle. If one of these groups of muscles is paralyzed and without tone, the other tilts the balance. Growth in the length of the bone accentuates this effect: the flaccid muscle fibers atrophy and the normal muscle, being unopposed, does not grow proportionately. In effect, the *normal* muscle, because it is too short, is the deforming force (Fig. 16-3).

CASE 1: An example of severe, unusual paralysis of the lower limbs was found in a boy born to a mother who was known to have a bicornuate uterus. One month before term, the child had stopped kicking. Heart sounds remained normal. At birth a constriction ring was present around the waist of the child, who had total anesthesia and flaccid paralysis of both legs, which were folded severely backward so that they touched the scapulas. In the early stages of treatment, lively wire splants were used (Fig. 16-4) to prevent ulceration of the anesthetic feet. Later, soft-tissue correction was required. The child has made a partial neurologic recovery. At 4½ years, he can run and attend a normal school, provided he wears appliances on both legs.

REFERENCE

1. Sharrard, W. J., and Grosfeild, I.: The management of deformity and paralysis of the foot in myelomeningocoele. J. Bone Joint Surg., *50B:* 456, 1968.

17 Neurologic Conditions of the Foot in Childhood

GEOFFREY WALKER

Although a large number of children with foot problems are referred for orthopaedic advice, the great majority of them have conditions that are simply variants of normal. These include flatfoot, curly toes, and toe-in gait associated either with resolving outward curved tibias (bow legs) or an increase in femoral neck anteversion. The management of these largely benign conditions has been dealt with elsewhere.[1] When foot problems occur in otherwise apparently healthy children, however, there is always the possibility of an underlying neurologic abnormality.

In addition, a small number of children are referred with foot disorders as part of an already established neurologic condition such as spina bifida aperta or cerebral palsy, and in the less favored parts of the world, anterior poliomyelitis is unfortunately still far too common. Where there is a definite underlying neurologic condition it is essential to try to establish whether this is likely to be progressive, but even when this is not so, the condition of the foot may alter and deteriorate during the child's growth and development.

While normal function without symptoms must be the primary aim and consideration in management, the availability of suitable shoes and the cosmetic appearance of the foot are important. A foot needs to be plantigrade, (i.e., all the specialized weight-bearing skin of the sole and heel should be used during weight bearing). The joints of the foot and ankle should have normal mobility. There should be normal and balanced muscle function, and the sensibility, especially of the sole, should be unimpaired. Where possible, the foot should have a pleasing appearance, and in unilateral conditions it should match its fellow. Feet should be shaped so that they may be fitted into normal shoes without producing symptoms or requiring excessive and abnormal shoe wear. Both progressive and nonprogressive neurologic disorders may interfere with any or all of these functions and require orthopaedic management.

"NEUROLOGIC FEET" IN AN OTHERWISE APPARENTLY NORMAL CHILD

In this category are included children who have been noted by their parents, grandparents, neighbors, physical education instructors, fitters in shoe shops, school medical officers, or others, to have an apparent blemish of one or both feet. The problems that must always be in our minds are spinal dysraphism; mild cerebral palsy, especially hemiplegia; missed mild anterior poliomyelitis; pes cavus; and peroneal muscular atrophy and Friedreich's ataxia.

It is important to take an accurate and detailed history from the child and parents.

187

This should include details of the pregnancy, ease or complications of the delivery, the attainment of milestones, the child's intellectual ability, the presence or absence of related symptoms, problems in obtaining or repairing shoes, and unequal or abnormal shoe wear, and whether or not the child enjoys full normal activities.

At no stage are the children handled by anyone other than the parents or myself. I find that this regimen reduces recalcitrance and other management problems to the minimum. On each visit every child is fully examined and asked to walk normally, on tiptoe, on the heels, and on the outer and inner borders of the feet. He then hops on each leg alternately, before jumping up to try and touch the ceiling. The neck, and particularly the back, is checked before the child lies on the couch. It is vital to examine the backs of all children at every opportunity, both for the insidious appearance of scoliosis and even more, for any significant abnormality or blemish in the lumbosacral region.

With the child on the couch, movements and power of the arms and of all the joints in the lower limbs are tested. The upper and lower limb reflexes are elicited, the joints are moved to detect spasticity, and if there is any possibility of a neurologic deficit, I perform the neurologic examination in greater detail.

It is important to enquire about similar problems of the feet in other members of the family. During the examination I often ask the attending parent or parents to show me their feet, and time and again, particularly when the child's feet are a normal variant, they will resemble closely those of the father or mother. If that parent's feet have been entirely asymptomatic and never given any trouble in the past, it is unlikely that the child will have significant trouble in the future.

It is important to try to make a positive diagnosis in every case, even though, with growing children, and for that matter in the early stages of progressive neurologic disease, a definite diagnosis may not be possible until the child has been seen again on one or more occasions. Probably the most common special

examination required is radiography, and, if there is even a faint hint of a spinal problem, radiographs of the lumbosacral region are mandatory. A full blood count and erythrocyte sedimentation rate estimation is a useful screening test. With children who have postural problems or variants of normal shape, the situation is explained to the parents. The family returns to the care of their general medical practitioner, on the understanding that the situation can be reviewed if the child, parents, or doctor is concerned about the feet at any time in the future. With children who were born after a difficult or prolonged labor (which raises the possibility of a neurological problem) but who show no supporting physical signs, I arrange to see the child again, usually in a few months, but I always offer to advance this date if there is parental or other concern.

Some neurologic disorders may take months or years to become manifest. Where, after further review, there is still "a neurologic aura" the advice of a pediatric neurologist is sought, and the signs to look out for are unequal shoe wear or size of the feet and legs and, in particular, a suspicion of a varus heel or retraction of the toes. In this way very few, if any, infants or older children with incipient "neurologic feet" or other problems, slip through the net of reasonably early diagnosis.

Spinal Dysraphism

Attention has been drawn to this fascinating problem by James and Lassman.[2] In essence, their message is to suspect a neurologic problem affecting the spinal cord or cauda equina in any child or adult who has or who develops an abnormal foot or feet. In practice this means examining the entire spine (especially the lumbosacral region) with the naked eye. The presence of hairy patches, scars, or swelling such as lipomata in or near the midline, may well be relevant and may suggest an underlying pathological problem (Fig. 17-1). In addition, there are children whose backs are clinically normal but in whom plain radiographs of the lumbosacral spine reveal an occult spina bifida of greater extent than can be considered normal, or diastematomyelia (and this may be in

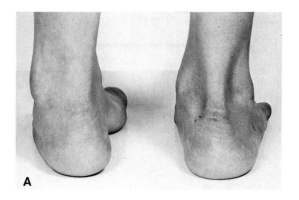

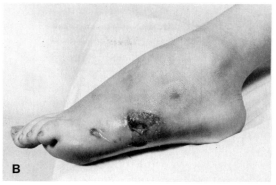

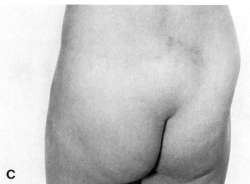

Fig. 17-1. (*A*) A "neurologic" left foot; note the heel varus and cavus deformities. (*B*) A pressure sore on the outer border. (*C*) A large lumbosacral lipoma with overlying skin markings.

the thoracic as well as the lumbar region). Where any of these conditions exist, or, indeed, where there is even a possibility of their presence, the child should have the benefit of a pediatric neurologist's opinion, and this should be followed by appropriate myelography and neurologic exploration.

From our point of view—and in this I include everyone dealing with children's feet—I must reiterate the importance of examining children's backs and remembering the possibility of an occult spinal canal problem when a foot or feet, leg or legs have a neurologic "flavor." In my experience such feet and heels often begin to develop varus deformity, and this is often best seen from behind. In addition, a decrease in length and in size of the entire affected limb may become apparent. In more advanced cases there is likely to be anesthesia or altered sensibility of part of (or the entire) sole, and indolent ulcers may develop. In addition, bladder function may be disturbed, with enuresis and incontinence. An early presenting feature is unequal shoe wear, with the

heel of one shoe being worn down on the medial margin rather than on the more usual posterolateral edge.

The management of these children depends first on the recognition of their condition and second, to some extent, on the underlying spinal problem. When the neurologic deficit is progressive, the majority will come to myelography and neurosurgical exploration. If the blemish is only slight, myelography is usually undertaken on neurologic advice, but occasionally neurologic intervention is considered inappropriate, and the child is simply observed closely during the remainder of the growth period. In addition to this attack on the primary problem in the spinal canal, the feet occasionally require orthopaedic management. Anesthesia of the sole in an otherwise mobile foot is unlikely to result in pressure sores,[3] but when there is both anesthesia and fixed deformity, sores occur under bone prominences where there is excess pressure. Often correction of the deformity (e.g., by heel cord lengthening for fixed equinus) will allow the pressure sore to heal. When the deformity is more advanced with marked varus, and weight is being borne only on the outer border of the foot, a triple arthrodesis after the age of 12 years achieves correction of the deformity and a reasonably plantigrade foot. Until the child is old enough for this fairly extensive bone surgery, surgical boots or shoes will be required with sponge rubber insoles, often made from plaster casts and occasionally supported by an inside iron and outside T-strap or a double below-knee caliper brace.

While many children who have these "neurologic feet and legs" have a demonstrable intraspinal lesion, there are some in whom full investigation fails to reveal any obvious problem. These are considered to be due to myelodysplasia, for want of a better diagnosis, but the condition of the feet and legs runs a similar course with a tendency to progression during growth (Fig. 17-2).

Further details of these interesting and important conditions, together with review of their first 100 cases, are given in that excellent book by James and Lassman.[2] My message is to stress the importance of remembering spinal dysraphism and spina bifida occulta with their associated neurologic lesions as a cause of foot and leg abnormalities.

Unrecognized Cerebral Palsy

While the feet of children with severe or established cerebral palsy are considered later, a small number of infants, children, and adolescents present with an apparently minor foot problem which is a result of an underlying mild, and hitherto unrecognized, cerebral palsy. Suspicion may well have been raised by the history, of delayed or difficult labor, prematurity, a long period spent in an incubator after birth, an Rh-factor problem or postpartum injury or disease such as meningitis.

Examining the naked child, particularly as he walks, often reveals the diagnosis. This is especially true in mild forms of hemiplegia. A lower limb on the affected side may appear a shade short, and the child will walk with an equinus gait. Examination of the shoe will show lack of heel wear, and further examination will confirm the presence of spasticity and probable loss of dorsiflexion at the ankle. In addition, the arm on the affected side is likely to be used less than the good limb, and may be carried in the classical "wing" position. Very minor degrees of cerebral palsy hemiplegia often escape detection for many years, but where there is any doubt about the diagnosis a pediatric neurologist should be consulted.

Many of these children have little more than a minor cosmetic blemish with a minimally disturbed gait of hemiplegic pattern. They function well, play football and other games without significant difficulty, and all that is required is regular parental stretching of the tight heel cord and calf muscles under the supervision of a physical therapist. Sometimes night splinting is helpful, and, on very rare occasions, heel cord lengthening or gastrocnemius recession may be indicated. The important thing to remember is that this condition may be present, and, when the foot or leg problem is unilateral the underlying neurologic lesion must be sought. Even when the cerebral palsy hemiplegia is minimal but the child is young, I usually refer the patient to our Cerebral Palsy Unit for assessment and total care, as well as keeping an eye myself on the affected foot and limb. Cerebral palsy, after all, is a general disease.

"Missed" Polio

Owing to immunization, anterior poliomyelitis is, fortunately, rare in the United Kingdom now. Even in immunized persons, however, very mild poliomyelitis can occur, and of course there are also missed cases among child visitors or those who have immigrated to Britain. In other words, a history of adequate immunization does not totally exclude a diagnosis of poliomyelitis; I see a small number of children, usually with minor foot or leg problems and reduced or absent tendon reflexes, in whom a positive diagnosis of paralysis from poliomyelitis can be made. Often they require little treatment other than careful observation during growth. The management of more florid paralysis is dealt with later in this chapter.

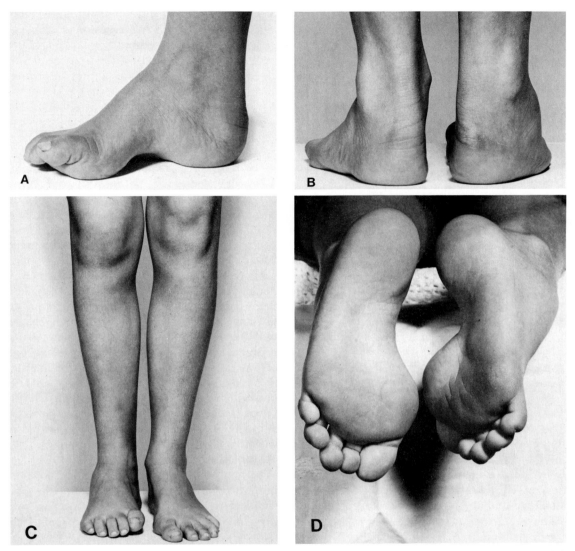

Fig. 17-2. (*A*) Neurologic cavus foot with varus heel. (*B*) Note the varus of the right heel. (*C*) The entire right limb is shorter and smaller below the knee with an obvious cavus foot. (*D*) Cavus foot seen from below. This child had a myelodysplasia.

Pes Cavus

Although "normal" flat feet with valgus heels and associated ligamentous laxity are exceedingly common, feet with high arches and retraction of the toes, a cavus deformity, are seen much less often. Usually the heel is relatively normal in the early stages. The deformity can best be considered a "fixed dropping of the forefoot." If the condition is progressive, retraction of the toes and a varus deformity of the heel may follow. Sometimes one sees a baby with high-arched feet; this is usually familial, and the more severe forms of cavus feet with fixed deformity occur later in life. Lloyd-Roberts believed those that occur at about 3 years of age are likely to be secondary to myelodysplasia; at seven, to peroneal muscular atrophy; and at fourteen, to either Friedreich's ataxia or spinal dysraphism.[4] Sharrard believed that Friedreich's

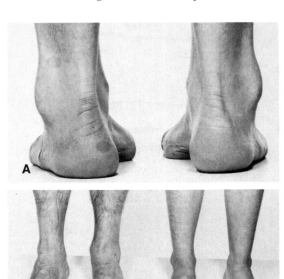

Fig. 17-3. (*A*) Neurologic cavus feet with varus heels in a child. (*B*) Feet of the same child photographed with similar feet in the father, who had the same underlying neurologic problem.

ataxia may produce pes cavus as early as 5 years of age.[5] While many cavus feet used to be considered "idiopathic," Brewerton, Sandifer, and Sweetman were able to demonstrate, in their classic paper, a disorder in the central nervous system in 66 per cent of 77 patients.[6] I believe that all children who present with or who develop cavus feet should be assessed by a pediatric neurologist, and a really thorough search in the family will often reveal similar problem feet (Fig. 17-3). Both points are important, as it is helpful to establish whether the child is suffering from a progressive or potentially progressive condition. Often the feet are asymptomatic when the child is first seen, but there may already be difficulty in obtaining shoes, and some cause for concern to ballet dancing teachers or physical education instructors. Pain from callosities under the metatarsal heads, or from corns on the retracted clawtoes, comes later and can be difficult to manage. As well as the neurologic conditions listed above, cavus feet occur in

poliomyelitis and the major forms of spina bifida with myelemoningoceles. The management can be considered both in the light of the underlying cause, when this has been elucidated, and also of the resulting foot deformity, particularly when symptoms have appeared. As with most children's foot problems, I do not believe that physical therapy has a very significant part to play.

Many of these cavus feet are comfortable in shoes with sufficiently high uppers, and, indeed, almost any foot deformity can be fitted into corduroy or suede chukka boots; in some respects, manufacture of this footwear in sizes suitable for children has been a notable advance. Later, many of these feet can be made comfortable in surgical shoes with sponge rubber insoles prepared from plaster casts, but a small number of these feet, particularly when there is severe and rigid deformity, will need bone surgery. Triple fusion is required, usually of the Elmslie type.[7] This involves a two stage procedure in which, a dorsally based wedge is first excised from the mid-tarsal region and the foot is put into extreme calcaneus in plaster; then, 3 or 4 weeks later, a posterior based wedge is excised from the subtalar joint, allowing the foot to be brought down from calcaneus to the plantigrade position (Fig. 17-4). Where there is additional heel varus as can occur with spinal dysraphism, peroneal muscle atrophy or Friedreich's ataxia, a more classical triple arthrodesis with internal fixation performed through an anterolateral incision will allow good correction. The transfer of tendons at the same time, or at a later stage, is rather more debatable, and the wisdom of these procedures must depend on the underlying cause. It is perhaps a matter of refined judgment for the surgeon and neurologist involved.

THE FEET OF A CHILD WITH A KNOWN NEUROLOGIC PROBLEM

The main conditions to be considered are spina bifida, cerebral palsy, anterior poliomyelitis and muscular dystrophy. While the latter two are not present at birth, problems with the feet are an integral part of these general

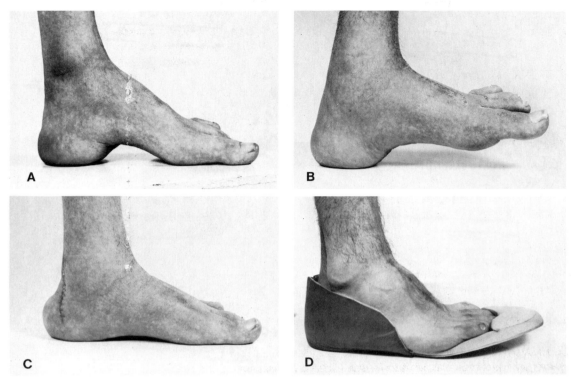

Fig. 17-4. (*A*) A cavus foot. (*B*) After first stage Elmslie with removal of a dorsal tarsal wedge. (*C*) After second stage Elmslie following removal of a posterior subtalar wedge. (*D*) Foot in a "false foot" insole which allows the child to wear a pair of equal-sized shoes.

diseases and are therefore unlikely to be the presenting symptom.

Spina Bifida Aperta

This is a condition in which deformities, both rigid and flail, are present in anesthetic feet and usually in a child who was born with an open myelomeningocele. Atrioventricular shunt for increasing hydrocephalus may well have been required, and the child may have gross bladder dysfunction, and quite possibly mental deficiency. Obviously, therefore, management of the feet, although important, must be considered in the light of the general picture.

While it is tempting to try and correlate the deformities that are found with specific levels of neurologic deficit, this is rarely either practical or, in my experience, helpful. From my experience with several hundred of these unfortunate children, it appears to me that any deformity, or combination of deformities can be found. There are various common patterns, but even so, it is important to establish and to remember the basic aims of management. The multiple problems of deformity and paralysis are compounded by the associated anesthesia, which is nearly always present. To a considerable extent the problems are often offset by the child's general state. The degree of paralysis and associated handicaps which reduce walking potential and may limit actual walking to such an extent that a foot which is neither anatomically nor cosmetically perfect may meet the needs of that specific spina bifida child. Again, it is important to remember that an anesthetic foot is unlikely to develop sores unless there is a fixed deformity (Fig. 17-5). When there is cause for pressure on the plantar skin of spina bifida children, damage to the skin occurs even faster than it does in normal children, possibly because the feet are small and the children tend to be obese.[8]

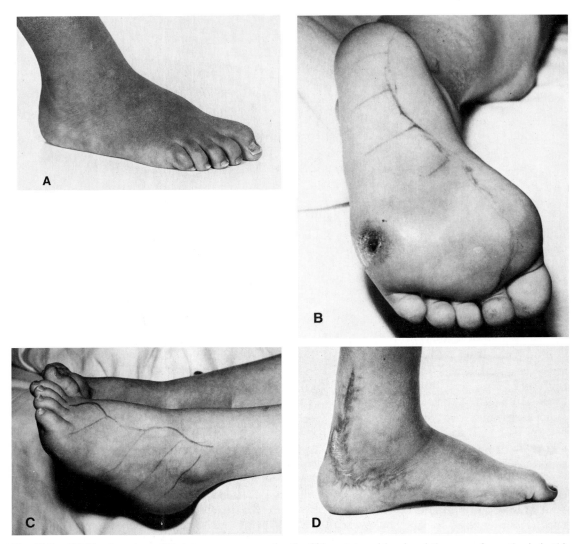

Fig. 17-5. (*A*) Fixed equinus. (*B*) A pressure sore under the fifth metatarsal head and the area of anesthesia in this rigid foot marked with crayon. (*C*) A posterolateral view of the same foot with the anesthetic area marked. (*D*) The same foot after posterior release, which allowed healing of the pressure sore without further surgery.

In this chapter detailed discussion of spina bifida feet problems will be limited to the deformities which most commonly occur. These are varus, with or without equinus; pronation of the forefoot with rogue evertors; calcaneus; valgus feet and ankles in the older spina bifida child, and failed primary surgery. Detailed management of the many toe deformities, and of those occurring less commonly in the foot, can be found elsewhere in the literature.[5,9]

Varus With or Without Equinus. This is probably the commonest severe problem, and may be related to a neurologic lesion at L3 or L4, with or without activity in the tibialis anterior muscle (Fig. 17-6). The deformity, which is present at birth, is rigid and severe and, from the practical point of view, there is total anesthesia of the foot. The object of treatment is to produce a plantigrade foot, but it is important to discard the methods of treatment used in congenital equinovarus, as the lack of sensation precludes wedging in plasters or strapping of Robert Jones type with nonelastic adhesive plaster. If these methods are employed, severe pressure sores may result, and amputations have had to be performed.

The method we have used, with some success, at Queen Mary's Hospital for Children, Carshalton, is a combination of conservative and operative. The physical therapist, reinforced by the parents and grandparents, stretches the varus deformity as often as possible, starting soon after the birth of the child. The foot and ankle are partially immobilized without tension, but with as much correction as possible, with elastic adhesive strapping.[10] When this has been applied it is possible to continue stretching regularly. In our experience this technique will overcome most, if not all, of the varus deformity. The equinus remains, or in fact is sometimes revealed when the heel has been moved from varus to neutral. It is not possible to overcome the tight posterior heel structures by closed means, and open operation is required. Until recently, I have used an extensive posterior release in which the heel cord and the tendons of the paralized muscles passing behind either malleolus are excised and the subtalar, the inferior tibiofibular, and ankle joints are opened widely. Postoperatively, the foot is maintained in maximum correction, but without pressure, using elastic adhesive strapping. In this way we have produced plantigrade feet which often function well, although they need external support because of the complete paralysis. Recently, a more formal heel cord lengthening, without sacrifice of tendons, has been used in order to avoid producing feet with a flail calcaneus deformity (see below).

When varus feet have proved refractory to this regimen, either on account of general problems or, in children who reach us at a later age and in whom it has been impossible to treat the feet in this fashion, I make no attempt at conservative management. Operation then consists, basically, of a very extensive, medial release, but there is a problem with closure of the skin. This has been solved

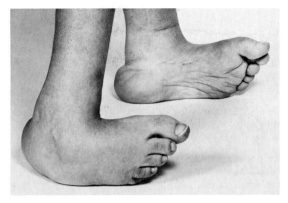

Fig. 17-6. Varus deformity with spina bifida; the feet bear weight along the outer borders.

largely by the use of an enormous dorsal flap which, based proximally, allows skin which becomes surplus on the lateral side of the foot to be used to cover the defect which appears on the medial side of the foot after correction.[10] During the medial release, all the mid-tarsal joints are opened, and it is usually also necessary to allow the talus to tilt in the mortise by dividing the medial ligament of the ankle. After this extensive procedure, the feet are immobilized in a series of plasters for 4 to 6 months. The results have been encouraging.

Unfortunately, in spite of every care, some of these feet relapse into varus, or present later on when other methods of treatment have been tried. These are a real problem, as there is often extensive scar tissue and there may have been loss of posterior tibial vessels in the primary procedure. I have tried repeating medial release, using the extensive flap incision, but I have had major vascular complications. Probably the best technique is to remove the talus and, as these feet are already rigid, the final result may be as good as in those following astragalectomy for arthrogryposis. I have no experience of supramalleolar osteotomies for relapsed varus feet, but the idea is certainly attractive, although it may result in a rather "off-set" foot. This, however, may well be acceptable in a child with very limited walking potential.

Pronating forefeet are usually associated with some calcaneus deformity and the condition appears to be due to spastic or reflex activity in the evertors and dorsiflexors of the foot. The child will bear abnormal weight on the heel, and unless this is corrected and use is made of all the specialized weight-bearing skin, pressure sores are likely to develop under the heel. While transfer of tendons around the foot in poliomyelitis is a well-established procedure, I have grave doubts as to its use in the majority of spina bifida feet. The muscles and tendons are often not working in normal fashion, and, apart from producing an effect of tenodesis, I have been singularly unimpressed with the result of transfers in this condition. For this reason I advocate excision of all the tendons producing eversion and pronation of the forefoot, a relatively simple procedure which allows the foot to adopt a more normal position. Even so, a below-knee caliper is required, and occasionally I have added a front- rather than a back stop which, with a slight rocker sole on the shoe, ensures that the child bears some weight on the forefoot.

Talipes Calcaneus. With paralysis of the calf, or after excision of all the tendons passing behind the ankle joint, the foot is likely to develop calcaneus. This may be either flail or fixed.[8] In the former, the forefoot will lie on the ground when the child stands but will not tolerate any weight bearing (Fig. 17-7). When fixed, the forefoot will not even reach the ground when the leg is vertical. Either of these conditions will allow excessive pressure to be borne on the heel, with resulting sores.

The management of calcaneus is difficult, and, in my experience, transfer of dorsiflexors to the heel cord has been ineffective. It is probably best to excise these tendons and then control the foot and ankle with external bracing. Strach has had some success with a spring implanted between the posterior surface of the upper tibia and the os calcis,[11,12] but often these children, with limited walking potential as a result of fairly severe paralysis and other problems, are best managed with calipers.

Valgus Feet and Ankles in the Older Spina Bifida Child. As the children grow and put on weight, some feet adopt an increasing valgus position. Radiography reveals that this is from tilting of the ankle joint and, for this reason, subtalar fusion of the Grice or Batchelor type is unsuccessful. Supramalleolar osteotomy, with a closing wedge, is a useful technique for improving both the function and the appearance of such feet.

Failed Primary Surgery for Spina Bifida. These are some of the most difficult spina bifida feet to manage. They are often rigid, almost inevitable anesthetic, and with abnormal or damaged blood vessels and multiple scars. Attempts at major, corrective procedures have resulted in necrosis and amputation, and this underlines the importance of using a proper operation and doing it adequately on the first occasion (Fig. 17-8). Astragalectomy is certainly useful, but bone, and hence size, nearly always has to be sacrificed in order to produce a plantigrade foot. Surgery usually has to be followed by prolonged plaster immobilization, and the surgeon must be certain that he will improve the child's mobility and function before picking up his knife.

Footwear. A great deal of the management of anesthetic feet, both those with and without deformity, depends on the provision of appropriate footwear. During recent years commercial manufacturers have produced an increasing range of special shoes and footwear, and most feet can be fitted from stock* (Fig. 17-9). Most of these allow attachment of sockets for the calipers, which are so often needed, both to control paralyzed and flail feet as well as other paralyzed joints in the lower limbs.

Vascular Problems. Finally, it is important to realize that the vascular supply of spina bifida feet appears abnormal. Spontaneous gangrene can occur and there may be skin or toe necrosis after relatively innocuous surgical procedures (Fig. 17-10). Everyone concerned, not least the parents and children themselves, must be made aware of the importance of avoiding pressure and burns. Skin which has once had a full-thickness sore will never return to normal, and therefore it is most important to avoid the first sore or burn. Constant vigilance, avoidance of pressure, and care with footwear are vital.

* See Appendix.

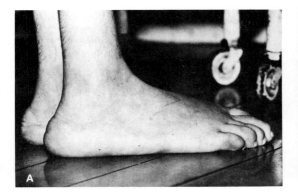

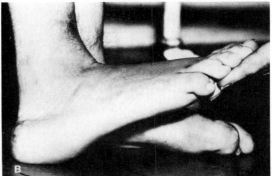

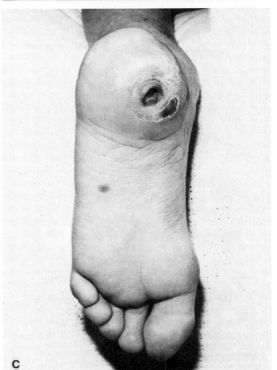

Fig. 17-7. (*A*) A flail calcaneus deformity. (*B*) Although the foot appears plantigrade, there is no muscle action or tone behind the ankle, and the forefoot can be easily elevated. (*C*) Virtually all weight is borne through the heel, with a resulting large pressure sore.

Anterior Poliomyelitis

Polimyelitis is now rarely a cause of "neurologic feet" in the United Kingdom (Fig. 17-11). Occasional cases are seen in immigrants, and in visitors from overseas. The experience of treating older children with problems resulting from the post-war poliomyelitis epidemics has proved helpful during consulting visits to developing countries where poliomyelitis is still rife. Usually the diagnosis is not in doubt, although often, in less well-developed areas, an injection into the buttock, given for a transient fever, is blamed for the limb paralysis which follows. This, of course, is not from direct involvement of the sciatic or other nerve, but is a result of the injection being given during the prodromal phase of the acute poliomyelitis infection.

The ultimate paralysis and residual muscle function has a direct bearing on the production of deformity which may itself alter and deteriorate during growth. While it may seem attractive to try and restore muscle balance around joints by tendon transfer, this is often

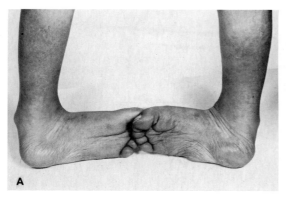
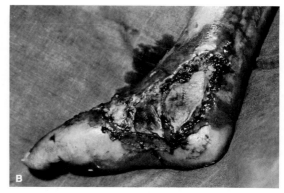

Fig. 17-8. (*A*) A pair of varus feet which had failed to respond to primary surgery. (*B*) One of the same feet after a second operation. Note the large area of skin necrosis.

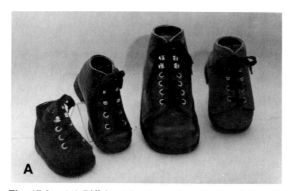
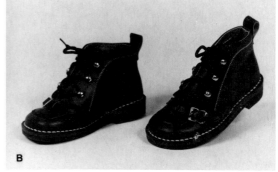

Fig. 17-9. (*A*) Biffabout boots can be supplied from stock, and adaptations can be made on them. (*B*) Piedro boots.

impossible, and little more than a holding procedure, with external bracing, can be arranged until the child is old enough to undergo definite joint fusion, with any necessary excision of bone. Such fusions, which may often be of the midtarsal joints or of the ankle joint, can occasionally be combined with a stabilizing tendon transfer. They are best performed between the age of 12 years and the point when the patient reaches skeletal maturity. The basic aim is to ensure the best possible limb function; cosmesis is of secondary importance. As these feet have normal sensibility, they rarely develop significant ulcers or pressure sores unless a great deal of weight is being borne on a very small area of skin. Readers are referred to standard orthopaedic textbooks for details

of specific problems and their suggested solutions.

Muscular Dystrophy

The primary diagnosis of muscular dystrophy (probably not a neurologic disease!) is rarely an orthopaedic problem, although the possibility of its presence in two patients during the last 13 years has first been suggested to me by a physical therapist. In one of these, the diagnosis unfortunately proved correct. Sharrard[5] gives an excellent description of the early gait abnormality with occasional toe walking.[5] Severe deformities of the feet can occur, in spite of assiduous physical therapy and splinting, and on a very few occasions I have been persuaded to operate on these

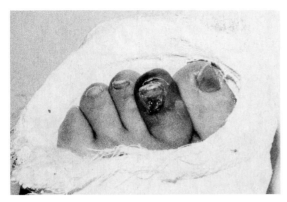

Fig. 17-10. Idiopathic necrosis of part of one toe following a simple corrective foot procedure.

deformed feet, largely for cosmetic reasons; the unfortunate patients already being confined to wheelchairs but wishing to wear more normal shoes.

Cerebral Palsy

While foot and ankle deformities are often found in children with cerebral palsy, in my experience many of these can be managed adequately with physical therapy and the provision of special footwear or modifications or ordinary shoes. I see regularly many of the children in our Cerebral Palsy Unit, and I always ensure that the relevant cerebral palsy therapist, as well as a parent, is available at the consultation. Orthopaedics, although important, is only one part of the general management of these handicapped children, and it is always valuable to be aware of the child's mental state and associated nonorthopaedic problems. As the orthopaedic surgeon grows older, he finds the results of surgery to be disappointing, with the exception of a small number of well-tried procedures, and his youthful enthusiasm is slowly eroded. Be that as it may, tightness of the heel cord and associated calf muscles can disturb gait, and, while most of this problem can be managed by regular parental and professional stretching reinforced by adequate night splinting, occasionally heel cord lengthening or, when indicated, gastrocnemius recession, can produce a marked improvement. These relatively sim-

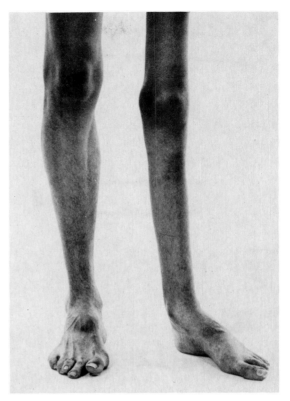

Fig. 17-11. The left leg of a patient who had polio. Note the wasting, valgus, and mild cavus deformity.

ple surgical procedures must be followed by intensive and prolonged physiotherapy and splinting, and I always warn the patient and the parents that recovery to the preoperative state may take a long time and that there will be an even greater interval before improvement is noted. I have had little experience with tendon transfers in cerebral palsy, but they have been used with enthusiasm elsewhere. Valgus feet, again often associated with tightness of the heel cord structures, may not be a grave, or even a significant, functional disability, although the feet are cosmetically undesirable. Very often they can be contained in appropriate shoes or boots, but heel cord lengthening or gastrocnemius recession will occasionally improve the appearance although less often the function.

The foot of the spastic hemiplegic, however, is in a different category altogether. If the

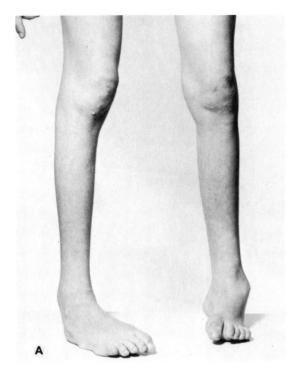 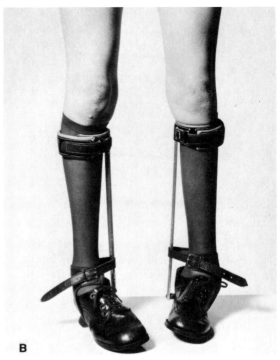

Fig. 17-12. (*A*) Varus feet in a mentally retarded child with cerebral palsy and spastic paraplegia. (*B*) The same feet deformed the child's shoes and calipers. In fact, these feet were scheduled for surgical correction although walking potential was limited by the child's general condition.

spasticity is at all marked, the foot may slowly move into varus, and this deterioration is often rapid during the child's second growth spurt. A foot which before could be managed in ordinary shoes begins to turn inward. Lateral heel floats are the first line of attack, and these must soon be followed by the use of a caliper with inside iron and outside T-strap, to be replaced in turn by a double below-knee caliper, Further deformity of the foot finally necessitates triple fusion at about the time of skeletal maturity, via an anterolateral approach, with excision of appropriate wedges and internal fixation before a plantigrade foot is produced. Triple fusion for these feet is well worthwhile (as, very occasionally, it can be with varus feet in spastic paraplegia; Fig. 17-12), but it is important to warn the child and the family that there will be a period of some weeks or months after the plaster is removed before definitive footwear can be fitted. If at all possible the position of the foot after surgery

should be such that normal, shop-supplied footwear is satisfactory, but if the foot has been reduced in size, both by the original problem and the surgery, then manufacture of an insole of false foot type will allow normal shoes of the same size to be worn (see Fig. 17-4D).

EDITOR'S NOTE. In fixed foot deformities Dwyer's osteotomy is a useful alternative to triple arthrodesis. (A.J.H.)

ODDMENTS

While I have concentrated on neurologic feet problems which occur commonly, there are a few other points worth mentioning. There is a large group of relatively rare neurologic disorders including peripheral neuropathies, some progressive and some not, which may be associated with orthopaedic foot problems (Fig. 17-13). From our point of view it is necessary to be aware of a possible neurologic flavor when an abnormal foot or, rarely, both

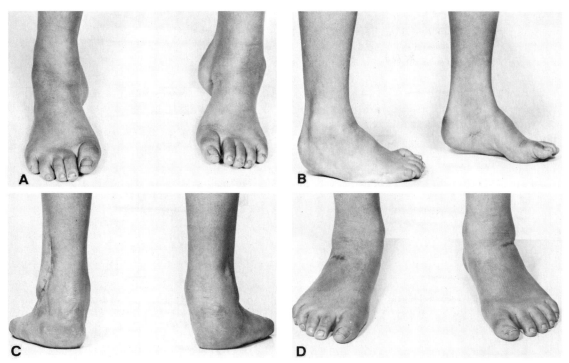

Fig. 17-13. (*A*) A pair of "neurologic" feet in which the deformity developed slowly and insidiously. (*B*) The eventual diagnosis was a peripheral neuropathy of unknown etiology. The same feet after triple fusion at skeletal maturity, posterior (*C*) and anterior (*D*) views.

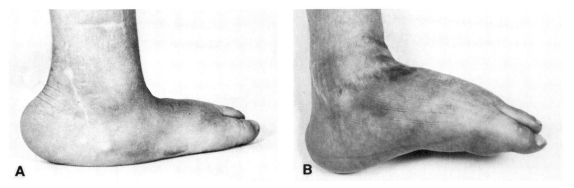

Fig. 17-14. (*A*) Paralytic vertical talus. Note the heel equinus, and prominence under the head of the vertical talus. (*B*) The same foot after surgical correction.

feet, are being assessed and, as previously mentioned, it is important, before planning management, to determine, whenever possible, whether or not the condition is progressive. The keynote in management, as with most orthopaedics, is to go for function as first priority.

Congenital vertical talus, which is a rare orthopaedic problem, may have an underlying neurologic basis, although this is as yet unproven. A very similar clinical picture, with paralytic vertical tali, occurs in spina bifida children, and this is often associated with an L5 or S1 neurologic level (Fig. 17-14).

In spite of extensive experience in the developing parts of the world where leprosy is rife, I have yet to see or to hear of a leprous child with a foot problem. I suspect that the absence of foot problems in leprous children is because of the extreme chronicity of this horrible disease, but provision of appropriate footwear for the anesthetic feet of leprous adults remains largely unsolved in most parts of the world.

Likewise, I have yet to see diabetic neuropathy producing orthopaedic foot problems in a child.

REFERENCES

1. Walker, G.: Minor orthopaedic problems of childhood. Practitioner, *208:*227, 1972.
2. James, C. C. M., and Lassman L. P.: Spinal Dysraphism, Spina Bifida Occulta. London, Butterworth, 1972.
3. Clawson, D. K. and Seddon, H. J.: The late consequences of sciatic nerve injury. J. Bone Joint Surg., *42B:*213, 1960,
4. Lloyd-Roberts, G. C.: Orthopaedics in Infancy and Childhood. London, Butterworth, 1971.
5. Sharrard, W. J. W.: Paediatric Orthopaedics and Fractures. Oxford, Blackwell Scientific Publications, 1971.
6. Brewerton, D. A., Sandifer, P. H., and Sweetman, D. R.: 'Idiopathic' pes cavus. An investigation into its aetiology. Brit. Med. J., *3:*659,1963.
7. Cholmeley, J. A.: Elmslie's operation for the calcaneus foot. J. Bone Joint Surg. *35B:*46, 1953.
8. Hay, Malcolm C., and Walker, Geoffrey: Plantar pressures in healthy children and in children with myelomeningocele. J. Bone Joint Surg., *55B:*828, 1973.
9. Menelaus, M. B.: The Orthopaedic Management of Spina Bifida Cystica. Edinburgh, E. & S. Livingstone, 1971.
10. Walker, G.: The early management of varus feet in myelomeningocele. J. Bone Joint Surg., *53B:*462, 1971.
11. Strach E. H.: The spring implant operation, a preliminary report. Develop. Med. Child Neurol. [Supp. 27], *14:*121, 1972.
12. Strach, E. H.: The Spring Implant Operation. J. Bone Joint Surg., *55B:*883, 1973.

SUGGESTED FURTHER READING

Huckstep, R. L.: Medicine in the Tropics, Poliomyelitis. London, Churchill Livingstone, 1975.
Sandifer, P. H.: Neurology in Orthopaedics. London, Butterworth, 1967.

18 Endocrine Disorders that Affect the Feet

W. P. U. JACKSON,
J. H. LOUW,
H. S. MYERS

PART 1 The Diabetic Foot*

W. P. U. JACKSON,
J. H. LOUW

The best definition of *the diabetic foot* is simply *the foot of a diabetic*. It implies that all diabetics have from the outset potential pathological changes in their feet which may lead to serious consequences such as corns, callosities and clawtoes, deformities and disarticulations (Charcot's joints), ulceration and necrosis, cellulitis and suppuration, and, above all, gangrene.

These various lesions are caused by ischemia (angiopathy), neurologic changes (peripheral neuropathy), and infection, or a combination of the three. Gangrene in the diabetic foot, to quote Catterall, usually follows "the addition of sepsis to a foot already desensitized by neuropathy and devitalized by ischemia."[1]

Marchal de Calvi in 1864 was perhaps the first to notice that gangrene of the foot occurred more frequently in diabetics than in nondiabetics.[2] In 1941 Dry and Hines found occlusive disease in the legs to be some 35 times more common in diabetics, while Bell found gangrene to be 156 times more common in the diabetic in the fifth decade of life, and 53 times more common in the seventh decade.[3,4]

* This work was supported by a grant from the South African Medical Research Council.

PATHOGENESIS

Ischemia

Peripheral ischemia in diabetics is due partly to atherosclerosis affecting large and medium-sized vessels, and partly to a microangiopathy of the skin and muscle capillaries.[5,6]

Atherosclerosis is more common in diabetics than in nondiabetics and tends to occur at a younger age. The cause of the high incidence of atherosclerosis in diabetics and its possible relation to changes in serum lipid levels remain unclear. It would appear to be related particularly to the age of the patient and to the duration of the diabetes rather than to the severity of the disease or to the standard of its treatment.[7,8] Ischemia of the feet is very rare in diabetics under the age of 40 years. The lesions also have a somewhat different distribution in diabetics, tending to affect the medium-sized and small arteries, with the result that there is an increased severity of occlusive disease as one proceeds distally from the aorta. Aortoiliac lesions do occur in diabetics but do not commonly advance to complete occlusion. On the other hand, changes in the popliteal, tibial, and foot vessels are so common that they are referred to as the "classical diabetic

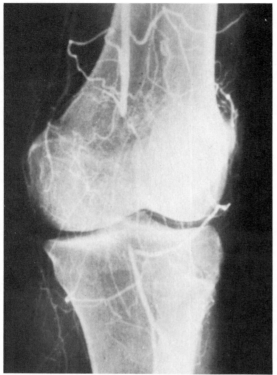

Fig. 18-1. The typical occlusion of the popliteal and anterior tibial vessels. Note the well-marked collateral vessels.

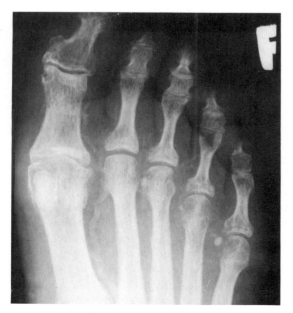

Fig. 18-2. Calcification of metatarsal and digital arteries. There are small areas of porosis in the bones.

occlusive pattern'' (Fig. 18-1), and this pattern is noted 20 times more frequently in long-standing diabetics (15 years) than in an age-matched non-diabetic group.[9] Involvement of the metatarsal arteries is also common, and medial calcification in these vessels can frequently be seen on x-rays of the foot (Fig. 18-2).

The delineation of a more specifically diabetic small vessel disease—diabetic angiopathy—has thrown further light on the development of ischemic lesions in diabetes. In 1959 Goldenberg and co-workers described PAS-positive thickening of the basement membrane and endothelial proliferation in small arteries and arterioles in tissues from the legs of diabetics.[10] In the same year Fagerberg reported similar thickening in intraneural arterioles of the sural nerves obtained from diabetics.[11] Subsequently, capillary lesions have been described in muscles, nerves, and skin of the legs which resemble the microangiopathic diabetic lesions of the retina, kidney, and other organs, but small artery occlusion seems to be the most important pathological disorder in the foot.[12]

The mechanism of production of small blood vessel disease and its relation to hyperglycemia in diabetics is unknown. One recent suggestion envisages excessive sorbitol deposition in the vessel walls (see under neuropathy), while Spiro has pointed to the increased production of glycoproteins in insulin-deficient states in vessel basement membranes—even chemically abnormal glycoproteins, at least in renal glomeruli.[13]

It should be pointed out that, although widespread small vessel disease is often present in the diabetic extremity, the lesions do not necessarily progress to complete occlusion, and Conrad has shown that there is no greater tendency toward occlusion of the small vessels in the arteriosclerotic diabetic than in the arteriosclerotic nondiabetic.[14]

Neuropathy

Neuropathic changes[15,16] involving the feet include chronic progressive symmetrical peripheral polyneuropathy, autonomic neuropathy, and occasionally a mononeuropathy of the common peroneal nerve that produces foot drop. Destructive joint lesions following sensory and autonomic nerve involvement are sometimes considered separately as neurogenic arthropathy (Fig. 18-3).

Segmental demyelination is an early histologic feature, corresponding to an early reduction in nerve conduction velocity. Axonal loss and degenerative changes in the spinal root ganglia also occur. The primary disturbance probably involves the lipid metabolism in the Schwann cell, but the precise defects are not clear. Similar changes probably occur in the autonomic nerves, but there have been few reliable observations.

There are two opposing main theories as to the etiology of diabetic peripheral polyneuropathy: (1) ischemia on the basis of angiopathy affecting the vasa nervorum, and (2) metabolic derangements in the nerve, and especially the Schwann cell, caused by the diabetic state, in particular hyperglycemia. There is no doubt, as clearly demonstrated by Fagerberg and others, that the small blood vessels supplying nerves are frequently affected in diabetics;[11] however, the relation of this to clinical neuropathy is unproven. On the other hand, while metabolic changes that might well affect nerves certainly occur in chronic hyperglyemia, yet there appears to be little if any relationship between the level of blood glucose and the presence or severity of chronic diabetic neuropathy.

Biochemical changes that occur in diabetics and are capable of affecting nerves include: abnormalities in pyruvate metabolism (not at present favored); impairment of fatty acid synthesis with reduced lipid levels in nerve tissue; myoinositol deficiency, which probably does occur in diabetics, and the accumulation of sorbitol and other polyols within the Schwann cell.[17,18] This latter mechanism is popular at the present time. In insulin-deficient states more glucose than normal is transformed into sorbitol and fructose in various tissues under the influence of the enzyme aldose reductase. These products diffuse poorly through the cell membrane and are only slowly

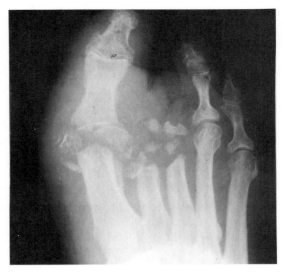

Fig. 18-3. Lytic destruction of the first metatarsophalangeal joint and decapitation of the second and third metatarsal heads with loose bone fragments. The second toe was surgically removed. This case was probably almost entirely a neuropathic lesion.

metabolized, so remaining entrapped within the cell and leading to damage by osmotic effects. This certainly appears to happen in the lens of the eye, but while sorbitol and fructose have been shown to accumulate in the nervous tissue of experimental diabetic animals, it is not yet clear that they produce serious damage. Chemical inhibitors of aldose reductase are at present being examined for possible therapeutic use.

Whatever the cause of the neuropathy, it is frequently seen in elderly diabetics at the apparent onset of their clinical disease, which, because of its insidious development, has actually been "smoldering" for several years without being diagnosed.

Infection[19]

Although there is some dispute over whether diabetics are more prone to infection than nondiabetics, there is no doubt that infections of the foot are very common in diabetic patients. There is some evidence to suggest that the leukocyte function of diabetics may be impaired (viz., there is an inability to utilize available glucose to produce bactericidal quantities of lactic acid), and this may be an important factor in increasing susceptibility to infection.[20] The microangiopathy may also impair resistance to infection, because the thickened basement membrane interferes with the transfer of nutrients and humoral factors to the tissues, and with the migration of leukocytes into the tissues.[5] Furthermore, the diabetic neuropathy which also affects the autonomic nervous system produces an autosympathectomy of the feet which interrupts vasomotor reflex pathways, so interfering with the normal vascular response to infection and resulting in poor reaction to invading organisms.[20] Finally, the increased dextrose content of the body fluids offers a more favorable situation for bacterial growth and for the production of gas in the tissues by nonclostridial organisms such as *E. coli, Proteus* and anerobic streptococci.[21]

In any event, the high incidence of areas of denuded skin from ischemic and neuropathic lesions clearly renders the diabetic foot more liable to infection than the normal foot. And, because of the devitalized tissues, any infection that does occur is more severe and more difficult to eradicate.

Bacteria may gain entry from any ulcerated area, from epidermal fissures resulting from interdigital dermatophytosis, and from the nail beds following fungal infection or paronychia. A mixture of organisms is frequently found in infected tissues, including coliforms, staphylococci, streptococci and *Klebsiella*. Several of these may give rise to gas in the tissues, which does not, therefore, necessarily indicate the presence of *Clostridia*. Gangrene results from the combination of the hypoxic state produced by vascular disease and the increased tissue demand for oxygen caused by the inflammatory reaction. Because of the diabetic's poor reaction to infection the septic lesion tends to spread to the deeper tissues and along tissue planes to involve muscles, bones, and joints, and along the flexor tendons into the sole of the foot.

Combined Lesions

The complex series of processes that occur in the diabetic foot are shown schematically in Fig. 18-4.[22] In many patients combined lesions exist and result in the more serious complications with ultimate gangrene. It is for this reason that gangrene is 30 times more

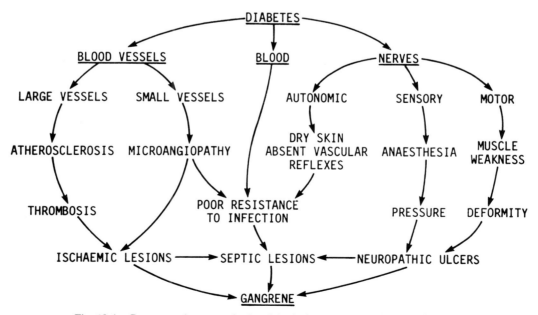

Fig. 18-4. Processes that occur in the diabetic foot. (Modified from Levin, 1973).

common in diabetics than in nondiabetic atherosclerotics, and the cause of death in 10 to 15 per cent of diabetic patients.

CLINICAL FEATURES

Three varieties of lesions are encountered: senile atherosclerotic ischemia, neuropathy, and infections.

Ischemia Without Neuropathy or Infection

In essence atherosclerotic ischemic manifestations in diabetics are simply those of atherosclerosis in a patient who happens to be a diabetic. The condition is frequently associated with extensive atheroma affecting other vessels, particularly the coronary and cerebral arteries. If large peripheral vessels are occluded with absence of the popliteal pulse, the patient will complain of calf claudication, and, if, in addition, the collateral circulation is impaired, the condition will progress to rest pain in the foot. Pain is the dominant feature, and so the patient is seen early. The foot is cold, often with dependent rubor (the pink, painful foot), slow venous filling, blanching on being elevated at 45 degrees for 1 to 2 minutes, and no pedal pulses. Later the skin becomes shiny and waxy-looking, cool, dry, and atrophic with thickened nails and loss of hair; finally ulceration and gangrene supervene, commencing at the extreme periphery (i.e., the tips of the toes, Fig. 18-5). However, if the collateral circulation is satisfactory tissue viability will be maintained. In this connection it should be pointed out that there are numerous instances in which patients are relatively asymptomatic in spite of calcification of the digital vessels and very extensive arterial occlusion on angiography.[9]

In practice the ischemic manifestations are usually altered by other factors. First, on account of the distribution of the atheroma to the more distal vessels, thrombosis in the major proximal arteries is uncommon. Consequently, claudication is seldom a presenting symptom. Second, the coexistence of diabetic microangiopathy often precipitates localized ulceration and gangrene over any part of the

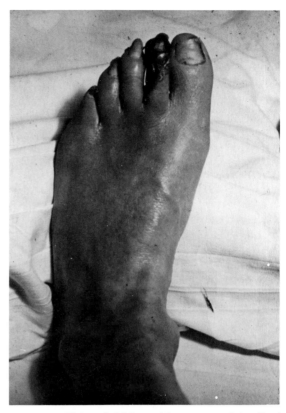

Fig. 18-5. Pink, painful foot with gangrene of the distal part of the second toe.

foot, and especially over the heel (Fig. 18-6) and the dorsum (Fig. 18-7). The prognosis tends to be worse than in the nondiabetic, and unless the circulation can be improved by surgery, the limb will be lost. In these cases angiograms may also be misleading, and patients with minimal angiographic occlusion may have rest pain or frank tissue necrosis.

Neuropathic Lesions

Neuropathic lesions are usually bilateral and symmetrical. They may occur in teenagers who have long-standing insulin-dependent diabetes, but are seen mostly in middle- and old age (the same applies to diabetic small blood vessel disease). Pain and paresthesias may be prominent or totally absent. The pain may be severe, shooting, burning, or knifelike, worse at night but, unlike vascular pain, relieved by walking about. Some patients have such gross

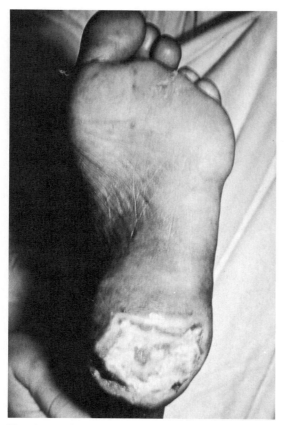

Fig. 18-6. Ulceration of the heel.

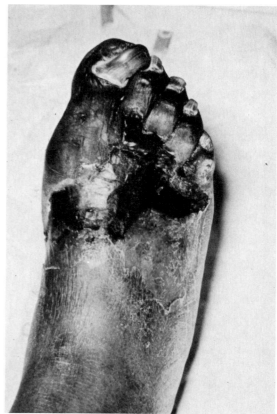

Fig. 18-7. Ulceration and gangrene of the dorsum of the foot.

hyperesthesia that they can scarcely bear the touch of bed clothes or trousers. On the other hand, a loss of pain and temperature sensation is common, and the patient may feel his feet are "dead" and that he is "walking on cotton wool." There is absence of pain appreciation as indicated by pin-prick testing. At the same time, the foot is warm due to autosympathectomy, and the peripheral pulses are often bounding. The ankle reflexes are usually lost. Vibration sense may be lost early on, but touch and position sense are usually retained, though in the rare pseudotabetic syndrome, with lightning pains and ataxia, gross proprioceptive loss occurs.

Blisters and small ulcers appear on pressure areas, largely from painless trauma, as from an unappreciated nail in the shoe, or from mild burns. The perforating plantar ulcer (mal perforans) is characteristic of diabetic neuropathy, having a small round mouth leading to considerable destruction of deeper tissues (Fig. 18-8). Pure neuropathic disease may lead to largely painless, disorganized, hypertrophic, Charcot-type joints (Fig. 18-9) in the metatarsophalangeal and mid-tarsal regions.[23] Indeed, the first sign of the development of diabetic neuropathy may be the appearance of a Charcot joint, because of the associated inflammatory swelling and heat secondary to repeated injury. Bony swelling from joint deformities may produce new pressure points.

Weakness of the intrinsic muscles of the foot leads to loss of extension at the proximal interphalangeal joints (lumbrical palsy) and loss of flexion at the metatarsophalangeal joints (palsy of interossei). The normal power of the long flexors and extensors is unbalanced. The

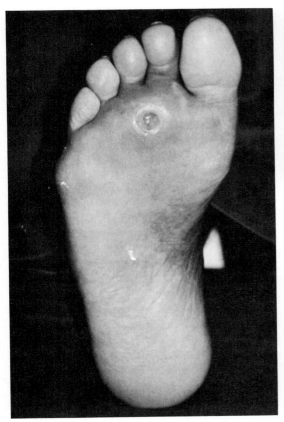

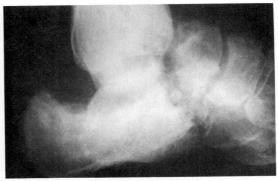

Fig. 18-9. Disorganization of the mid-tarsal joints with osteosclerosis and new bone (Charcot-type). Several bone fragments are present. There is destruction of the tarsal bones and the upper part of the calcaneum, with porosis and sclerosis.

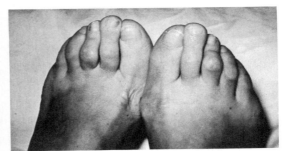

Fig. 18-10. Clawtoes.

Fig. 18-8. Perforating plantar ulceration (mal perforans).

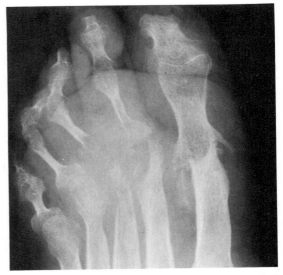

toes are thus cocked-up and clawed (Fig. 18-10), with subsequent uncovering of the metatarsal heads. Here is another site for the formation of callosities and ulcers. The development of a hallux valgus provides yet another pressure point.

Radiography may reveal not only a Charcot joint but also osteolysis, particularly of the heads of the metatarsals and ends of the phalanges, and attenuation of the phalanges and metatarsals, especially at their necks (Fig. 18-11).[24,25] This bone resorption indicates that adequate circulation must be present, so helping to distinguish ischemic from neuropathic lesions.[26] Infection may also cause bone destruction with patchy rarefaction and, later, piecemeal fragmentation.

Autonomic nerve involvement diminishes sweating and leads to a dry, scaly, cracked,

Fig. 18-11. Selective destruction of the metatarsophalangeal joints with some osteoporosis and thinning of the shafts of the proximal phalanges. Again, the lesions are largely neuropathic.

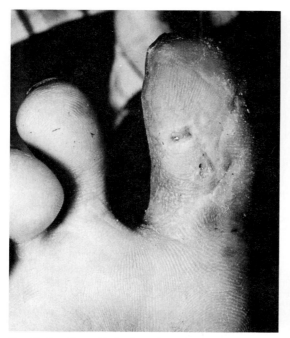

Fig. 18-12. Fungal infection of the great toe.

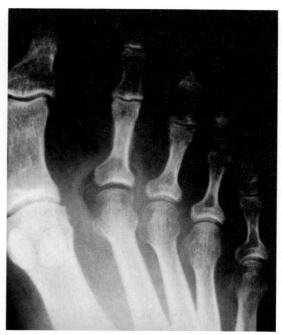

Fig. 18-13. A penetrating ulcer in the soft tissues in the neighborhood of the second metatarsophalangeal joint, with periostitis of the shaft of the second proximal phalanx. The joint itself appears to be intact.

and fissured skin. Vasomotor involvement causes changes in skin temperature resulting in a warm rather than a cold foot. Further trophic degenerative changes in skin, nails, and bone may be in part related to autonomic disorder.

Infection

This often commences at the site of injury, either accidentally or as a result of injudicious treatment of corns, calluses, or toenails. Sometimes the infection starts between the toes, secondary to fungal infections, which are very common in diabetics (Fig. 18-12), or in pressure sores over bony deformities (Fig. 18-13). Once infection is established it tends to spread to the deeper tissues along tissue planes with involvement of muscles, bones and joints, and along the flexor tendons into the sole of the foot.

The clinical presentation depends largely on whether there is arterial insufficiency or not.

Infection Without Evidence of Ischemia—Neuropathic Gangrene. Such infection occurs in careless, alcoholic, neglected, or derelict patients who develop painless neuropathic ulcers over abnormal pressure points. Because of the absence of pain both the patient and the medical attendant may be unaware of spreading infection, and the only clue may be swelling of the foot (Fig. 18-14), crepitus on moving the affected joint, or bone erosion or gas in the soft tissues on radiographs (Fig. 18-15). The foot is warm, and often peripheral pulses are present. However, a clean defect soon becomes purulent, and with a free blood supply, large amounts of pus form and track backward along the fascial planes and tendons of the sole. Gangrenous lesions of the foot accompanied by clinical or radiographic evidence of subcutaneous gas are common and usually due to mixed gram-negative bacilli and enterococci.[27] Clostridial gas gangrene is extremely uncommon. In other cases the heel is

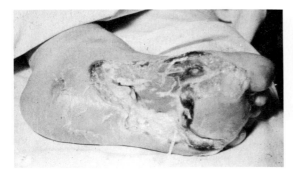

Fig. 18-14. Deep infection of the sole of the foot.

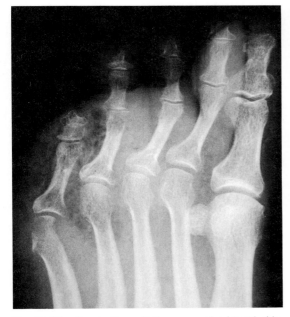

Fig. 18-15. Gas in the soft tissues on the lateral side. Mottled lucencies in the soft tissues on the lateral side are caused by gas bubbles. Partial destruction of the heads of the lateral metatarsals and phalanges is secondary to osteitis.

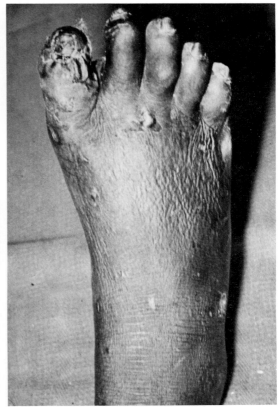

Fig. 18-16. Infection with gangrene of the first and second toes.

affected with extensive sloughing of the skin, osteomyelitis of the calcaneus, and even tracking of pus into the calf. Nevertheless, the skin of the foot remains pink, warm, and dry, and pedal pulses may be bounding. The constitutional disturbance is often minor, out of all proportion to the gravity of the situation.

Infection With Added Ischemia—Ischemic Gangrene. In patients with infection and is-chemia (Fig. 18-16), who almost always have neuropathic damage, the blood supply is insufficient to meet and overcome the infection, which, therefore, spreads rapidly and precipitates early gangrene. Because of the neuropathic element, the foot is not cold, despite impaired blood supply, and the sepsis remains apparently indolent with less pain and tenderness than would be expected. Often the skin of the affected side is warmer because of open collateral channels, autosympathectomy, or inflammation. The pedal pulses are often absent (on both sides), but more important is absence of the popliteal or superficial femoral pulses.

Absence of the popliteal pulse must be recognized as a warning signal that particular care will be required to save the limb. Careful assessment of the vascular status by special investigations is, therefore, necessary. In this regard Doppler ultrasonography is useful, in that it may demonstrate patent pedal vessels. Another useful device is the quantitative segmental pulse volume recorder developed by Darling and co-workers in 1972.[28] By combining the data from this and the measurement of ankle pressure by ultrasound, important prognostic conclusions can be drawn. Both Raines and Jacobs have found that ankle pressures of at least 90 torr. are necessary for healing of the diabetic ulcerative lesion, and that ankle pressures greater than 75 torr will prevent rest pain.[9,29]

PREVENTION

Knowledge, understanding, and education are of primary importance. All diabetics must know that their feet are in danger—young people after 10 years of diabetes, and older people from the time of diagnosis. As well as explanations, diabetics should receive written instructions and advice. At Groote Schuur Hospital we include printed instructions on foot care in our booklets for diabetic patients, and a more detailed handout is available from the Peripheral Vascular Clinic.

Foot Care for Diabetic Patients

1. Socks must be warm, soft and undarned. No elastic around legs.
2. Shoes must be well-fitting and wide enough not to compress the toes. Pointed toes are anathema. Fashion may be fun, it may also be fatal.
3. Care must be taken with any source of heat. Hot water bottles, over-hot baths, and open fires must be avoided.
4. Injuries of all kinds must be avoided. Barefoot is banned.
5. Toenails, corns and callosities call for a chiropodist;[30] regular attendance is preferable.
6. Athletes foot must be treated and then prevented (e.g., with clean, dry toes and medicated foot powder).
7. If a minor injury does occur the part should be cleaned gently with soap and water, and bed rest for a few days is advisable. Strong disinfectants, chemical compounds, ointments, corn cures, or adhesive plasters should

be avoided. No medication is better than taking chances.
8. Any open ulcer that does not rapidly heal should be treated by a physician.

MANAGEMENT

Neuropathic Lesions

Pressure ulceration over a hallux valgus, clawtoe, or other foot deformity can be prevented by proper modifications to the shoes. Extra-deep shoes with quarter-inch insoles are useful for the prevention of plantar callosities over the heads of the metatarsals and "mal perforans" ulcers. If bed rest has been prescribed for the healing of an ulcerated or gangrenous area, or for the treatment of Charcot's joints, care should be taken to prevent rubbing of the heel and sides of the neuropathic foot against the bedclothes, lest a new area of ulceration develop. This can be achieved by suspending the calf in a wide and soft foam rubber padded sling from an overhead beam, but it tends to immobilize the patient too much.[8] A more practical alternative is to wrap the foot in a very large mass of cotton wool to create a protective boot and to nurse the patient on sheepskin underblankets.[31] Charcot's joints are caused by repeated injuries, and, as in the treatment of all injuries, the most obvious and effective remedy is rest to allow healing to occur. After initial bed rest the simple application of a short-leg walking cast is usually all that is required, but it may take 2 to 3 months for healing.

A simple neuropathic ulcer should heal on its own wiht expectant treatment. If the ulcer is small or superficial it may be treated by limited local debridement in the Outpatient Department. This should be followed by regular bathing of the feet with Betadine soaks twice daily and protection of the ulcer from further pressure. If the ulcers are somewhat larger, a short-leg plastic walking cast with an insole should be applied. In the case of deeply penetrating ulcers with secondary infection and involvement of the underlying bone, thorough debridement is necessary (see below).

Ischemic Lesions

If a main vessel is occluded and the collateral circulation is inadequate, gangrene will result and a major amputation will be required unless the main vessel flow can be restored or the collateral circulation significantly improved. Since occlusion of the popliteal and proximal tibial arteries is so common in diabetics, the standard method of lower leg revascularization (viz. femoropopliteal bypass) can rarely be used. However, direct revascularization of the leg and foot may be achieved if the distal tibial and peroneal arteries are patent and communicate with the arterial arches of the foot. This may be demonstrated by arteriography (Fig. 18-17). Operations for bypass of these distal vessels are tedious and technically demanding, because they involve quite small vessels, a considerable discrepancy between the graft and the recipient vessel, and unfamiliar anatomical approaches. Reichle and co-workers claim that satisfactory results can be obtained if there is direct communication between the recipient vessel and the plantar arch, but we have found the procedure disappointing.[32]

However, these bypasses may be of value in promoting healing of open lesions and thereby avoiding spreading infection. In such cases failure of the bypass after healing has been achieved does not inevitably lead to loss of the foot or even to renewed tissue breakdown.[9]

Limbs with superficial femoral and popliteal occlusions will often remain viable and comfortable, provided that adequate flow in the distal smaller vessels can be maintained through the main collateral to the lower leg, the profunda femoris. Arteriograms should, therefore, include special views of the origin of the profunda (Fig. 18-18), and if an occlusive lesion is demonstrated, it can be corrected by profundoplasty. In patients with noninfected lesions this may be sufficient to restore adequate circulation to the foot.

It is generally agreed that lumbar sympathectomy does not have much to offer the diabetic with a neuropathic foot, because he is likely already to have had an autosympathectomy. However, Jacobs and colleagues

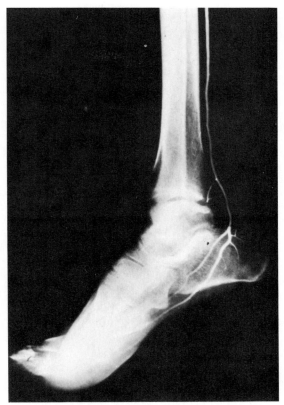

Fig. 18-17. A patent posterior tibial vessel communicating with the plantar arch.

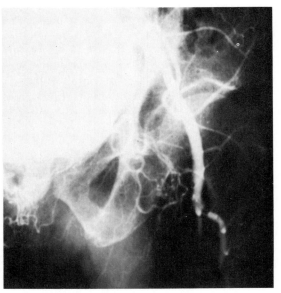

Fig. 18-18. Occlusion of the superficial femoral artery and stenosis of the origin of the profunda femoris.

maintain that 30 per cent of diabetics who had sympathectomies as "last ditch" procedures showed a significant improvement in blood flow to the skin and healing of indolent ulcers.[9] We have found that the procedure is only of value in the occasional cases where appropriate tests such as plethysmography confirm that an autosympathectomy has not taken place. Clinically, this is suggested by sweating of the foot.

If direct arterial surgery is impossible, local surgery is permissible for gangrenous toes, provided the collateral circulation is reasonable. However, apart from drainage of abscesses, no local surgery should be carried out while there is rest pain and no clear line of demarcation. Once demarcation has occurred the gangrenous soft tissue can be excised through the line of demarcation, together with enough bone to allow the soft tissues to approximate. Conservative treatment of a single dry gangrenous toe while waiting for spontaneous separation is feasible and can be undertaken if the patient is totally unfit for surgery, but it takes a long time, and infection is always likely to occur.

If local surgery fails or infection supervenes, further delay should be avoided and a major amputation performed. Catterall said ". . . when man is increasingly tending to outlive his arteries . . . a properly designed amputation and limb-fitting may be the quickest way of restoring the painless locomotion which was the patient's birthright."[33] In purely ischemic lesions this usually amounts to an above-knee amputation.

Infective Lesions

In diabetics, simple drainage of abscesses and regular dressings are not enough, because the impairment of blood supply leads to late separation of sloughs and delayed healing, while the infection tends to spread without warning because of reduced pain sensation due to neuropathy. Moreover, it is difficult to judge how far the infection has spread because of the poor inflammatory reaction.

The primary object of local treatment is to remove all the necrotic tissue, but because of the risks of spreading infection, this can be done only after the acute infection has been controlled by antibiotics and surgical drainage.[34] In the desloughing process, sufficient bone should be removed to allow the edges of the wound to fall together, but the balance of the foot should not be upset.

Superficial Lesions. If it is certain that the lesion is superficial, appropriate antibiotics and drainage of abscesses with subsequent strictly aseptic dressings will usually suffice. Sloughs should be softened with regular sterile soaks and petrolatum dressings and then snipped away.

Deep Lesions. The approach to deep infections with tissue necrosis depends upon the degree of coincident ischemia. If the foot is cold, with no popliteal pedal pulses, and particularly if there is rest pain proximal to the lesion, it is unlikely that local surgery will succeed. In such cases a major amputation is inevitable unless the circulation can be improved by a bypass graft. However, the urgency of the situation and the presence of sepsis usually preclude grafting procedures. The ultimate outcome is, therefore, often an above-knee amputation.

On the other hand, if the foot is warm and the circulation apparently adequate, and especially if the popliteal pulse is present, the approach must be that of "aggressive conservatism," (i.e., major amputations should be avoided, but drainage must be established by generous incisions and necrotic tissue removed by bold excisions of soft tissues together with removal of sufficient bone to allow skin approximation without tension). It must be borne in mind that the operation is essentially a drainage and deboning procedure (Fig. 18-19). Viable toes or rays should not be sacrificed merely to accomplish primary closure; and as much healthy skin as possible should be preserved.

The infection should be followed wherever it has spread, usually along the flexor tendons into the sole of the foot. The wound is left unsutured but Steristrips may be used to approximate the edges. After five days a second look under general anesthesia is necessary, to

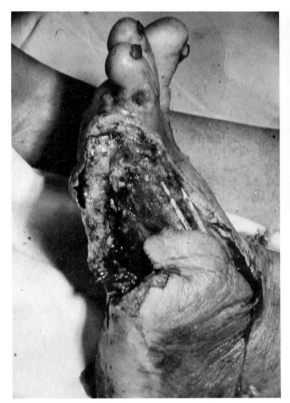

Fig. 18-19. Note the extent of debridement.

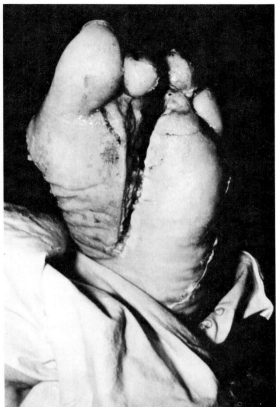

Fig. 18-21. Ray excision of the third toe.

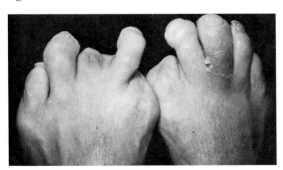

Fig. 18-20. Distortion is caused by removal of more than one toe.

detect and deal with pockets of pus and residual necrotic tissue. Thereafter, dressings should be changed weekly in the operating room and antibiotics should be continued until healing is sound. The patient is allowed up on crutches, but weight bearing should be avoided for 5 to 6 weeks.

AMPUTATIONS. Various local amputations may be necessary. If a single toe is affected, simple disarticulation at the metatarsophalangeal joint will suffice. However, if more than one toe has to be removed, a transmetatarsal amputation of the foot is usually necessary to avoid strain on the remaining toes (Fig. 18-20). Sometimes removal of the two lateral toes may leave a useful foot, provided the incision is carried well onto the sole of the foot to ensure adequate drainage of pus; very rarely, two middle toes may be removed with a reasonable functional result. If the infection has spread proximally to the metatarsophalangeal joint and flexor tendon, a ray excision of the toe and distal part of the metatarsal bone will be necessary (Fig. 18-21). Although this is not generally recommended for the great toe because of consequent instability of the foot, we have found that some patients manage very well afterward. Transmetatarsal operations of the foot are probably the ideal for

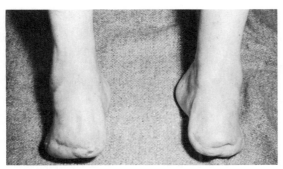

Fig. 18-22. Bilateral transmetatarsal amputations. This patient walks comfortably, but there is some inversion of the left foot.

lesions of the feet in diabetics, because extensive removal of damaged tissue is possible and the most vulnerable areas are removed (e.g., the bony pressure points over the heads of the metatarsals).[34] The wounds heal, and the patients can walk quite well even with bilateral amputations (Fig. 18-22).

If infection has spread to the proximal part of the foot or if a transmetatarsal amputation fails, a major amputation will be required. This also applies to gangrene of the dorsum of the foot with involvement of the tendons and to ulceration of the heel. In infected neuropathic lesions with minimal ischemia a below-knee amputation is often possible, even if the popliteal pulse is coincidentally absent. However, if there is a pronounced ischemic element, an above-knee amputation will be necessary, unless the Doppler pressure in the popliteal artery is above 90 torr. It should be remembered that at least one third of diabetic amputees will require amputation of the other extremity within 3 years, and therefore major ablations should not be undertaken lightly.[35] At the same time the objective is to restore the patient to nearly normal activity as soon as possible (i.e., to early independence so that he can care for his own needs). A patient who is not walking (with or without a prosthesis) on discharge from hospital will either never walk at all, or will walk with crutches and put an excessive strain on the remaining foot and risk ending up as a double amputee in a wheelchair.

PART 2   *The Acromegalic Foot*

W. P. U. JACKSON,
H. S. MYERS

Acromegaly

Acromegaly is a condition produced by an excessive amount of active circulating growth hormone in an adult, or at least in a person whose epiphyses are closed or nearly closed. It is caused by an adenoma of the acidophils of the pituitary gland and typically occurs within a few years of puberty. The hormonal effects are many and varied and include a drive toward overgrowth of all tissues of the body, particularly the connective tissues, skeleton, internal organs, skin, and blood vessels.

Acromegaly means "large extremities," and so it is fitting that we should consider the acromegalic foot. The hand, however, is more characteristically affected and more important diagnostically (except for the foot-pad thickness as discussed below). After epiphyseal fusion the skeletal system can be affected in the following ways:

Increased bone formation in areas still capable of this (i.e., subperiosteally, especially in acral bones; the mandible and the anterior aspects of vertebral bodies)
Paradoxically, a thinning of some bones with reduced cortical thickness and density; actual osteolysis and cyst formation may occur. The mechanism of this is not understood.
A revival of cartilaginous growth leading to increased width of joint spaces on x-ray, ossification of articular cartilage, and secondary arthritis.
Calcification at the sites of attachment of ligaments, cartilage, and tendons to bone.

Characteristic features in the acromegalic hand therefore include thickening of skin and subcutaneous tissues with redundancy of skin folds, frequently an increase in the width (but not length) of phalangeal bones, but sometimes narrowing and wasting with rarefaction and osteolysis, increased size and coarsening of the terminal phalangeal tufts, increased interphalangeal joint space, and variable small bony excrescences at various sites at the points of attachment of connective tissues. There is considerable increase in hand width but very little in length (comprising only the sum of the increases in joint spaces).

The acromegalic foot shows similar but usually less prominent changes (Fig. 18-23A); several are particularly interesting:

> *The greater tendency for slimming,* reduced width and wasting of the metatarsal and phalangeal shafts
> *Irregular enlargement of bone ends,* especially metatarsals, increasing the appearance of thinning of the shafts
> *Irregular enlargment of sesamoid bones,* especially striking at the great toe
> *The enormous increase in thickness of the heel pad* (Fig. 18-23B)

This is measured on a standard lateral film, taken at a 40-inch tube-to-film distance, as the perpendicular distance between the inferoposterior aspect of the calcaneus and the skin surface, as defined by Kho and colleagues.[36] The heel pad should normally be less than 22 mm. in width, and as far as we are aware no condition other than acromegaly causes any considerable widening to occur. The sign is therefore of diagnostic importance. Other simple historical features of diagnostic value result from the general widening of hand and foot tissues (e.g., rings no longer fit, glove and shoe sizes increase).

Peripheral nerves may also become involved in acromegaly in two ways:

> *Compression from the overgrowth of surrounding connective tissues*—an entrapment neuropathy most frequently seen as the carpal tunnel syndrome
> *True peripheral neuropathy*[37] with paraesthesias, absent tendon reflexes, muscle wasting, and sensory loss. The mechanism of production of this is unclear.

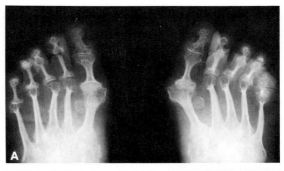

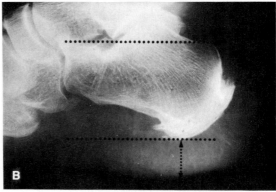

Fig. 18-23. (*A*) Several features characteristic of acromegaly are shown in this radiograph: (1) Extreme thinning of the shafts of the metatarsals and proximal phalanges; (2) irregular enlargement of bone ends and sesamoids; (3) increase in joint spaces (second and third metatarsophalangeal on the left); (4) bony excresences (e.g., on metatarsal shafts). (*B*) Thickened heel pad and the method of measurement. There are prominent spurs at the insertion of the plantar fascia and the achilles tendon.

Gigantism

Excessive growth hormone secretion before closure of the epiphyses leads to greatly increased bone growth in length, but no hastening of bone maturation. The large feet are in proportion with the rest of the skeleton. Features of acromegaly may be added to those of gigantism if the disorder starts at about the same time as the beginning of puberty.

Eunuchoidism

Eunuchodism may occur together with gigantism if the gonadotropins of the pituitary gland are damaged by the A-cell adenoma. In this condition the acral bones are excessively long and slender, out of proportion to the height of the subject.

PART 3   The Foot in Disorders of the Thyroid

W. P. U. JACKSON

Pretibial Myxedema

Seldom actually on the foot, this rash is most common on the front of the legs, sometimes all round the legs and sometimes in other areas. It occurs usually in adults, who have been treated for thyrotoxicosis and who may be mildly toxic, euthyroid or (less commonly) hypothyroid when the rash starts. It appears as multiple, painless, more or less rounded swellings, plaques or indurations in the subcutaneous tissue, shiny and reddish-brown in color, firm and non-pitting, enlarging up to 10–20 cm and becoming bilateral, accompanied by hyperkeratosis and fissuring, with coarse skin and prominent hair follicles. Sometimes diffuse firmness of the subcutaneous tissues is present and sometimes pitting edema of leg and foot may be present.

The rash is of no importance other than cosmetic and tends slowly to diminish over months or years. It may accompany thyroid ophthalmopathy ("malignant exophthalmos") and thyroid acropachy (see below).

Thyroid Acropachy

This occurs under the same conditions as pretibial myxedema but is probably less common. Sausagelike swelling of the soft tissues of the phalanges occurs, with clubbing of fingers and toes. The diagnostic feature on x-ray is a raising of the periosteum in metaphyseal areas adjoining peripheral joints, especially of the small long bones, and it may resemble "bubbles" on the bony surface. It is similar to hypertrophic pulmonary osteoarthropathy, but is painless.

Primary Hypothyroidism

In childhood (cretinism, juvenile myxedema), the most important skeletal feature is retardation of development—delay in appearance and in closure of the epiphyses, most clearly seen in the hand. The abnormal development of the epiphyses from multiple calcifying centers is usually confined to the hip joint.

The skin in primary hypothyroidism tends to become coarse, thick, dry, and cold. Some patients may complain of cold feet, but more commonly "feel the cold" in general and pile on blankets in bed at night, even in summer. (The skin in hypothyroidism secondary to pituitary disease tends to be thin and finely wrinkled). Two other features may occasionally be seen on the skin in myxedema, namely *carotenodermia* (carotenemia, xanthosis) and *eruptive xanthomatosis*. Untreated hypothyroidism apparently delays the conversion of carotene to vitamin A, so allowing enough of this pigment to accumulate in the blood to impart a yellow tinge to the skin, particularly well seen in the palms and soles.

Eruptive xanthomas may occur with gross hyperlipidemia, especially involving the triglycerides. The skin lesions consist of bright yellowish-red papules, up to 5 mm. in diameter, appearing particularly on buttocks, forearms, elbows, and knees. They subside on treatment of the underlying condition (which is more frequently diabetes than myxedema). Other forms of xanthoma—tuberous, planus, and tendinous (often around the ankles)—may also occur.

A very helpful clinical feature in the diagnosis of hypothyroidism is a delay in relaxation of the achilles tendon after elicitation of the ankle jerk. While this can be accurately quantitated using a modified electrocardiograph machine, it can generally be clearly appreciated by the operator after a little practice.

Thyrotoxicosis

The feet are not outstandingly affected in active thyrotoxicosis but may share in the general process of loss of bone substance (Osteoporosis). In some instances of longstanding, unrecognized hyperthyroidism the femurs and tibias may be markedly porotic.

REFERENCES

1. Catterall, R. C. F.: The diabetic foot. Brit. J. Hosp. Med. 7:224, 1972.
2. de Calvi, M.: Recherches sur les accidents diabetique. Paris, P. Asselin, 1864.
3. Dry, T. J., and Hines, E. A.: Role of diabetes in development of degenerative fascular disease

with special reference to incidence of retinitis and peripheral neuritis. Ann. Intern. Med., *14:* 1893, 1941.

4. Bell, E. T.: Artherosclerotic gangrene of the lower extremities in diabetic and non-diabetic persons. Am. J. Clin. Pathol., *28:*27, 1957.

5. Banson, B. B., and Lacy, P. E.: Diabetic microangiopathy in human toes. Am. J. Pathol., *45:*41, 1964.

6. Siperstein, M. D., Norton, W., Unger, R. H., and Madison, L. L.: Muscle capillary basement membrane width in normal diabetic and pre-diabetic patients. Trans. Ass. Am. Phys., *79:* 330, 1966.

7. Lundbaek, K.: Diabetic angiopathy. A specific vascular disease. Lancet, *i:*377, 1954.

8. Oakley, W., Catterall, R. C. F., and Martin, M. M.: Aetiology and management of lesions of the feet in diabetes. Brit. Med. J., *2:*953, 1956.

9. Jacobs, R. L., Karmody, A. M., Wirth, C., and Vedder, D.: The team approach in salvage of the diabetic foot. In Nyhus, L. M., (ed.) Surgery Annual.

10. Goldenberg, S., Alex, M., Joshi, R. A., and Blumental, H. T.: Nonatheromatous peripheral vascular disease of the lower extremities in diabetes mellitus. Diabetes, *8:*261, 1959.

11. Fagerberg, S. E.: Diabetic neuropathy. A clinical and histological study on the significance of vascular affections. Acta Med. Scand. [Suppl. 345], *164,* 1959.

12. Stary, H. C.: Disease of the small blood vessels in diabetes mellitus. Am. J. Med. Sci., *252:*357, 1966.

13. Spiro, R. G.: Search for a biochemical basis of diabetic microangiopathy. Diabetologia, *12:*1, 1976.

14. Conrad, M. C.: Large and small artery occlusion in diabetics and non-diabetics with severe vascular disease. Circulation, *36:*83, 1967.

15. Eliasson, S. G.: Neuropathy and the diabetic foot. Levin, M. E. and O'Neal, L. W., (eds.): The Diabetic Foot. St. Louis, C. V. Mosby, 1973.

16. Thomas, P. K. and Ward, J. D.: Diabetic neuropathy. In Keen, H., and Jarrett, J., (eds.): Complications of Diabetes, London, Edward Arnold, 1975.

17. Winegrad, A. I., and Greene, D. A.: Diabetic polyneuropathy: the importance of insulin deficiency, hyperglycaemia and alterations in my-oinositol metabolism in its pathogenesis. N. Engl. J. Med., *295:*4, 1976.

18. Gabbay, K. H.: Role of sorbitol pathway in neuropathy. *In* V. H. T. James, (ed.): Endocrinology. New York, Excerpta Medica, 1976.

19. Little, J. R.: Bacteriology and the diabetic foot. *In* Levin, M.E. and O'Neal, L. W., (eds.): The Diabetic Foot. St. Louis, C. V. Mosby, 1973.

20. Martin, S. P., McKinney, G. R., Green, R., and Becker, C.: The influence of glucose, fructose and insulin on the metabolism of leucocytes of healthy and diabetic subjects. J. Clin. Invest., *32:*1171, 1953.

21. Spring, M., and Kahn, S.: Non-Clostridial gas infection in the diabetic. Arch Intern. Med., *88:* 373, 1951.

22. Levin, M. E.: Medical evaluation and treatment, *in* Levin, M. E. and O'Neal, L. W., (eds.): The Diabetic Foot. St. Louis, C. V. Mosby, 1973.

23. Ellenberg, M.: Diabetic neuropathy: Clinical aspects. Metabolism, *25:*1627, 1976.

24. Staple, T.: Roentgenography of the diabetic foot. Levin, M. E. and O'Neal, L. W., (eds.): The Diabetic Foot. St. Louis, C. V. Mosby, 1973.

25. Martin, M. M.: Involvement of autonomic nerve fibers in diabetic neuropathy. Lancet, *i:* 560, 1953.

26. Naide, M., and Schnall, C.: Bone changes in necrosis in diabetes mellitus. Arch. Intern. Med., *107:*380, 1961.

27. Bessman, A. N., and Wagner, W.: Non-Clostridial gas gangrene. J.A.M.A., *233:*958, 1975.

28. Darling, R. C., Raines, J. K., Brener, B. J., and Austen, W. G.: Quantitative segmental pulse volume recorder: a clinical tool. Surgery, *72:*873, 1972.

29. Raines, J. K., Darling, R. C., Buth, J., Brewster, D. C., and Auster, W. G.: Vascular laboratory criteria for the management of peripheral vascular disease of the lower extremities. Surgery, *79:*21, 1976.

30. Lippard, O. L.: Podiatry. *In* Levin, M. E., and O'Neal, L. W., (eds.): The Diabetic Foot. St. Louis, C. V. Mosby, 1973.

31. du Plessis, D. J.: Lesions of the feet in patients with diabetes mellitus. S.Af. J. Surg., *8:*29, 1970.

32. Reichle, F. A., Shuman, C. R., and Tyson, R. R.: Femoro-tibial bypass in the diabetic patient for salvage of the ischemic lower extremity. Am. J. Surg., *129:*603, 1975.

33. Catterall, R. C. F.: The surgeons viewpoint. Postgrad. Med. J. [Supplement], 969, 1968.

34. Wheelock, F. C., McKittrick, J. B., and Root, H. F.: Evaluation of the transmetatarsal amputation in patients with diabetes mellitus. Surgery, *41:*184, 1957.

35. Kritter, A.: A technique for salvage of the infected diabetic gangrenous foot. Orthop. Clin. North. Am., *4:*21, 1973.

36. Kho, K. M., Wright, A. D., and Doyle, F. H.: Heel pad thickness in acromegaly. Br. J. Radiol., *43:*119, 1970.

37. Low, P. A., McCleod, J. G., Turtle, T. et al.: Peripheral neuropathy in acromegaly. Brain, *97:*139, 1974.

19 The Swollen Foot

Very few adults manage to go through life without developing swollen feet at some time. Mild swelling may cause little bother, but with increasing tissue turgor the patient develops a throbbing sensation that may progress to constant burning, accompanied by an unpleasant feeling of tightness within the shoes or stockings. Eventually, swelling leads to foot fatigue and increasing symptoms on standing or walking.

GENERAL DISEASES THAT CAUSE LIMB EDEMA

Swelling of the feet may be the first signal of general disease. Three conditions, in particular, may manifest themselves in this way.

CONGESTIVE CARDIAC FAILURE

Whatever the cause of right-sided heart failure, by definition there is an increase in venous pressure, causing peripheral capillary congestion. Fluid is forced from the small vessels into the extracellular space, until enough is present in the soft tissues to constitute clinical edema. The collection of fluid in significant amounts is also dependent on gravity. The patient in bed first develops edema at the base of the spine; the ambulatory patient, in his feet. Many apparently quite healthy old people are in a state of incipient cardiac failure, as revealed by elevated jugular venous pressure and edema of the ankles.

RENAL FAILURE

Whatever the cause of failure of the kidneys to excrete sufficient fluid and whether it be acute or chronic, potentially serious or merely transient; edema is the inevitable accompaniment and may be the presenting symptom of the condition.

MYXEDEMA

Inadequate thyroid function in the adult is so often accompanied by a brawny edema of the front of the shins, extending to the feet and ankles, that the name, *myxedema,* implying a particularly "gelatinous" soft-tissue fluid swelling, has been given to the condition (see Chap. 18). The disease is of very slow onset and, although accompanied by a gain in weight, general sluggishness of body reactions, loss of hair of the outer third of the eyebrows, and intolerance to cold, it may easily be overlooked.

LOCALIZED CAUSES OF EDEMA WITHIN THE LIMB

The majority of swollen feet are the result of factors within the lower limb itself. To understand these it is necessary to consider the mechanism of blood flow through the limb, bearing in mind that an increase in capillary pressure results in the collection of extracellular fluid.

VENOUS STASIS

Left ventricular cardiac output provides the hydrostatic pressure required to deliver arterial blood to the limbs and from there to the capillaries, where the normal interchange of fluids takes place for oxygenation, feeding and the replacement and clearing of metabolites. Under normal conditions, a proportion of this blood is shunted from the arterial to the venous circulations by arteriolar contraction.

Anything that brings about arteriolar relaxation increases the capillary hydrostatic pressure and tends to increase extracellular fluid. Increased environmental temperature is a common cause; hence the almost universal complaint of swelling of the feet and ankles in hot weather. Local tissue trauma, whether effected by injury or the surgeon's knife, has a similar result because of the release of histamine.

Gravity, similarly, causes pooling of capillary blood in the dependent parts. High G-forces, whether in fighter pilots or astronauts, may reduce venous return so severely in the short term as to lead to cerebral anoxia. Repeated exposure to such forces may induce edema of the legs.

It is a common complaint of those taking long flights on jet aircraft that, on arrival at their destination, their feet are swollen. If they have been unwise enough to remove their shoes at the beginning of the journey, they may find difficulty in putting them on again. Normal gravity, especially in a hot atmosphere, may cause venous stasis; an effect to which generations of theatre- and film-goers can bear witness.

Lack of movement of the feet is a potent cause of edema. Much physiological research has been required to explain the mechanism of venous return of blood to the heart, for it is not immediately obvious how this is achieved. Capillary hydrostatic pressure, transferred to the venous system, plays a small part, but certainly not enough to counteract the effect of gravity. To accomplish the feat, two venous pump systems are involved.

The Calf Pump

The deep venous plexus lying between the layers of the calf muscles, especially the soleus and gastrocnemius bellies, constitutes the distal pump. Each contraction of these two layers of muscle during dorsiflexion and plantar flexion of the foot squeezes the blood in the sandwiched venous plexus. The constituent veins are amply supplied with flap valves that allow the blood to move in one direction only. Each time the muscles contract, the blood they contain is moved up the leg toward the heart, to be replaced by blood from the foot and, in particular, from the subcutaneous tissues of the leg. Similar valves between the superficial and deep venous systems ensure that the flow is always one way.

If the normal function of the valves breaks down—if movement of blood is no longer exclusively one-way—severe venous stasis results (Fig. 19-1), and swollen feet occur: high venous pressure in the deep veins is the main cause. Whether this is the result of extreme muscular effort in weight lifters; habitually raised, central venous pressure in patients with chronic smoker's cough; extrinsic pelvic pressure on the veins due to expanding intrapelvic masses or a pregnant uterus, or even to congenital or acquired inadequacy of the valves themselves; in the end, the walls of the veins are permanently stretched and the valves suddenly lose their competence. The one-way flow of the pump has failed, and capillary stasis results. The patient develops swollen feet and, in extreme cases, breakdown products of the red blood cells appear extracellularly. Such substances, usually hemosiderin from the breakdown of hemoglobin, are deposited subcutaneously and are a potent cause of venous ulcers in the leg.

Venous blowouts, described above, are known clinically as varicose veins. The principle of treatment consists of breaking the column of blood and so reducing the hydrostatic pressure. This can be performed surgically by tying the superficial veins or stripping

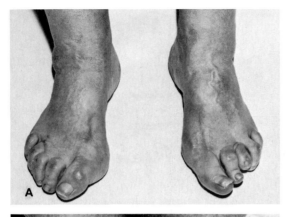

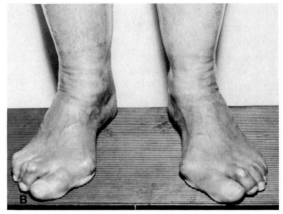

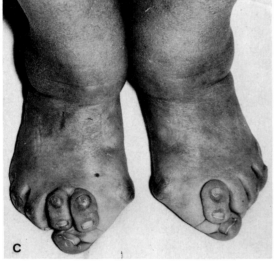

Fig. 19-1. The stages of venous stasis. (*A*) Venous engorgement in a patient with pes cavus and consequent lack of muscle development. (*B*) Hallux valgus and hammering of the toes. The telltale rings around the ankles indicate dependent edema. (*C*) In a case of deformities of the toes with collapse of the arches of the foot, gross edema of the legs has resulted in chronic subcutaneous induration of the ankles.

them. The injection of sclerosant fluids into an affected vein will cause the formation of a clot within the lumen. In time the injected vein is completely obliterated. All such treatments depend on the patency of the deep veins. If they have been blocked by deep-vein thrombosis, the superficial veins may be the only path for the return of venous blood from the leg. Removal in such cases could be catastrophic.

The Abdominothoracic Pump

The calf pump is by no means the only mechanism for draining the blood from the legs against the force of gravity. A second, and perhaps more important, pump exists in the inferior vena cava, at the level of its passage

from the abdominal- to the chest cavity through the diaphragm. As the dome-shaped muscle, the diaphragm, contracts during the inspiratory phase of respiration, its fibers are shortened and it is pulled downward, thus expanding the chest cavity. At the same time the intercostal muscles pull the ribs apart and widen the bony cage of the thorax. This increase in size of the thoracic cavity lowers the pressure in the intrapleural space and expands the elastic lung tissue, so drawing air into the bronchi. The thoracic part of the inferior vena cava and the right atrium expand equally. Since blood is prevented from being sucked back from the right ventricle by the tricuspid valve, blood is drawn up from the abdominal portion of the inferior vena cava. Simultaneously, the contraction of the diaphragm increases intraabdominal pressure, adding to the effect.

A failure of this pump, whether due to poor abdominal musculature; diaphragmatic weakness, due to hiatal hernia, for example; or poor thoracic expansion, tends to result in edema of the legs on standing.

Normal physiologic causes of fluid retention, such as changes in estrogen levels in pregnancy or during the premenstrual part of the cycle, may facilitate the formation of edema.

Treatment of the Venous Stasis Syndrome

Gravity may be used to decrease venous stasis instead of aggravating it. Simple elevation of the limb after surgery or following an injury plays a large part in the prevention of swelling. Firm compression of the subcutaneous tissues of the leg is similarly effective. Elastic bandaging, whether by crepe (Ace), true elastic bandages, or the modern variant called Tubigrip,* prevents edema in patients when they first leave their beds.

Repeated contraction of the calf pump prevents edema by overcoming the effect of gravity. This is why London policemen are traditionally known to go up and down on their toes while standing on duty. It is also why Guardsmen, in the annual ceremony known as "trooping the colour" before the Queen on her birthday, are notoriously liable to faint: having to stand quite still on parade, they develop venous pooling in the lower limbs until cerebral circulation fails. The policemen, in contrast, return venous blood to the heart by their repeated calf exercises.

The point is not merely academic. Foot exercises will prevent postoperative edema and reduce the chance of deep venous thrombosis following sluggish circulation in the deep veins of the leg. Exercise, especially in conjunction with firm bandaging, will also prevent edema when the patient is able to walk. Healthy people who complain of swollen feet should similarly be instructed to perform foot movements on sitting or standing and should

be advised to elevate the feet whenever possible.

All patients after operation, and those whose only complaint is edema of the dependent feet, should also be instructed in deep breathing exercises.

Varicose veins must be dealt with; those patients who cannot be treated because of deep venous obstruction need permanent, properly fitted, elastic stockings.

LYMPHEDEMA

Swelling of the foot may be due to lymphedema. Part of the drainage of extracellular fluid and protein from the lower limb is via the lymphatic system. It is filtered through the regional lymph glands to the main lymph channels and thence to the superior vena cava.

Any disease in the proximal part of the limb can cause lymphatic obstruction, be it infective lymphadenitis or neoplastic infiltration of the glands. The resultant swelling of the leg is only part of a severe acute or chronic illness.

Lymphedema can occur without any associated disease of the glands. It is common; more so in women than in men. The condition rarely begins in childhood, but is often well-established in adolescence and persists for life. It varies from slight puffiness of the dorsum of the feet and ankles after standing, to very severe, indurated, subcutaneous edema of a brawny type. The condition is congenital. Kinmonth has shown by lymphangiographic studies that the lesion in the lymphatic channels may be one of hypoplasia or hyperplasia.[1]

Treatment consists of the wearing of elastic stockings for life. In mild cases the modern fashion for elastic nylon tights has been a great boon, since they are elastic enough to prevent edema in many cases.

SUDECK'S ATROPHY

One form of swelling that may complicate an injury or operation to the lower limb is Sudeck's atrophy. First described by Sudeck in 1900, the condition is also known as reflex sympathetic dystrophy in the United States, and perhaps most graphically, as algodystro-

---

* The Jobst venous pressure gradient stocking.

phy, since the latter term implies pain as well as dystrophy.[2]

It has been considered a rare complication of trauma or surgery. Hannington-Kiff has pointed out that the full-blown syndrome is really a series of complications of the original disorder, and that the latter is by no means uncommon.[3]

The primary mechanism is sympathetic overactivity manifesting as vascular instability in the foot. The condition usually occurs in the distal part of the lower or upper limb, but cases confined to the knee joint have also been seen. Sympathetic changes in the small vessels of the foot cause blushing and capillary stasis. This is accompanied by other signs of sympathetic overactivity, including piloerection. (Often, the first sign of the onset of Sudeck's atrophy is the hair on the dorsum of the foot standing on end.) Later the hair grows thicker and coarser, so that the condition has been called "the hairy swollen foot." Excessive sweating is present in at least 30 per cent of cases; it may be copious enough to warrant the term, "the leaking foot."

The symptom that characterizes the condition is pain, which is severe and of a particularly unpleasant nature. It is probable that, for some unknown reason, the sympathetic afferent nerves within the limb are abnormally sensitive to the chemical noradrenergic drive of the sympathetic system. There are three aspects of such autonomic sensation: pain itself, which is severe; hyperesthesia, or increased sensation, amounting to a distressing symptom; and hyperpathia, the interpretation of all sensation as pain. Associated with the pain is stiffness. This may be present early in the onset of the syndrome and increases with time.

Anxiety is an integral part of the condition. There has been debate about whether it is a cause or a result of the condition. The authors hold the view that there is a psychological element in the onset of Sudeck's atrophy; that is to say, some patients are vulnerable to the condition because of their personalities, and others may develop it at a critical stage in their lives. Anxiety may well cause constant sympathetic stimulation, and if there is superadded trauma, Sudeck's atrophy ensues.

Hannington-Kiff cites the case of a dirt-track motorcycle rider who had suffered many fractures of his ankles and feet without complication, yet who developed a severe case of algodystrophy after twisting his ankle on a polished floor at a time of crisis in his life.

One of the authors (D.G.L.) has seen a case of a 32-year-old woman of a highly nervous disposition and artistic temperament who required an operation on the toes of both feet. A note was made to the effect that she seemed a likely candidate for Sudeck's atrophy. Fortunately it did not occur postoperatively, but some years later she developed the condition in a severe form after suffering an undisplaced fracture of the lower end of the radius.

Once established, the condition is complicated by the effects of disuse. There is marked, subcutaneous swelling and shiny, atrophic skin. Muscle shortening and wasting add to capsular adhesions in causing severe stiffness and disuse of the limb. Atrophy of the bone is common, frequently leading to severe demineralization. This is present in established cases so often as to constitute a pathognomonic sign of the disease. Many instances are thus diagnosed by the radiologist.

Diagnosis

Sudeck's atrophy should be suspected in any patient who complains of severe pain in the foot which starts 1 to 3 weeks after injury, particularly if the trauma was mild.

The foot should be inspected closely for the early signs—piloerection, capillary stasis and engorgement, and copious sweating. The latter can often best be appreciated by running the hand over the part. The foot must be seen daily; not at the usual weekly or monthly fracture clinic visits. The condition develops quickly and becomes progressively more severe.

The patient should be questioned about anxiety and psychological stress. Radiographic changes are not usually present for some weeks. Recently it has been found that radionucleide scans (using radioactive technetium (^{99}Tc) uptake by the limb) have a diagnostic value, since the osteoporosis has been shown to be of the high-turnover variety due to highly active osteoclasts. The test is most useful for prognostication and to assess the results of treatment. Since technetium has a short half-life, the test is not dangerous in the long term.

Treatment

Sudeck's atrophy has a tendency to resolve naturally. It may take up to 2 years for the process of recovery to be complete. In severe cases some permanent stiffness may be present from muscle and capsular fibrosis, but the pain and swelling disappear.

Movement—whether active, by forced exercise or passive, by manipulation—increases the pain, sometimes to a marked degree. Rest is indicated.

The naturally anxious patient is considerably helped if his doctor has made the diagnosis and can explain it. If the symptoms are inexplicable to the medical practitioner, his unease communicates itself to the patient, and the stage is set for a loss of confidence on both sides. Patients who, owing to temperament or circumstance, might be vulnerable to the syndrome at the time of an operation that cannot be delayed, should be warned about the condition: this may even prevent its occurrence.

In 1974, Hannington-Kiff reported on his experience with an antinoradrenergic drug for the treatment of Sudeck's atrophy.[3] Guanethidine is a sympathetic-neuron-blocking agent that was previously used as an antihypertensive drug; so it was a logical choice for use in the condition. It has proved effective in many cases.

Guanethidine is injected directly into the venous circulation of the leg. A sphygmomanometer cuff is inflated around the thigh to block arterial blood from entering the leg and, at the same time, to prevent all venous return. The veins of the leg are not emptied first. Twenty mg. of guanethidine, diluted in 40 to 50 ml. of saline, is injected into the venous system of the leg via a butterfly needle. The tourniquet is kept inflated for 10 minutes after the injection, to allow the drug to be fixed completely by the neural tissue in the leg.

Guanethidine has a profound effect in Sudeck's atrophy. Its sympathetic blocking effect lasts for up to 21 days, and improvement is often permanent. Pain is relieved within a few minutes and, interestingly enough, the stiffness usually decreases as quickly. The long-term blockage of sympathetic pain allows movement to be regained in the limb, and remineralization to begin.

The technique has its dangers. It should be employed only by an experienced doctor, and only in a hospital adequately equipped for emergencies. Were the tourniquet to fail before 10 minutes were up, a large dose of guanethidine might be dumped into the general circulation. This would induce a transient hypertension which, in a patient with vascular damage, could precipitate a vascular catastrophe such as a stroke due to cerebral bleeding. Severe postural hypotension would probably result, after a few minutes, from the antinoradrenergic action of the drug, and might be persistent.

An alternative, but equally logical, method of treatment is by repeated lumbar sympathetic block with a long-acting local anesthetic agent. The result is not always transient, and progress may be sustained, but the treatment is less effective than guanethidine, and requires more skill; however, it has the advantage of fewer dangerous general reactions.

THE ANTERIOR TIBIAL COMPARTMENT SYNDROME

Direct injury to arteries in the leg may cause ischemic necrosis of muscle (see Volkmann's contracture, below), but death of muscle can occur without such arterial injury. In the anterior tibial compartment, strenuous or unaccustomed exercise, such as that to which new recruits in the military service are exposed, may cause ischemia. The syndrome may be acute or chronic.[4-6]

The Acute Condition

Pain usually begins soon after exercise but may be delayed for a few hours. It starts as a dull ache, but becomes increasingly severe, especially when the foot is moved. Within a short time there is paralysis of the anterior tibial compartment. There is marked swelling of the muscles of the compartment, with redness, warmth, and tenderness. The condition might easily be misdiagnosed as cellulitis.

Paralysis is pathognomonic, and there may be an area of sensory loss between the first and second toe. The patient is in great pain and may be pyrexial. The leukocyte count may even be raised. Although many other conditions produce pain and swelling, in none other is paralysis present.

The Chronic Syndrome

The syndrome also occurs as a chronic condition in which normal walking does not cause pain, but marching or running does. The physical examination reveals pain, tenderness, and some swelling. Transient paresis may be found. Differentiation from intermittent claudication, shin splints, or stress fractures may be more difficult than in the acute syndrome.

The etiology is one of arterial compression within the unyielding walls of the anterior compartment. In chronic cases swelling causes transient ischemia, but in the acute syndrome, necrosis of muscle and ischemia of the nerve may result. Unless it is treated immediately, the paralysis may be permanent.

Treatment is by adequate surgical decompression of the compartment by splitting the fascia along its length. In severe cases, this should be performed wihin 8 hours of the injury, to avoid permanent disability.

VOLKMANN'S CONTRACTURE

Arterial obstruction in a limb may precipitate ischemic necrosis of the muscles dependent on that blood vessel.[7] The condition has been recognized in the upper limb for many years, but recently there have been an increasing number of reports in which it is pointed out that avascular necrosis is by no means rare in the leg.

Arterial blockage may be due to direct injury to the artery. Usually this follows a fracture just above, or just below, the knee joint, when the popliteal artery is damaged. The artery is seldom torn completely, but endarterial damage is complicated by thrombosis within the lumen. Often the viability of the limb is threatened and urgent operation is required, either by endarterectomy[2] or by the insertion of a lateral vein graft to widen the vessel at the point of damage, which usually is the more successful alternative. In other cases, muscle necrosis alone occurs, leading to Volkmann's ischemia and, finally, contracture.

Soft-tissue damage in the limb may be extensive without direct arterial injury. Any form of constriction around the limb may precipitate necrosis. Unpadded plasters are well-known to be dangerous, especially as a primary treatment, and are therefore seldom used. What is not so well recognized is that any circumferential bangage may have a similar effect. Even orthopedic cotton or gauze bandages that have become blood-stained and wet, and so shrink, can be responsible.

Avascular necrosis of muscle causes severe pain. This should never be forgotten. The patient's complaint of unexpected pain following a reduction of a fracture is always significant, and the surgeon disregards it at his peril. All circumferential bandaging must be split down to skin and along its full length. If the pain is not relieved, the arterial supply to the limb should be further investigated without delay.

Capillary filling time, Doppler ultrasonic recording, or arteriography may be needed. If the situation does not improve, fascial decompression or arterial exploration may be required.

Early diagnosis depends upon recognizing the cause of pain and observing loss of movement. Any attempt to move the toes passively increases the pain.

Within a short time, untreated ischemia progresses to necrosis of muscles. The condition is irreversible and inevitably leads to contracture of the muscle bellies.

Diagnosis now depends upon the *phenomenon of constant length*. In the normal foot, passive extension of the toes can be followed by passive extension of the foot and ankle. If, for example, the flexor muscles of the calf are replaced by fibrous tissue, the normal elasticity of the muscle bellies is lost. As a result, passive dorsiflexion of the toes results in forced plantar flexion of the ankle.

The fibrous tissue may affect the nerves of the compartment, due to ischemia of the nerve itself. The worst examples of chronic Volkmann's ischemic contracture are of stiff, swollen feet with atrophy of the skin; stiff clawtoes; and pes cavus. Sensory loss may be present, and the function of the leg is very poor. Such a result, after a major compound fracture of the femur with arterial injury, is unfortunate; after a simple, spiral fracture of the tibia, it is catastrophic. Delay in diagnosis and treatment is the cause.

REFERENCES

1. Kinmonth, J. B.: Primary lymphoedemia of the lower limit. Proc. Roy. Soc. Med., *58:*1021, 1965.
2. Sudeck, P.: Uber die acute entzyndliche Knochenatrophie. Arch. Klin. Chir., *62:*147, 1900.
3. Hannington-Kiff, J. G.: Intravenous regional sympathetic block with guanethidine. Lancet, *1:* 1019, 1974.
4. Horne, C. E.: Acute ischaemia of the anterior tibial muscle and long extensor muscles of the toes. J. Bone Joint Surg., *27:*615, 1945.
5. Hughes, J. R.: Ischaemic necrosis of the anterior tibial muscles due to fatigue. J. Bone Joint Surg., *30B:*581, 1948.
6. Paton, D. F.: The pathogenesis of the anterior tibial syndrome. J. Bone Surg., *50B:*383, 1968.
7. Seddon, H. J.: Volkmann's ischaemia in the lower lib. J. Bone Joint Surg., *48B:*627, 1966.

20 Orthotics of the Foot and Ankle

DAVID W. HOLMES

There is nothing new in the use of orthoses for deformities of the lower limb, and more particularly of the foot and ankle. Ever since shoemakers first plied their trade, patients have required specially measured shoes or boots for their abnormalities. Good shoemakers have always been held in high esteem. Traditionally, the reigning monarch invariably had his personal bootmaker. The trade even had its own patron saint, St. Crispin.

Today, too, a good craftsman in making footwear is worth his weight in gold. Despite the trend toward ready-made shoes which can be adapted to suit various shapes of foot, there will always be an important place for the shoemaker and his custom-built shoes.

In recent years, many advances have been made in the field of orthotics. With new materials and techniques, as well as research into normal and abnormal gait patterns, the orthotist is keeping pace with the demands of modern medicine.

The aim of this chapter is not to catalogue the various splints in use today but to explain the principles of the appliances that can be used in the treatment of deformities and other conditions of the foot and ankle.

ORTHOSES FOR CHILDREN
The Infant's Foot
Most common conditions at this age are congenital. Denis Browne probably made the greatest single contribution in the treatment of such problems. Today the original splints designed by him, with minor modifications and some change in materials, are still being used to great effect. After the initial treatment by strapping, followed if necessary by soft-tissue correction, the hobble splint (Fig. 20-1), or in some cases the individual equinus night splint, can be used with good results, provided it is applied so as to maintain the correct position.

Calcaneovalgus deformity requires a different approach. To begin with, it is a less common problem for the orthotist, since it does not, as a rule, require splinting. Even severe cases are usually treated surgically: consequently, there is no established device that has been used for this condition. Occasionally, a severe case may need a succession of release procedures, and a splint is provided to maintain or even to improve the position of the foot over a relatively long period of time. The orthosis should, therefore, be designed to provide maintenance of the *postoperative position,* and ideally to exert some further corrective pressure.

Metatarsus varus, a common condition, is less of a problem and can usually be treated conservatively by splinting alone. A valgus night bootee (Fig. 20-2) shaped to overcorrect the deformity is all that is required for treatment at this age. Later, when the child begins to walk, shoes with straight inner borders

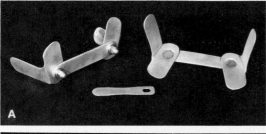

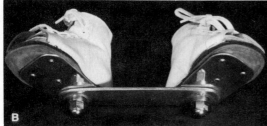

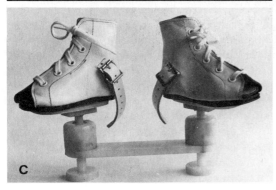

Fig. 20-1. (*A*) The Denis Browne hobble splint. (*B*) The Denis Browne hobble splint with bootees attached. (*C*) A modified Denis Browne hobble splint with polypropylene universal joints.

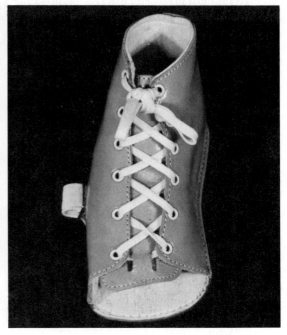

Fig. 20-2. A metatarsus varus night splint. The curve of the sole is into valgus, to reverse the original varus curve of the foot. There is a strap to hold the foot to that curve.

should be worn: an ordinary shoe worn on the opposite foot will achieve the same effect.

Metatarsus valgus is seldom seen and is usually due to ill-fitting shoes; when they are abandoned, it is resolved.

The Child's Foot

The most common condition the orthotist has to deal with in children is pes planus, whatever the cause. Whether it has its origin in ligamentous laxity causing a hypermobile foot, or valgus heels, the appearance is similar and, at one time, so was the treatment. The child would probably have been fitted with valgus arch supports or medial wedges to the sole or heel of the shoes. There are still occasions when a medial wedge should be fitted, perhaps in combination with an elongation to the heel on the same side; but this is best kept for mild cases of flatfoot. The orthosis of choice is a properly fitted heel cup, such as the one designed by Helfet.

Valgus arch supports should not be used in the treatment of valgus heels in children, nor in the treatment of pes planus, except, perhaps, in the more severe cases of ligamentous laxity. They restore the foot to a more normal position, but at the expense of the intrinsic musculature, which is encouraged to become lazy, so that the longitudinal arch cannot be supported once the orthosis is removed.

In pes cavus valgus arch supports are helpful, sometimes combined with metatarsal pads. The aim is to relieve symptoms such as midtarsal strain or pain under the metatarsal heads. Gross deformities may need surgery or the provision of adequate footwear to accommodate the high instep and clawtoes.

Medial and lateral wedges are usually pre-scribed to prevent excessive wear of the child's shoes, rather than for the foot itself.

The "Neurologic" Foot in Childhood

The anesthetic foot presents some problems of its own. The obvious one, that of the child's having no sensation, means that particular attention must be paid to the correct fitting of any orthosis. Most children need special foot-wear, and with the vastly increased rate of survival of patients with conditions such as spina bifida a number of ready-made boots are available for the purpose. It is important that the lining should be soft and that there is adequate room for the toes, and also for the general "podginess" of the paralyzed foot. They should be easily adaptable to take cali-pers.

Where specially made shoes are required, the same criteria should apply. The ultimate aim of the orthotist in this sort of case is to improve the function of the foot; that is, to provide a plantigrade base on which the child may stand. The foot is invariably flat, but this should be accepted, provided any ankle de-formity is corrected. Heel cups or valgus supports are of little use, except in the mildest cases. The simplest form of fixed ankle or-thosis, made of a thin polyprypolene material with a Velcro strap, is all that is required to achieve a mechanically sound base on which to stand. Depending on the level of the lesion and the severity of the neurologic involvement, more complex splints may be necessary, ex-tending to full-length calipers and even, in some cases, hip joints. For the purpose of this chapter, I shall confine may discussion to ankle and foot deformity only.

The flail foot is mechanically unstable. It is usually unilateral, and may be smaller than the contralateral normal one (as in the case of anterior poliomyelitis). The aim of the orthotist is to improve the mechanical stability and function of the foot. It can be done by fitting a double-bar caliper with either toe-spring or plantar-flex stops, together with a medial or lateral T-strap; but more recently it has been found that the provision of a splint made of one of the modern plastics, which fits inside the shoe, is more acceptable to the patient (Fig. 20-3). It also gives a more positive control of the foot. When the affected foot is smaller, a full-length footpiece, with perhaps a toe block, can be fitted, thus enabling the patient to wear normal footwear.

The trimlines of a plastic ankle- or foot orthosis may be altered to provide a variety of different effects. By leaving more material anteriorly, a fixed ankle orthosis can be ob-tained, while progressive trimming will pro-duce a flexible and lively splint. It is obviously important to obtain as much movement in the joints as possible, but mechanical stability must be the prime objective. If there is no lateral deviation or, at most, mild pronation of the foot, the leaf-spring type of appliance is sufficient to provide active dorsiflexion while restricting excessive plantar flexion. This type of appliance allows a more normal gait pattern and should be used whenever practicable. Where there is excessive ankle deformity, or in those cases with abnormal inversion of the foot and eversion of the ankle, a splint that allows little or no ankle movement should be fitted, to stabilize the joint. In this case care must be taken to assure that minimal pressure is exerted on any particular point and that relief areas are provided for any bony promi-nence. An inherent problem in the use of plastics in orthotics is that the surfaces are not porous, and skin will become necrotic if it is exposed to these man-made materials under pressure for more than a short time.

The spastic foot presents a different prob-lem. Any appliance fitted to this type of foot should be designed to maintain it in as good a position as possible for function. Springs of any sort should be avoided, as muscle spasm will overcome a spring of any strength that could possibly be tolerated by the patient under normal conditions. Any double-bar cal-iper, therefore, must be fitted with plantar-flex stops, together with a strong, lace-up shoe or boot to prevent the heel rising out of the footwear as a result of the tone in the muscle or the spasms which occur. A polypropylene fixed ankle-foot orthosis could also be used.

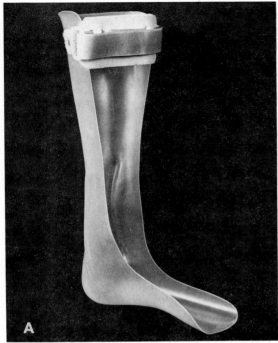
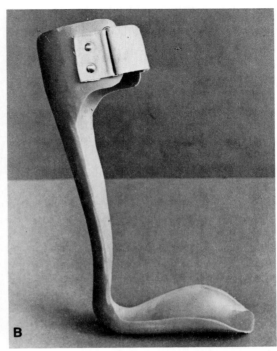

Fig. 20-3. (*A*) Polypropylene drop-foot splint with Velcro closure. (*B*) Ortholen leaf-spring type of drop-foot splint with Velcro closure.

With the addition of an instep or ankle strap, it can be fitted in most types of shoes.

Other less common conditions occur in children, and these are treated symptomatically. Postcalcaneal bursitis ("winter heel") is usually treated initially by relieving pressure over the tender area. This can be achieved by cutting out the back of the shoe and replacing it with sponge.

The symptoms of calcaneal apophysitis can be relieved orthotically by raising the heel of the shoe to reduce the pull of the calcaneal tendon. The fellow shoe should be raised equally to balance the patient and prevent strain on the hips and even the spine.

The patient with hemophilia presents special difficulties to the orthotist. This blood disorder manifests itself most commonly in spontaneous bleeding into joints and muscles. Although the knees and elbows mainly are affected, the ankle joint is occasionally involved. Recurrent bleeding into any joint (hemarthrosis) provokes degenerative changes causing pain and limitation of movement. The

management of a bleeding episode includes not only replacement therapy and symptomatic treatment, but either plaster-of-Paris or other immobilization. Here the orthotist becomes involved.

Similarly, he plays a part in the prevention of bleeding. Splinting of the vulnerable joint to reduce the possibility of excessive strain is often necessary. When the ankle is involved, its orthotic management can be quite difficult. In recent years it has been found to be unnecessary to prevent plantar- and dorsiflexion, provided the limb is stabilized to prevent medial or lateral movement. To this end, a rather foreshortened type of splint has been used, made either of block leather or polypropylene. The fastenings on any splint fitted to the hemophiliac patient should always be made from Velcro or lacing, since buckles or clips will cause bleeding or severe bruising of the opposing limb.

There is, finally, the problem of dealing with the grossly misshapen foot with fixed deformity in the child. When the orthopaedic surgeon has done all that he can to improve the appearance, it is left to the orthotist to provide adequate footwear. This will be dealt with in a later section; suffice it to say here that each patient must be treated individually, and by definition this means by the provision of custom-made footwear.

ORTHOSES FOR ADULTS

Insoles

When exercise fails to relieve symptoms in adults' flatfoot, arch supports are often prescribed. A well-fitting longitudinal support can overcome the pain of foot strain, which is due to malalignment of the bones and joints of the arch. Supports are ineffective when the natural arch is completely flat. The support should be made of leather and sponge rubber or plastic molded to a plaster cast of the foot.

Foot strain does not necessarily indicate a flat longitudinal arch. The pain may arise from the mid-tarsal region, or, in plantar fasciitis, from the under-surface of the calcaneus. These conditions are usually transient. They can be helped by a support that reduces pressure on the affected part until healing is complete. Tarsal ligament strain responds to a properly fitted valgus support, while plantar fasciitis may be treated by the provision of a Rose's insole. This consists of a full-length leather-base insole with a low sponge pad fitted between the anterior edge of the calcaneus and the posterior edge of the metatarsal heads. The effect is one of cushioning the mid-tarsal region and reducing the stretching of the plantar ligament.

Relief from pain associated with a calcaneal spur (''policeman's heel'') can usually be achieved by wearing a sponge heel pad excavated directly under the painful spot.

Metatarsalgia is a common problem in both orthopaedic and rheumatoid clinics. There are many causes, and the orthotist must know the precise diagnosis, as the design of the insole will vary accordingly.

With a dropped transverse arch, the pad should be shaped to restore the arch to a more normal position, to relieve excessive pressure on the metatarsal heads and the associated callosities, and to provide a better distribution of weight. The pad should be positioned just behind the metatarsal heads and should extend the full width of the foot at this point. It should be fuller in the center than at the medial and lateral borders and can be combined with a valgus pad to provide support for both the transverse and longitudinal arches. Wherever possible it should be fitted to a full-length insole, provided there is room in the shoe. This will ensure that the position of the pad within the shoe is maintained.

The flexibility of the foot should be considered when deciding on the position of the pad. A stiff, arthritic foot will slide forward on weight bearing, and the pad will have to be placed further forward to obtain the same weight relief.

In the case of stress fracture of a metatarsal bone, the important feature of the pad should be to restore the natural arch to a comfortable and, if possible, normal position. It should be shaped like the one described above, but it does not have to provide weight-bearing relief.

Morton's metatarsalgia is a more localized problem. The aim of the insole is to increase the affected interdigital space and to provide some degree of weight relief to the painful area. It must be emphasized that standard pattern metatarsal arch supports made to shoe sizes are seldom satisfactory. Each should be made individually, according to the patient's particular needs. Excavations should be made to accommodate callosities, and a variation in the consistency of pad material will provide more support or less, as required.

For those patients whose work demands that they spend long hours on their feet, a firmer material will give a longer-lasting support.

The use of thermoplastics in orthotics has increased dramatically in the past few years. Amongst these, Plastizote has become one of the most popular. Low- or medium-density Plastizote is an ideal material for making insoles.

A length of the material, either 6 mm. or 13 mm. in thickness, is cut to the approximate shape of the foot. It is then preheated in an oven to a temperature of 140 degrees C. It is removed from the oven and remains malleable for some minutes. The heated material is placed on a block of sponge or Plastizote.* The patient immediately places his foot on the material and bears full weight. The Plastizote can be molded by the orthotist's fingers to obtain the desired shape, and the foot is held in position for 3 or 4 minutes, until the plastic has cooled and hardened. The insole can then be trimmed and finished. It retains its shape unless reheated. Extra material can be added under the longitudinal or transverse arch, to give extra support in these areas.

There is a disadvantage in the use of Plastizote. Being thermoplastic, it retains heat from the foot. It is hot to wear, and may cause sweating. On the other hand, there may be a definite advantage for patients with circulatory deficiency.

The Metatarsal Bar

Ideally, any support for the metatarsal arch should be fitted inside the shoe, but occasionally there is too little room for this to be done. An external metatarsal bar may be fitted. If possible this should be concealed by placing it between sole and welt, but on cemented-construction shoes it may have to be fitted to the outside of the sole.

Adaptations of Footwear

Adaptation of shoes is often required. Many such alterations are in common use (Fig. 20-4). A few important points are worth mentioning. The first, and most important, consideration is that the shoe must be suitable for the required alteration, as well as affording the necessary support for the foot. Some modern methods of shoe construction can present the

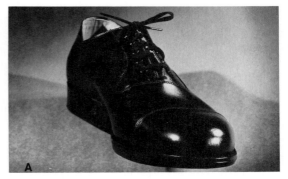
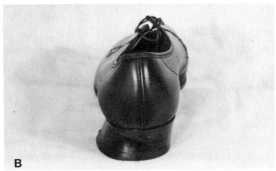
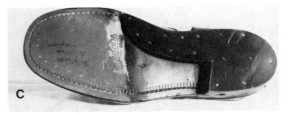

Fig. 20-4. Adaptations of the heel and sole. (*A*) Medial wedge added to the heel and sole of an ideal welted shoe. (*B*) Lateral flare of a leather heel. (*C*) Fully elongated heel on the medial side.

technician with problems, even for the most simple adaptation such as fitting a wedge.

Metal sockets in the heel of a shoe for the insertion of calipers put an enormous strain on the heel and waist of the shoe, particularly those sockets with backstops, or the box-section type. The shoe must be strong enough to stand the strain, especially in the vulnerable areas.

Elevations (Fig. 20-5) of up to $\frac{1}{2}$ inch may be fitted to the heel, and microcellular synthetic material, leather, or rubber can be used for this. For shortening between $\frac{3}{4}$ inch and one inch, the raise should be fitted to the sole

---

* Plastizote is patented by Bakelite Xylonite, Ltd., available from Smith & Nephew, Ltd., Bessemer Rd., Hertfordshire, England; or The Knit-Rite, Inc., Paramedical Distributors, 1121 Grand Ave., St. Louis, Missouri 64106; or Apex Foot Products Corp., 118 West 22nd St., New York, N.Y. 10011. Two similar materials are: Pelite, available from Apex, or Ali Plast, available from Ali Med, 11 Concord Square, Boston, Massachusetts 02118.

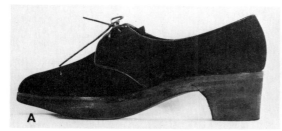 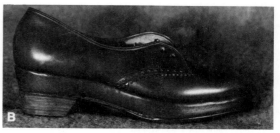

Fig. 20-5. (*A*) A microcellular raise added to sole and heel; the sole is in the form of a rocker to allow a normal gait. (*B*) Cork elevation fitted between upper and sole tapers toward the toe.

as well as the heel; the sole raise being lower than that of the heel, to take account of the pitch of the shoe. For shortening of 1 inch and more, a cork elevation should be fitted. This involves stripping the sole and heel from the upper, inserting a cork wedge of the required height at the heel, and tapering it forward again to the pitch of the shoe. The toe end should be "rolled-off," especially for patients who have had arthrodesis of the ankle. The cork is then covered with a matching leather, and the sole and heel are replaced.

Rocker Sole. Hallux rigidus can be a very painful condition, but by fitting a rocker sole, sometimes with the addition of a metal sole plate inserted between sole and rocker, extension of the affected joint can be stopped and the pain relieved.

Valgus and Varus Splints. Valgus and varus neurologic deformities nearly always present problems for the orthotist, the former more particularly, perhaps, than the later. The well-tried and long-established medial iron and lateral T-strap are usually effective in controlling a varus deformity, but the valgus foot quite often defies all efforts at correction. I am sure that, in more cases, this is owing to bad design of the orthosis.

Research into this problem by Mr. G. K. Rose, F.R.C.S., and his bioengineering department at the Robert Jones and Agnes Hunt Orthopaedic Hospital in Oswestry, has produced a modified orthosis.[1] The success of this apparatus relies on repositioning and correction of the talus, with mobilization of the subtalar joint an integral part. The force vector produced by the conventional T-strap is horizontal and medial, which all too often produces

pressure above the malleolus and a gap below. A Y-strap is used to overcome this by producing a rotary force. Because of the angle at which the strap meets the iron, it tends to slip down. A loop fitted to the iron, through which the strap passes, prevents this. The third adaptation to the conventional design consists of the fitting of a wedge under the lateral aspect of the heel. This provides the reaction point to produce the couple of forces which rotates the foot in the long axis. Absence of this wedge would allow the foot to move laterally, eventually distorting the shoe, producing pressure against the iron, and ejecting the spur from the socket. Rose's final modification is made to the iron itself. Single irons are notorious for breaking at the junction of side stem and spur, a consequence of the dynamics of the forces which obtain at the beginning of the stance phase.

Often a medial wedge is fitted in conjunction with this type of orthosis, and the subsequent angle at which the socket is fitted also produces a strain on the junction of the stem and spur. To overcome both these problems, and also to cope with wear and tear on the heel during use, a self-aligning joint has been designed. It permits limited angulation between spur and stem, eliminating the bending moment which frequently causes recurrent fracture at this point but also allows any heel modification actually to have some beneficial effect.

With such an arrangement a small axial force may be created along the spur, causing it to withdraw from the socket. To avoid this, the spur should be continued right through the heel and secured on the inside with a lock nut.

Improvements made since the introduction of the orthosis include padding added to the Y-strap where it crosses the front of the ankle and the Achilles tendon, and a medial float-out of the heel for the rheumatoid foot to provide support beneath the deformity (Fig. 20-6).

Orthoses for Hemiplegia

Orthotic problems in hemiplegia can be divided broadly according to the needs of the patients: those who will achieve a full, or almost full, recovery and those who will make some recovery but will remain partly or severely disabled. The purpose of providing splints and aids is different for each type, and this should be borne in mind when the initial assessment is made.

Let us consider the patient who has suffered a mild cerebrovascular accident and who presents with a typical weakness of arm and leg, the latter associated with foot drop and ankle inversion. For this patient the prognosis is usually good, provided rehabilitation is started as early as possible. This should now include the orthosis to control the ankle and foot drop. Fortunately, today there are a number of ready-made splints for the purpose, which can be supplied almost immediately. They should be used whenever possible. The polypropylene ankle-foot splint controls the foot drop and at the same time provides some stability for the ankle. The patient's own footwear can be used—adapted, if necessary, to provide a more stable foundation, for example by wedging or floating out the heel. The splint can be used for mild spasticity only.

I have used a molded foot-drop splint made of polypropylene or medium-density polyethylene and find that it controls the foot drop successfully. Because of the inherent resistance to torsion in the material, it also provides some lateral stability. Velcro closure (one strap only is required) enables the patient to apply the splint without help (a happy contrast to the days of straps and buckles).

The second category of patient, who has suffered a more severe injury or whose disability is long-standing, requires a different

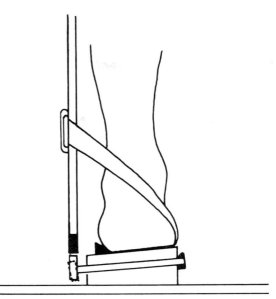

Fig. 20-6. This diagram shows the essential features of Rose's single lateral iron apparatus—the oblique Y-strap, the self-aligning joint between the side-stem and the spur (which extends across the width of the heel), and the lateral wedge on the outer side of the heel to prevent the foot from sliding laterally.

approach. Rehabilitation will go some way toward enabling the patient to cope with daily living, but aids of various kinds will be needed to provide some degree of independence. These include adaptations in the home as well as walking aids and splints for the arm and leg.

In the more severe cases a long-leg brace may be required, but quite often a below-knee caliper is sufficient. Stabilization of the ankle and control of the foot drop are the important factors. The presence of spasticity in the majority of these cases means that molded polypropylene splints are not suitable. Toe springs shorten the gastrocnemius muscle and so increase the tendency for the foot to drop. Perhaps this encourages a fixed deformity (Fig. 20-7).

The alternatives that should be considered are a double iron with plantar-flex stop, or a single or double iron with ankle joint and dorsiflex spring attached. The former should be combined with a T-strap, usually lateral, and care must be taken to set the stop to allow

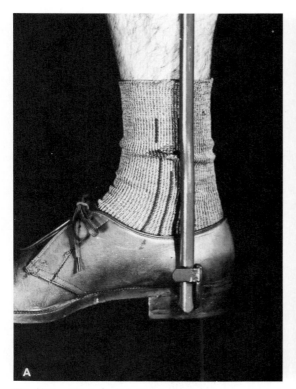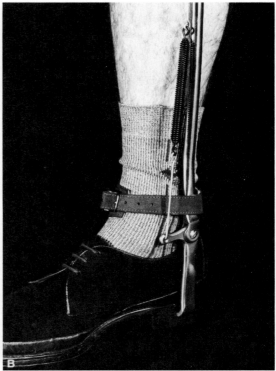

Fig. 20-7. (*A*) A single below-knee medial iron with a plantar-flex stop and a retaining ear. (*B*) A single medial below-knee iron with ankle joint and dorsiflex spring. It is combined with a lateral T-strap.

maximum dorsiflexion. The height of the heel may have to be increased if the foot cannot be raised sufficiently for the heel to reach the ground on weight bearing. The fellow shoe will then have to be raised to match.

The ankle-jointed caliper tends to be heavier than the one described above but nevertheless is an effective brace. It can be supplied as a single- or double-sided splint and can be worn in conjunction with a T-strap. It should be fitted to a strong shoe; one fitted with a stout metal shank (as should also the other caliper).

The ankle joint is designed to allow approximately 20 degrees of dorsiflexion and has a stop which prevents the foot from dropping below 90 degrees. Despite the extra weight, it provides a motion that is anatomically closer to normal ankle flexion than the type with plantar-flex stops.

Experience has shown that many severely hemiplegic patients tend to develop a fixed ankle deformity with the foot in equinus. The orthotist can help delay the progression by accurate assessment and fitting of a correct splint.

Anterior Poliomyelitis

The adult flail foot resulting from poliomyelitis or other lower motor neuron lesions can be treated orthotically in a way similar to the hemiplegic foot. In the absence of spasticity, the task becomes simpler. Any of the established or recently developed ankle-foot orthoses may be used, and the orthotist can exert his skill and judgment in choosing the one best suited to the particular patient. Provided the splint is functional, the simplest, lightest and cosmetically most acceptable kind should be used.

Surgical Footwear

The provision of orthopaedic footwear requires special skills, both from the orthotist and the shoemaker. Once the orthopaedic surgeon has done what he can for the patient, it is up to the orthotist to make his contribution. The first and most important measure is to assess the foot: to take note of the deformities; to estimate the possible range of motion; to ascertain whether the foot swells; and to record the age and level of activity of the patient.

Without this background knowledge, the provision of truly adequate footwear is impossible. Only then may measurements or plaster casts be taken. An outline sketch of the foot should be made, and while the foot is still in position, four circumference measurements are taken. The exact position of these measurements should be recorded on the outline. Girth measurements are taken at the joints, waist, instep, and around the heel. For boots, an additional "short" heel measurement should be taken, plus circumferential measurements around the ankle (at the level of the malleolus) and around the leg at the level of the top of the boot. The following measurements should also be recorded: overall length of the foot, using a size stick; length from heel to first metatarsal joint; and the height, individually recorded, of any clawtoes. Any other abnormalities, such as prominent bones, swollen ankles, callosities, or exostoses, should be recorded. Arch supports and excavations which may be required can be noted at this time and their position marked on the outline. When it is necessary to take plaster casts, the above measurements and details should be taken in the same way.

A plaster-of-Paris cast will give a very accurate, three-dimensional model of the foot and should always be used for a grossly deformed foot. The method of taking a plaster cast is as follows: the foot is prepared by spreading oil or petrolatum over it to form a barrier. A plaster slab is then cast to a suitable size, soaked, and placed on a board pitched at the required height. The foot is placed on the plaster slab, which should be molded up to approximately halfway. The edges are turned out and trimmed to about 6 mm. This slipper cast is allowed to dry, and the outturned lip is spread with oil. A second plaster slab is soaked and molded to the dorsal aspect

of the foot, and the edges are turned out and gently pressed onto the flange from the bottom section. When this has dried it is a simple matter to remove both sections from the foot and refit the two pieces together to form a negative shell. From this, the shoemaker is able to make his last, or positive, mold, either from wood, plaster-of-Paris, or expanding hard foam. Wood is the traditional material, usually maple or beech, but hard foam is becoming more popular as it is easier to form and lighter to handle. The last should be hinged to enable the shoe to be slipped off without breaking the back seam.

Choice of leather is vitally important. Consideration should be given to the patient's age, level of activity, general condition of the skin, and particular foot problems (e.g., prominent bones, local tenderness). The types of leather used include calf of various grades (from stout chrome calf to soft), glacé, suede, pigskin, and foam-lined leathers. An active man with minor foot deformities would obviously require a shoe made of a fairly stout calf leather, whereas a patient with rheumatoid disease and associated deformities and tenderness needs something much softer, such as glacé, suede, or foam-lined leather (Fig. 20-8). It is worth mentioning here that the type of fastening is very important. Quite often someone with foot deformities is also handicapped in other ways. He may have stiff or fused hips, limited spinal flexion, or impaired use of the fingers and hands, so consideration must be given to the type of fastening. In many cases a slip-on style might be preferable, or a Velcro closure. The ideal lace-up is often not practical, and a compromise may be necessary, for instance, foregoing a little support to allow the patient to don the shoes more easily.

Once the patient's feet have been measured or a cast has been taken; the material for the uppers decided upon (including the color and the type of fastening); the style of shoe, gibson or oxford (Fig. 20-9) selected; there are a few more details to note before the order is complete.

The insoles must be designed. All too often, a well-fitting shoe is spoiled by an inadequate

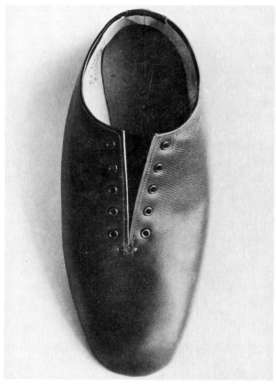

Fig. 20-8. This foam-lined leather shoe was custom-made for a patient with rheumatoid disease.

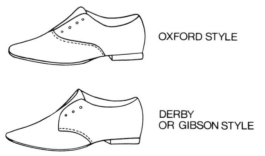

OXFORD STYLE

DERBY OR GIBSON STYLE

Fig. 20-9. Diagram to show the oxford and derby or gibson styles of shoes.

or poorly designed insole. The same criteria apply for insole design for surgical footwear as for insoles to fit into the patient's own shoes, except that the choice is a little wider, since the made-to-measure shoes can be made larger to accommodate them. Most frequently the need is for an insole that will redistribute body weight, thus relieving areas of pain and stress. It is therefore plain to see that a molded insole is preferable, with relief areas built in. Plastizote and other thermoforming materials are eminently suitable for this purpose. The mistake should not be made of trying to fit too many pads and supports, when quite often all that is necessary is some sort of soft insole, made, perhaps, of Dunlopillo or similar sponge.

The rigid foot with fixed deformity is, by definition, impossible to reform by arch supports. Accommodation and comfort are the prime needs. Care should be observed to ensure the foot is pitched and balanced correctly. The insoles may be designed to provide a plantigrade base on which to stand, or conversely, a foot which is already plantigrade should not be forced into an unnatural or uncomfortable position. It should be accommodated in that plane.

Finally, a decision must be made on the construction and associated adaptations of the soles and heels. The choice ranges from the traditional leather or rubber to the more recently developed synthetic materials such as microcellular material and polyvinyl chloride. The construction may be of the welted or cemented type, and again, due regard should be given to the amount of wear that the shoes are likely to undergo. Microcellular has the advantages of being light, more durable, and more spongy; complementing a soft insole to give more comfort to the painful or tender plantar aspect of a foot. A disadvantage is that, because of its inherent sponginess, it tends to be unstable laterally, affording little support for the already unstable foot or ankle. This is particularly evident when adaptations are added, such as wedges or a floated-out heel. Preference hould be given to another material in this instance, such as leather. Welted construction is preferred for patients who do a lot of walking or who require frequent shoe repairs, but the lighter, cemented or bonded construction can be used for the less-active patient.

Also at this stage, outside adaptations should be noted. Shoe elevations, wedges, extended heels, rocker soles, sockets and T-straps for

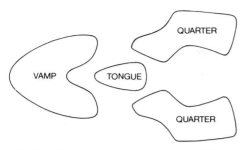

Fig. 20-10. Diagram showing the parts of the upper before closing.

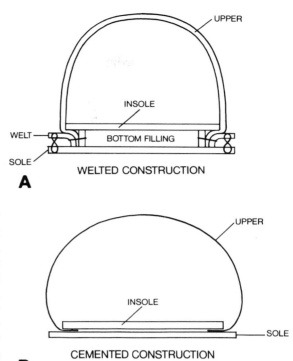

Fig. 20-11. (*A*) Diagram showing a cross-section of a shoe to indicate the method of welted construction. (*B*) A similar diagram showing the cemented construction method.

caliper fitting should be ordered as required, and lastly, the height of heel most suitable for the patient's needs. Heels should be of a height to give a balanced and secure base. Where a fixed ankle deformity is present, the heel height is predetermined, but in other cases it should be assessed according to the general condition. A patient suffering from a valgus deformity which can be corrected is often more comfortable, and the foot is certainly more easily corrected, with a slightly higher heel of perhaps 1¼ to 1½ inches, whereas someone suffering from a forefoot disorder might be more comfortable in a flatter heel of ¾ inch or less. The order is now complete, and the shoemaker has all the details required to produce the special shoes.

His first task, after making the last and selecting the appropriate leather and lining material, is to cut the working patterns for the uppers. It is necessary that these patterns should be molded to the exact shape of the last and yet be capable of being flattened and kept as a permanent record for future use. Impregnated cloth of soft plastic, vacuum-formed, is used for this purpose, and from this mean forme a paper pattern is produced. The leather uppers and linings are cut, using these paper patterns, after which they are filed for further reference. The different parts of the shoe are cut separately, and these are shown in Fig. 20-10. The parts are then assembled and stitched together or "closed." Eyelets, perforations or stitching as necessary are added, and the upper is now ready for lasting. The toe puffs (stiffness fitted at the toes to retain the shape), side-stiffeners, and insoles

should be cut in preparation for the lasting process.

Lasting is a term used to describe the molding (or, more accurately, the stretching) of the upper around the last and securing it to the bottom of the last over the insole with stitching, or, more commonly, tacks or adhesive.

The toe puffs and stiffeners are stuck between upper and lining during this process, and the lasted shoe is left to stretch for approximately 1 week. It can be safely removed at the end of this period without fear of the shape being lost. A metal shank is secured to the insole, using tacks, and the shoe is ready for the finishing process.

There are basically two methods of finishing surgical footwear. First, the traditional one of welting, giving a much stronger, more waterproof shoe; and the more recently used method of cemented construction (Fig. 20-11). The latter produces a somewhat lighter shoe, but it is more difficult to repair and does not withstand such hard wear as the welted shoe.

Welted Shoe. The welt is a narrow strip of leather running around the edge of the shoe. It is stitched to the insole, and the sole in turn is stitched, to the welt. The process is sometimes known as indirect attachment. Repairing a shoe with this type of construction is simply a matter of removing the sole, leaving the welt intact and attaching a new sole to it.

Cemented Shoe. Cementing, sometimes known as direct attachment, is a much quicker and easier method of finishing. More frequently, the upper has been lasted using an adhesive to secure it rather than tacks. It is now a simple matter to cement the sole directly to the upper and insole.

The shoe is now ready for the heel to be fitted, and finally the arch supports, if required. It is advisable to try the shoe on the patient before the sole and heel are fitted, so that any minor modifications can be made. Cork elevations, T-straps, etc., are also added between lasting and finishing.

RECENT TRENDS

Conventionally made shoes and boots have, of necessity, seams and stitching, and these can have a disastrous effect on sensitive feet or those prone to skin breakdown, for example the diabetic or rheumatoid patient. The space shoe has gone some way towards providing an answer to this problem. It is a seamless design and therefore stitching is absent in areas likely to cause pressure or rubbing. The uppers are of a synthetic material, sometimes foam-lined, or of Plastizote, with a more durable covering. They are molded over plaster-of-Paris casts of the patient's feet, and then bonded or cemented to microcellular soles and heels. Molded insoles are fitted inside, having been molded to the plantar aspect of the cast, thus providing a greater weight distribution. Velcro closure facilitates fastening for the disabled patient. This type of shoe is far less robust than the normal surgical footwear, but then the patients for whom they are usually

prescribed tend to have limited activity levels, and comfort is the primary requirement.

This type of footwear can be obtained much more quickly than can conventional surgical shoes, but despite this, there has been found to be a need for ready-made, easily modified, Space-type shoes. One such shoe, developed in England, is the DRU-Shoe (Fig. 20-12). It is made up of a one-piece upper, formed from a complex laminate of polyvinyl chloride, nylon, and Plastizote cemented to a special wedge sole unit of polyurethane material. Inside, it contains two 6-mm. Plastizote insoles, the lower of medium density and, on top, one of low density. Both insoles are loose, to allow heating and molding to individual needs. Velcro closure on the front flap provides ease of fastening and adjustment. This bootee has been found to be extremely versatile, adjustments being simply made. The uppers may be cut to provide relief areas, or they may be heated, using a hot-air blower at 140 degrees C. If necessary, the whole shoe may be heated in an oven to the same temperature, the patient's foot inserted, and the upper will assume the overall contour of the foot. The insoles may be molded in a similar way, and pads may be added to provide support in important areas. Rebalancing the foot may be achieved by grinding the insoles. The bootee has been successfully used by those suffering from insensitive foot conditions, where it has been found to promote healing of "hot spots," blisters, and ulcers. Its use is also indicated for hypersensitive foot conditions such as rheumatoid arthritis and gout, and postoperative application, where adjustments may be required after reduction of edema. It is suitable for a mildly deformed foot, and geriatric patients find it light and comfortable. As a consequence it eases walking and encourages it. The upper material is hypoallergenic and therefore can be used by patients who are unable to tolerate harsher materials.

New Concepts in Orthotics

Depth Shoes. Dr. Arnold Kratter, D.P.M., has written to us on the subject of depth

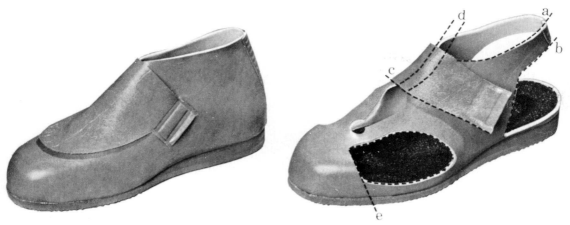

Fig. 20-12. The **DRU**-Shoe. (*Left*) A boot with soft thermoplastic one-piece upper closed by a Velcro front flap. The sole is a wedge design to give support, combining spring with resilience. Two 6-mm. Plastizote insoles are supplied in each boot, a medium-density lower to give firm support covered by a low-density insole to cushion the foot. (*Right*) The boots can be cut to make a sandal. This photograph shows the standard bootee cut down to below the malleoli to shoe height (cut a). Further cutting of the upper (i.e., removal of the heel "quarters" and "back strap") to the extent required (cut b). Ventilation can be increased by removing the front of the flap (cut c), taking care to avoid cutting the Velcro closure, and removing part of the "facing" and opening the "throat" of the shoe (cut d). Further, the "vamp" can be cut away to relieve pressure on the metatarsal joints, if needed (cut e). Thus the shoe becomes an individually formed sandle. (See Appendix for the address and the manufacturer of this shoe.)

shoes.[2] For many years, conventional long-counter oxford shoes with steel shanks, Thomas' heels, and the preferred Goodyear welt construction in a variety of lasts and upper leathers have provided some degree of room to accommodate prescriptions. In most instances, however, shoes had to be oversized to accommodate these insoles.

Such oversized shoes, instead of flexing at the metatarsophalangeal joints, crease and bend proximally and distally to the desired hinge area. This can result in postural imbalance as well as forepart irritation, slipping of the heel, and other distortions.

Space shoes are not a panacea, and need to be prescribed very selectively because of their rigidity and weight. The one-piece construction does not readily lend itself to modifications.

A group of orthopaedic shoe manufacturers cooperated to produce overlasted shoes providing increased depth of between $\frac{1}{8}$ and $\frac{1}{4}$ inch. Specific lasts were developed in an attempt to fit accurately most common foot shapes, as well as to provide the necessary depth to accommodate various insoles. Examples of such shoe manufacturers in the United States are shown in Fig. 20-13.

The Bow-String Foot Support. Dr. C. W. Coplans has put forward an idea for a new type of support for mobile, everted flat feet:[3]

"This device consists of a stainless steel plate (Fig. 20-14) inserted into the medial wall of the heel counter of the shoe upper, at the level of the talonavicular joint. It is connected to the inner sole or floor of the shoe by a flat strap, composed of a layer of thin brass shim, sheathed in canvas and leather, the width and length of which is related to the size of the shoe. The medial end of the strap or bow-string is attached firmly to the plate at an angle of 45 degrees at the level of the head of the talus, which lies upon it. The lateral end is nailed into the inner sole or floor of the shoe at the junction of the inner sole and lateral wall of the counter.

If the foot becomes everted, the head of the talus descends as the talonavicular joint widens and the bow-string is deformed. The reinforced medial wall of the shoe is consequently pulled

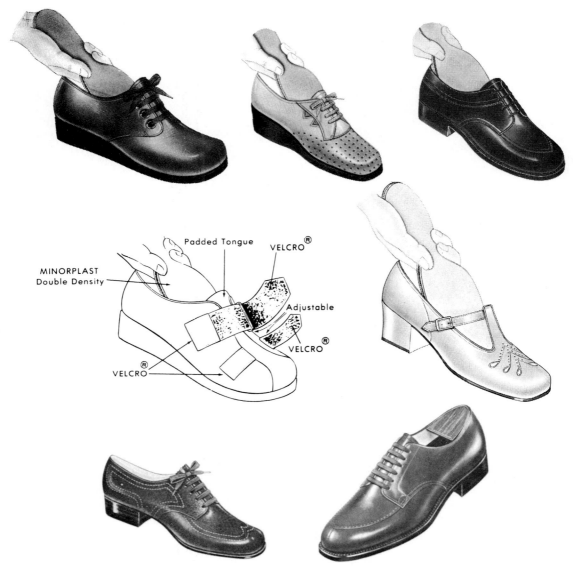

Fig. 20.13. Illustrations showing types of depth shoes commercially available. Of particular interest is the shoe that makes use of Velcro closures, which allow infinite adjustment of the straps, even by people who cannot handle conventional laces. (See Appendix for the address of the manufacturer of these shoes.)

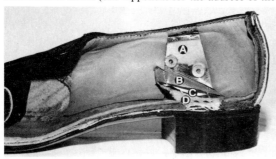

Fig. 20-14. A metal plate (*A*) stiffening the medial wall of the shoe and the bow-string strap which is shown here in three layers from above downward, (*B*) leather, (*C*) brass shim, (*D*) canvas. The bow-string is nailed into the lateral border on the inner sole, the nails passing through all three layers of the strap.

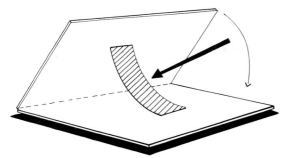

Fig. 20-15. Two hinged plates on the bow-string support are connected by the strap. The lower plate is fixed, representing the floor of the shoe. When a force is applied to the superior surface of the strap, the medial wall is approximated to the floor of the shoe.

laterally with a force equal to that which causes eversion of the foot (Fig. 20-15). The foot is thus corrected and remains so, as long as weight bearing takes place.

This device effectively corrects the mobile everted feet and the shoe no longer becomes deformed (Fig. 20-16). Heel wear now takes place over the center of the posteroinferior margin of the heel instead of the lateral aspect of the lateroinferior margin. The device is comfortable and well tolerated.''

REFERENCES

1. Rose, G. K., and Henshaw, J. T.: The Design and Mechanics of a Below Knee Single Lateral Iron. Paper presented at the International Society for Prosthetics and Orthotics Meeting, April, 1975, at Keele University in Stoke-on-Kent, U.K.
2. Kratter, A.: Personal Communication, 1978.
3. Coplans, C. W.: Personal Communication, 1978.

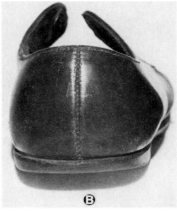

Fig. 20-16. (*A*) Shoe worn by a flat-footed child shows the typical deformation. (*B*) A shoe containing bow-string support which was worn by the same child. Each shoe had been worn for a period of 3 months. Note the central wear of the heel in the bow-string shoe, as well as lack of deformation.

APPENDIX

Alden Shoe Company
Taunton Street
Middleborough, Massachusetts 02346

John Drew (London) Limited
433 Uxbridge Road
Ealing, London W5, England

Marlin Orthotics, Limited
Gunstore Road
Hilsea, Portsmouth, PO3 5JP
Hampshire, England

Miller Shoe Company
4015 Cherry Street
Cincinnati, Ohio 45223

Musebeck Shoe Company, Inc.
Forest & Westover
Oconomowoc, Wisconsin 53066

P W. Minor & Sons, Inc.
3 Treadeasy Avenue
Industrial Park
Batavia, New York 14020

Index

Numerals in *italics* indicate a figure; "t" following a page number indicates a table.